THE MANAGEMENT OF THE MENOPAUSE

THIRD EDITION

THE MANAGEMENT OF THE MENOPAUSE

THIRD EDITION

Edited by
John Studd

Chelsea & Westminster Hospital, London, UK

The Parthenon Publishing Group
International Publishers in Medicine, Science & Technology

A CRC PRESS COMPANY
BOCA RATON   LONDON   NEW YORK   WASHINGTON, D.C.

Published in the USA by
Parthenon Publishing Inc.
345 Park Avenue South, 10th Floor
New York
NY 10010
USA

Published in the UK and Europe by
The Parthenon Publishing Group
23–25 Blades Court
Deodar Road
London SW15 2NU
UK

ISSN 1460-1397

Library of Congress Cataloging-in-Publication Data
The management of the menopause / edited by J. Studd. – 3rd ed.
    p. cm.
  Includes bibliographical references and index.
  ISBN 1-84214-137-6 (alk. paper)
    1. Menopause.   I. Studd, John

RG186.M287 2003
618.1'75–dc21

2003051286

British Library Cataloguing in Publication Data
The management of the menopause. - 3rd ed.
  1. Menopause   2. Age factors in disease
  I. Studd, John W. W.
  618.1'75

ISBN 1-84214-137-6

Typeset by AMA DataSet Ltd., Preston, UK
Printed and bound by Bookcraft (Bath) Ltd., Midsomer Norton, UK

Contents

List of principal contributors   vii

Foreword   xi

1   The future of hormone replacement therapy   1
H. G. Burger, S. Davison and S. R. Davis

2   National Osteoporosis Society statement, February 2003: hormone replacement   13
therapy and the Women's Health Initiative study
D. Barlow

3   Estrogen therapy for cardiovascular disease   17
G. Samsioe

4   Urogenital atrophy   27
D. Robinson and L. Cardozo

5   Urogenital collagen turnover and hormone replacement therapy   41
C. Falconer

6   Progestins in premenopausal women   51
A. E. Schindler

7   Effects of progestogen on the breast   59
E. Lundström and B. von Schoultz

8   Mammographic density and breast cancer   67
G. Svane

9   Estrogen replacement therapy in the endometrial- and breast-cancer patient   77
W. T. Creasman and M. F. Kohler

10   Oral contraceptives and ovarian cancer: a review   85
C. La Vecchia

11   Mood and the menopause   95
P. Klein

12   Premenstrual syndrome and the menopause   111
S. O'Brien, K. M. K. Ismail and K. Jain

13   Women, hormones and depression   119
J. Studd

14   The use of hormonal intrauterine systems in menopausal women   131
     C. Ng, J. Hockey and N. Panay

15   Clinical use of bone density measurements   139
     J. A. Kanis

16   Prevention and correction of osteoporosis   151
     D. I. Crosbie and D. M. Reid

17   Bleeding patterns and hormone replacement therapy   159
     F. Al-Azzawi and M. Wahab

18   Immunological changes after the menopause and estrogen replacement therapy   175
     S. Ocampo de Ruiz

19   Contribution of assisted reproduction technology to the understanding of early   185
     ovarian aging
     D. Nikolaou and G. Trew

20   Efficacy of and tolerance towards different kinds of hormone replacement therapy   199
     J. Donát

21   Vaginal estrogens: is there a role for their use?   213
     W. H. Cronje and J. Studd

22   Pulsed estrogen therapy: a new concept in hormone replacement therapy   221
     N. Panay and J. Studd

23   Dyspareunia: clinical approach in the perimenopause   229
     A. Graziottin

24   Menopause and the internet   243
     H. Currie and G. Cumming

25   Nutrition and the menopause   253
     S. Palacios and C. Rueda

26   Alternative therapies for postmenopausal women   261
     L. Speroff

Index   275

List of principal contributors

Farook Al-Azzawi
Gynaecology Research Unit
Department of Obstetrics and Gynaecology
Leicester Warwick Medical School
University of Leicester
RK Clinical Sciences Building
Leicester Royal Infirmary
Leicester LE2 7LX
UK

David Barlow
Nuffield Department of Obstetrics and
    Gynaecology
Level 3, The Women's Centre
The John Radcliffe Hospital
University of Oxford
Oxford OX3 9DU
UK

Henry Burger
Prince Henry's Institute of Medical
    Research
Level 4 Block E
Monash Medical Centre
246 Clayton Road
Clayton
Victoria 3168
Australia

Linda Cardozo
King's College Hospital
Denmark Hill
London SE5 9RS
UK

William T. Creasman
Department of Obstetrics and
    Gynecology
Medical University of South Carolina
Charleston SC 29425
USA

Wilhelm H. Cronje
The Menopause and Premenstrual Syndrome
    Trust
Academic Department of Obstetrics and
    Gynaecology
Chelsea and Westminster Hospital
369 Fulham Road
London SW10 9NH
UK

David I. Crosbie
Department of Rheumatology
Aberdeen Royal Infirmary
Foresterhill
Aberdeen AB25 2ZN
UK

Heather Currie
Department of Obstetrics and Gynaecology
Dumfries and Galloway Royal Infirmary
Bankend Road
Dumfries DG1 4AP
UK

Josef Donát
Department of Obstetrics and Gynecology
School of Medicine of Charles University
500 05 Hradec Kralove
Czech Republic

Christian Falconer
Division of Obstetrics and Gynecology
Karolinska Institute
Danderyd Hospital
SE-182 88 Danderyd
Sweden

Alessandra Graziottin
Center of Gynecology and Medical Sexology
Hospital San Raffaele Resnati
Milan
Italy

John Kanis
Centre for Metabolic Bone Diseases at
  Sheffield
(WHO Collaborating Centre)
University of Sheffield Medical School
Beech Hill Road
Sheffield S10 2RX
UK

Pavel Klein
Department of Neurology
Georgetown University Medical Center
Bles Building-1
3800 Reservoir Road NW
Washington DC 20007
USA

Chun Ng
The Menopause and Premenstrual Syndrome
  Centre
Department of Obstetrics and
  Gynaecology
Queen Charlotte's and Chelsea Hospital
Du Cane Road
London W12 0HS
UK

Dimitios Nikolaou
Chelsea and Westminster Hospital
369 Fulham Road
London SW10 9NH
UK

Shaughan O'Brien
Women and Children's Division
Maternity Unit
City General Hospital
North Staffordshire NHS Trust
Stoke on Trent ST4 6QG
UK

Santiago Palacios
Instituto Palacios Salud y Medicina
  de la Mujer
Calle Antonio Acuña 9
28009 Madrid
Spain

Nick Panay
The Menopause and Premenstrual Syndrome
  Centre
Department of Obstetrics and
  Gynaecology
Queen Charlotte's and Chelsea Hospital
Du Cane Road
London W12 0HS
UK

Sonia Ocampo de Ruiz
Sociedad Boliviana del Climaterio
Av. Moñoz Reyes No. 100 Cota Cota
La Paz
Bolivia
South America

Goran Samsioe
Department of Obstetrics and
  Gynecology
Lund University Hospital
S-221 85 Lund
Sweden

Adolf E. Schindler
Director of Institute of Medical Research and
  Education
Department of Obstetrics and Gynecology
University of Essen
Hufelandstrasse 55
D-45147 Essen
Germany

Bo von Schoultz
Department of Obstetrics and Gynecology
Karolinska Hospital
SE-171 76 Stockholm
Sweden

Leon Speroff
Department of Obstetrics and Gynecology
Oregon Health Sciences University
3181 Sam Jackson Park Road
Portland OR 97201
USA

John Studd
Chelsea and Westminster Hospital
369 Fulham Road
London SW10 9NH
UK

Gunilla Svane
Mammography Section
Department of Diagnostic Radiology
Karolinska Hospital
S-171 76 Stockholm
Sweden

Carlo la Vecchia
Instituto di Ricerche Farmacologiche Mario
    Negri
20157 Milan
Italy
and
Instituto di Statistica Medica e Biometria
Università degli Studi Milano
20133 Milan
Italy

Foreword

Five years ago, consensus concerning hormone replacement therapy (HRT) and the menopause was fairly straightforward. Estrogens helped symptoms, prevented osteoporosis, prevented heart attacks and probably prevented strokes and Alzheimer's disease. There was a problem with a possible small increase in breast cancer, but this was somewhat nullified by the view that the prognosis was so much better and that fewer HRT users died of breast cancer than a comparable group of non-users. It was all good news.

The Heart and Estrogen/progestin Replacement Study (HERS) secondary prevention study removed much optimism that estrogens would improve the prognosis of women who already had coronary artery disease. Stopping the trial at 5 years was certainly a wasted opportunity as the slight increase in cardiovascular events in the first year compared with placebo was being replaced by a clear benefit in years 3 and 4. Such is the wisdom of epidemiologists.

But it gets worse: the Women's Health Initiative (WHI) study has had a devastating effect upon patients' confidence in HRT. The media, quite correctly, made a great issue of these results. In spite of warnings from many clinical 'menopausologists', the WHI proceeded with a vastly expensive study using a standard dose of HRT whether the women were aged 50 or 79. They used, in my view, the wrong estrogen, probably the wrong route, and certainly the wrong population with an average age of 63 (range 50–79). Sixty-eight percent of patients were recruited over the age of 60 and 22% over the age of 70, with some recruited aged 79. Seven-point-seven percent had a past history of cardiovascular disease and 35% were taking hypertensives, but they were still prescribed 0.625 mg Premarin® and 0.25 mg Provera®. Only a clinical optimist would do this but this was the standard treatment in this group.

At \$100 million and still spending the WHI trial is the most expensive, and in my personal opinion, the most inappropriate and probably the worst clinical trial in the history of medicine. Approximately 40% of American and European women have stopped taking HRT and the North American Menopause Society Advisory Panel (03.10.02) recommend that estrogens should be reserved for the treatment of severe vasomotor symptoms and atrophy and should not be first choice for the prevention or treatment of osteoporosis.

The British Medical Research Council (MRC) spent almost £10 million reproducing the WHI study which was already underway using the same estrogen despite protests from individual experts from the British Menopause Society, and from some members of the Council of the Royal College of Obstetricians and Gynaecologists. Epidemiologists certainly know how to spend money whether they are American or British. The MRC WISDOM study was discontinued with hardly a murmur of protest nor a hint of apology.

I am constantly amazed at the reaction of the commentators to this study. Although recognizing its faults, their reaction is to advocate very-low-dose estrogens on the assumption that this must be safer and perhaps even better. We must be aware that our responsibility to peri- and postmenopausal women is to be sure that specific symptoms are treated correctly and that these women feel better without side-effects. The message is so simple: if women feel better, they will continue with estrogen therapy but they are unlikely to achieve this with a quasi-homeopathic dose of the fashionable American oral estrogen.

Older women certainly need a very low starting dose, perhaps given on alternate days. The recently postmenopausal woman will need a low-to-moderate dose with the appropriate progestogen for relief of symptoms and prevention of osteoporosis. The woman with osteoporosis needs estrogen that will produce plasma estradiol levels of at least 300 pmol/l. The perimenopausal woman with depression and even premenstrual syndrome symptoms requires moderately high doses of transdermal estrogens which will produce plasma estradiol levels of at least 600 pmol/l (note the normal range is 150–1500 pmol/l so we are not going too high), together with cyclical progestogen. Women with libido problems need higher doses of estrogen with the addition of testosterone, and those with estrogen-responsive depression with progestogen intolerance need moderately high doses of transdermal estrogens, probably with the use of a Mirena® intrauterine system. All these patients do not need the standard low dose of estrogen. None of these patient groups needed the standard low dose of estrogen as used in the WHI study.

Not surprisingly, a subsequent paper from the WHI showed that there was no improvement in quality-of-life scores on this dose of Premarin® in this age group. Once again this was the wrong dose for the wrong patient.

This is such an important issue that I am grateful for the chapters on this subject from Henry Burger and colleagues, David Barlow and Goran Samsioe in the early pages of this volume. Passing on quickly to the end of the book, Santiago Palacios and Leon Speroff have produced scholarly accounts on the value – or lack of it – of alternative therapies for the postmenopausal woman.

I am grateful to all of the authors for their timely contributions and I can reassure my friends who haven't quite been able to make the deadline that they will not be forgotten for the Fourth Edition next year. I must also acknowledge my thanks to the staff at Parthenon who are, at whatever level, always totally reliable. I particularly thank Jean Wright and Stephen Nicholls for their work on this volume.

John Studd, DSc, MD, FRCOG
Chelsea & Westminster Hospital, London
www.studd.co.uk

1

The future of hormone replacement therapy

H. G. Burger, S. Davison and S. R. Davis

INTRODUCTION

The future of hormone replacement therapy (HRT), more appropriately described as postmenopausal hormone therapy (PHT), has become an extremely topical issue with the recent publication of the first report from the Women's Health Initiative randomized controlled trial of estrogen plus progestin in 'healthy' postmenopausal women[1]. The field had been thrown into substantial controversy by the earlier publication of another prospective randomized controlled trial, the Heart and Estrogen/progestin Replacement Study (HERS)[2], in which the benefit of PHT for the secondary prevention of cardiovascular disease in women was shown to be lacking.

The latter, combined with major recent reports of the increased risk of breast cancer, had already begun to cast significant doubts about the advisability of long-term hormone therapy in particular. This chapter aims to give a current perspective on the future applications of PHT by considering the indications for such therapy, the preparations available now and likely to be modified in the future, dosages, methods of administration and availability of compounds such as tibolone and the selective estrogen receptor modulators (SERMs). Other potential new methods are mentioned briefly, and the potential role of androgens in future PHT is considered.

INDICATIONS FOR POSTMENOPAUSAL HORMONE THERAPY

Currently available preparations and dosages of estrogen with or without a progestin are prescribed both for the short-term relief of symptoms associated with the peri- and early postmenopause and for long-term risk reduction, specifically for osteoporotic fracture and, until recently, for cardiovascular disease. Other possible reasons for long-term therapy have included reduction in the risk of cognitive decline and prevention of Alzheimer's disease, and reduction in the risk of colorectal cancer. Each of these indications is reviewed in the light of current knowledge.

Short-term use for symptom relief

The vasomotor symptoms of hot flushes and night sweats, which are characteristic of the peri- and early postmenopause, can be satisfactorily relieved with an estrogen or an estrogen plus a progestogen. Appropriate attention to life-style factors such as exercise, diet and stress reduction may also contribute to relief. Urogenital atrophy occurs commonly and responds to local estrogen administration as well as systemic therapy. Other symptoms that are commonly experienced, but are not specific to the menopause, include depression, anxiety, palpitations, headaches, insomnia, lack of energy, fluid retention, backache, difficulty in concentrating and dizzy spells. These are usually not highly correlated with menopausal status, although they are strongly correlated with each other and are more common among women who experience severe flushing[3,4]. The severity of menopause-associated symptoms varies widely between women within the same culture, and even more widely among those from different cultures. Hormone therapy is effective for symptom relief and is indicated when a woman seeks this for moderate or severe complaints. With appropriate choice of dose and regimen, such therapy is generally regarded as non-controversial. The only significant risk of such short-term therapy is a small increase in the incidence of thromboembolism, estimated as an excess of about 1 in 5000 events per year in women early in their sixth decade. The results of studies such as the Women's Health Initiative (WHI)[1] and HERS[2] are not generally relevant to consideration of the short-term use of hormones, as the subjects were predominantly substantially older than women with symptoms. Once symptom relief has been obtained, it is common practice to continue therapy for 2, 3 or 4 years. The possibility of long-term therapy arises if symptoms recur when treatment is withdrawn. Treatment withdrawal should be staged and not abrupt, as the latter is more likely to cause recurrence. If symptoms persist each time hormone therapy is withdrawn, women may request ongoing therapy. However, the benefits and risks of long-term therapy must then be carefully considered so that each woman can make an informed choice to continue, as discussed below.

Long-term therapy

Results of the Women's Health Initiative randomized controlled trial

Long-duration PHT would generally be regarded as therapy lasting for more than 5 years. In that context, the results of the WHI to some extent become relevant. The WHI was initiated to define the risks and benefits of long-term PHT with particular reference to the incidence of heart disease and breast cancer, but with reference to other outcomes such as fracture and colorectal cancer. The study enrolled 161 809 postmenopausal women aged 50–79 years for various trials including PHT, low-fat diet and supplementation with calcium and vitamin D. One arm of this study was prematurely terminated in 2002 because the preset limit for the occurrence of invasive breast cancer 'exceeded the stopping boundary for this adverse effect'[1]. This randomized controlled primary-prevention trial included 16 608 postmenopausal women recruited in 40 American clinical centers between the years 1993 and 1998. Women were recruited by population-based direct mailing campaigns, were required to be postmenopausal and to have an intact uterus, and not to have medical conditions likely to be associated with only short-term survival. Some women were using postmenopausal hormones at their initial screening, and for these a 3 month wash-out period was required. The regimen evaluated consisted of conjugated equine estrogen (CEE) 0.625 mg and medroxyprogesterone acetate (MPA) 2.5 mg or a matching placebo.

The average age of participants at screening was 63.2 years. One-third were in the age group 50–59, 45% were 60–69 and 21% were 70–79. The majority were White women, but the study included small numbers of Blacks, Hispanics, American Indians and Asians/Pacific Islanders. Almost 20% of the subjects were past users of hormones, and a further 6% were current users. The majority of these had used hormones for less than 5 years, although 19% of the previously treated women in the active treatment arm and 17% of the controls had used hormones previously for 5–10 years and 12% in each group for more than 10 years. Average body mass index (BMI) was 28.5 kg/m^2, and fewer than one-third of women had a normal BMI < 25 kg/m^2. One-third of the women were overweight, and one-third had a BMI >30 kg/m^2, i.e. they were obese. Yet, overall, the subjects were described by the authors as 'healthy' postmenopausal women. Fifty per cent of the women had never smoked,

40% were past smokers and 10% current smokers. In each group 4.4% had been treated for diabetes, and 7% in each group had used statins at baseline, while approximately 20% had used aspirin. A very small number of women had a history of either coronary artery disease or prior thromboembolic events. The latter is generally considered a strict exclusion criterion for studies of postmenopausal estrogen therapy. The group were in general not at increased risk of breast cancer.

At the time of the report all women had been enrolled for at least 3.5 years and the average duration of follow-up was 5.2 years, with a maximum of 8.5 years. Forty-two per cent of women had stopped using hormones, and 38.5% had stopped using placebo at some time; 10.7% of the placebo group initiated hormone therapy. The authors provided data about the absolute numbers of various clinical outcomes by randomization assignment and presented their results in particular as annualized percentages, from which annual rates per 10 000 women were calculated. For purposes of clarity, the results from this study have been recalculated, as shown in Table 1, as events per 1000 women over the average 5.2 years of follow-up, together with the increased or decreased number of cases in the active group compared with placebo in that interval.

Many of the results in this first report from the WHI were in accord with the results of previous observational studies. Somewhat unexpected, however, was an increase rather than a decrease in the frequency of coronary heart disease events, with an excess risk of 4.2 cases per 1000 women over 5.2 years. It is noteworthy that the excess of coronary heart disease events occurred primarily in the first year of the study when the ratio of events in the treated versus placebo arms was 1.78, comparable to what was seen in the first year of the HERS trial[2]. There was also an excess of cases in year 5, 23 of 5964 participants compared with nine of 5566, although the trend was negative over time.

Stroke risk was somewhat higher than anticipated, while the risks of venous thromboembolism and pulmonary embolism were relatively high, but not unexpected for a group of women of average age 63 years, of whom most were overweight. The rate of increase in cases of invasive breast cancer was in line with the results of previous studies[5], and again showed an excess of 4.2 cases per 1000 women over 5.2 years. This can also be expressed as an excess risk of 1 : 240 over 5 years. Of considerable importance, but not highlighted in the publication, is that there was no increase in breast cancer risk among the 6280 women treated with active therapy for a mean duration of 5.2 years who had not used hormone therapy prior to commencing the study, compared with the 6204 prior non-users treated with placebo (hazard ratio for active therapy being 1.06, 95% confidence interval (CI) 0.81–1.38). This reconfirms the results of previous studies indicating that hormone therapy for less than 5 years is not associated with increased breast cancer risk[5].

Table 1 Women's Health Initiative[1]: events per 1000 women over 5.2 years (average)

	Active treatment	Placebo treatment	Excess/deficiency in active groups
Coronary heart disease	19.3	15.1	4.2 more
Stroke	14.9	10.5	4.4 more
Venous thromboembolism	17.8	8.3	9.5 more
Pulmonary embolism	8.2	3.8	4.4 more
Invasive breast cancer	19.5	15.3	4.2 more
Colorectal cancer	5.3	8.3	3 fewer
Total fractures	76	97	21 fewer
Hip fractures	5.2	7.7	2.5 fewer
Total deaths	27	27	—
Global index	88.3	76.9	11.4 greater

In contrast, in those who had used hormones for less than 5 years previously, the hazard ratio was 2.13 with 95% CI 1.15– 3.94.

Of interest was a reduction in colorectal cancer risk by three cases, and a reduction in total fractures by 21 and hip fractures by 2.5. Total deaths in both arms of the study were identical, but a global index comparing risk with benefit proved to be in the adverse direction in the actively treated women.

It was noteworthy that the absolute excess risks attributable to the therapy were low, and that the trial tested an oral drug therapy regimen usually used for symptomatic treatment in early postmenopausal women, not in women 10–25 years postmenopausal. The authors and other commentators have indicated that this combined hormone therapy regimen should not be initiated or continued for the primary prevention of coronary heart disease, and that the substantial risk for coronary heart disease and breast cancer must be weighed against benefit for fracture, in selection of the available agents to prevent osteoporosis. Recommendations have been made that clinicians should stop prescribing this combination for long-term use. A limitation of these recommendations is that event rates were not published per decade of age. One would strongly suspect that cardiovascular events would have been rare in women under 65 years of age in this study, and thus recommendations may not be applicable to younger women.

The authors were careful to point out that 'this trial tested only one trial regimen, CEE 0.625 mg per day, plus MPA 2.5 mg per day, in postmenopausal woman with an intact uterus. The results do not necessarily apply to lower dosages of these drugs, to other formulations of oral estrogens and progestins, or to estrogens and progestins administered through the transdermal route. It remains possible that transdermal estradiol with progesterone, which more closely mimics the normal physiology and metabolism of endogenous sex hormones, may provide a different risk–benefit profile'[1]. The authors also pointed out that the trial was unable to distinguish the effects of estrogen from those of progestin, the latter perhaps being particularly important for breast cancer and perhaps atherosclerotic disease. A separate trial within the WHI is testing the hypothesis of whether oral estrogen alone will prevent coronary heart disease in 10 739 hysterectomized women. The latter trial is continuing at the time of this writing.

Primary prevention of cardiovascular disease

The results of the WHI, as discussed in detail above, have been interpreted as indicating that long-term PHT has no place in the primary prevention of cardiovascular disease. This conclusion had also been drawn by some writers from the results of the HERS trial[2] and a limited number of other randomized trials. It may be argued that this is too strong a generalization on the basis of the published data. Women in the HERS trial were chosen deliberately to evaluate the place of PHT in secondary prevention, i.e. they were women with existing, clinically manifest coronary artery disease. Women in the WHI were chosen to be 'healthy postmenopausal women', as only 7.7% of the participants reported having had prior cardiovascular disease. However, this study population cannot realistically be characterized as 'healthy' considering the high rates of obesity and current and past smoking, that 35% were being treated for hypertension, 12% had hypercholesterolemia requiring therapy and 20% had an indication for aspirin use. Although the participants were in general free of clinical coronary artery disease, it seems highly probable that many had significant subclinical disease. That there were more coronary events in the treated group than in the controls is consistent with this interpretation. It could be argued that true primary prevention of coronary heart disease involves the treatment of women at risk, but without significant coronary disease at the time such preventive therapy is initiated. There is substantial literature indicating that modification of endothelial function plays a major role in the cardioprotection afforded by estrogen[6], but that this is attenuated in women with pre-existing endothelial dysfunction[7]. This, in turn, may in part explain the disappointing results of prospective estrogen intervention studies in women at high cardiovascular risk.

The work of Clarkson's group in the cynomolgus monkey model of postmenopausal atherosclerotic vascular disease[8] suggests strongly that, in animals in which advanced atherosclerosis has been allowed to develop, sex-steroid therapy is ineffective in reducing progression. In animals with moderate disease, some reduction in progression can be anticipated, but the striking results in terms of primary prevention are seen in animals with minimal or absent lesions[9]. A large body of evidence indicates that estrogen influences vascular function via genomic and non-genomic mechanisms, and therefore that sex-steroid administration to postmenopausal women should clearly be cardioprotective[6]. Extensive epidemiological data also indicate that current usage of PHT is associated with a reduction in the relative risk (RR) of cardiovascular events (current users RR 0.56, 95% CI 0.4–0.8; past users: RR 0.83, 95% CI 0.65–1.05)[10]. The women most likely to benefit are those with the most significant cardiovascular risk factors[11]. At best, in the WHI, this criterion might have applied to the group of women aged < 60 years at the time therapy was initiated. It could be postulated that a true primary-prevention trial should randomize women within the first 3–5 years after the menopause, and should perhaps use the most physiologically relevant type of hormone, namely estradiol itself, given parenterally, preferably associated with progesterone, a progestin closely resembling it, or a progestin administered directly to the uterus (for example by an intrauterine device) and thus avoiding systemic exposure. Only in those circumstances could true primary prevention be evaluated. This type of study is one which the authors would hope to see carried out in the context of the 'future of HRT'. Thus, although such observational studies are known to be limited by various biases, the design of the WHI is not such that it would allow an unequivocal conclusion that long-term PHT has no place in primary cardiovascular protection. The issues of dosage are considered below.

Secondary prevention of cardiovascular disease

While the results of the HERS trial[2] have been widely interpreted as indicating that long-term PHT has no place in the secondary prevention of heart disease, it is again noteworthy that observational studies such as the Nurses' Health Study[10] have suggested that some long-term protection may be afforded, as have several studies of women undergoing surgical procedures for coronary disease[12]. The HERS trial was conducted among volunteers of average age 68 years who were commenced abruptly on a regimen of CEE 0.625 mg per day and MPA 2.5 mg per day. Most clinicians would regard as inappropriate clinical management the abrupt initiation of therapy with doses actually appropriate for early-postmenopausal women, but not for those 10–25 years past the menopause. It could be postulated that such abrupt hormone dosage might have adverse effects on pre-existing atherosclerotic plaques, thus accounting for the increased event rate in the first year of active therapy. While it may be that extensively diseased arteries could never be affected favorably by long-term hormone therapy, a trial in which very low doses of therapy were administered initially and gradually built up to low therapeutic levels could be worthwhile if the issue was to be studied rigorously. Nevertheless, the availability of several other measures for cardiovascular protection makes it most unlikely that such a trial would ever be conducted. On current evidence, the appropriate measures for secondary prevention of coronary disease include life-style changes, avoidance of smoking, regular exercise, and specific treatment of hypertension and dyslipidemia[13].

Osteoporosis prevention and management

A major dilemma posed by the WHI findings[1] concerns the long-term use of PHT for women at increased risk of osteoporotic fracture, including those who have already suffered such an event. A woman may be considered at sufficient risk to warrant intervention, for example with PHT, if her bone mineral density indicates a T-score below −2.5 standard deviations from the mean in the absence of other risk factors, or a T-score at −1.5 to −2.5 standard deviations in the presence of other risk factors such as a maternal history of osteoporotic fracture. For such women, many clinicians have prescribed PHT for a period of at least 5–10 years postmenopausally, and some would consider such therapy appropriate lifelong. The findings of the WHI, particularly in respect of confirming the small increase in the risk of breast cancer, require that a decision about long-term PHT be properly assessed in terms of relative benefit and risk. The WHI report indicated benefit for fracture prevention. Because the risks of PHT become apparent after only 4–5 years, it may be reasonable to propose 5 years of therapy, particularly where risk for breast cancer is less, such as in women with a body mass index > 24–25 kg/m^2, where evidence suggests that exogenous hormones do not substantially increase risk[5]. This aspect of the data from the WHI is not evident in the initial report. Whether therapy should be continued for longer periods must be weighed up against the small increase in breast cancer risk. For many women, a substantial increase in fracture risk would justify long-term PHT. Previously, the belief that long-term therapy also provided primary protection against the development of heart disease was a factor supporting the decision to use therapy long-term. As indicated above, it is unclear whether the WHI results have really contradicted this supportive evidence. Other options for long-term fracture prevention include the use of agents such as tibolone, raloxifene and bisphosphonates. However, there are no long-term safety data available for any of these alternatives. Raloxifene in particular appears to have become an increasingly attractive option to women no longer suffering postmenopausal vasomotor symptoms[14]. In addition to a substantial reduction in the risk of breast cancer in osteoporotic women[15], a recent report indicates that raloxifene may reduce cardiovascular risk in

women with a substantially increased baseline risk[16]. In some countries, such as Australia, only PHT is reimbursed for long-term use, while agents such as raloxifene and bisphosphonates are reimbursed only when fracture has already occurred. The findings of the WHI may lead to changes in reimbursement policy in such situations.

Prevention of cognitive decline

Two large analyses published during the past 4 years have provided a systematic review of PHT and cognition[17,18]. Le Blanc and colleagues[18] concluded that observational studies indicate an overall reduction in risk of development of dementia of 34%. The majority of studies used CEE, and there is insufficient evidence to assess whether associated progestin use influences the response to estrogen. Many of the observational studies have the problem of confounding and compliance bias, given that users of PHT tend to have higher levels of education and better health, making them all at lower risk of developing dementia. Adequate long-term, prospective, randomized controlled data are awaited in this area. Long-term PHT cannot be recommended at present for Alzheimer prevention, but may become an indication in the future.

Management of estrogen deficiency in women with a history of treated breast cancer

A highly controversial area in contemporary menopause management is the approach that should be used to the management of estrogen deficiency in women living with a diagnosis of breast cancer. This has been the subject of an international consensus conference[19]. Selective serotonin reuptake inhibitors have been shown to be useful for the management of vasomotor symptoms in the short term, although not all women can tolerate this therapy[20].

No prospective, randomized controlled trial data exist to provide adequate guidelines for the use of hormones after breast cancer, but a number of observational studies, particularly using a case–control design, have suggested that hormone therapy may, if anything, be beneficial in terms of both recurrence and mortality[21]. Until randomized trials have been completed, no firm policy can be adopted, although the authors believe that it is appropriate to use PHT in the lowest effective doses for the minimal requisite time in women in whom other methods of treatment have failed to improve a markedly impaired quality of life arising from unrelieved menopausal symptoms.

HORMONE PREPARATIONS FOR THE FUTURE

The two major estrogens in current use are CEE and various preparations of estradiol. Much of the world literature on the benefits and risks of PHT arises from US studies, and, in particular, from the two randomized controlled trials, HERS and WHI[1,2]. CEE with or without progestin is clearly beneficial for menopausal symptoms, but carries the risks and benefits already discussed. Whether CEE will remain an estrogen preparation of choice in the future, in the light of the recent adverse reports, is a matter for speculation, but the demonstrable safety of this preparation, at least for short-term use, suggests that it will remain an acceptable therapeutic option. Estradiol preparations are also highly effective, and it seems unlikely that there will be any major shifts in choice with the European preference being for estradiol and its derivatives, while the American preference is for CEE.

New developments are occurring in the progestin field, however. The use of progesterone itself has not become widespread, although the results of the Postmenopausal Estrogen/Progestin Interventions (PEPI) trial[22] indicated that progesterone was metabolically the most favorable of the progestins evaluated in that prospective randomized study. Dydrogesterone is a progestin often preferred in Europe, which resembles progesterone closely and appears to be metabolically favorable[23]. Drospirenone is a new progestin with antimineralocorticoid and antiandrogenic properties[24], which has not so far been extensively evaluated, but could be a PHT progestin of the future. Trimegestone is another new progestin likely to be used more extensively in the future[24]. The two progestins most widely used currently are MPA and norethisterone (norethindrone). Data regarding an appropriate choice between these two agents is not clear-cut, and the choice again seems to be largely nationally determined. It is difficult to see what major changes will occur in the future. The other new progestins that have been evaluated mainly in Europe may become more widely used if initial favorable findings are confirmed.

A major area likely to develop substantially in the future is the therapeutic use of androgens, which are considered below. An important need is for appropriate preparations of testosterone, and various transdermal testosterone preparations including a patch and gel are currently under intensive evaluation prior to more widespread commercialization. Testosterone creams and perhaps troches for buccal use may also find application in the future. In some countries testosterone implants have found popularity, although it seems likely that they will be replaced by newer formulations.

More controversial is the question of whether dehydroepiandrosterone (DHEA) will become a widely used preparation in the future. DHEA is metabolized to testosterone and estradiol, and has been shown to be therapeutically effective in some studies[25]. Its theoretical advantage is that the degree of metabolism is controlled in peripheral tissues, and the agent may therefore be therapeutically more physiological.

HORMONE DOSAGE

A major trend in the therapeutic use of estrogens and progestins is to apply lower doses than have previously been regarded as standard and optimal. The dose of CEE chosen for the WHI and HERS is one usually recommended for the management of peri- and early postmenopausal symptoms, and, even in that setting, lower doses are currently under evaluation. Recent trials have compared that dose of CEE with two lower doses, 0.3 and 0.45 mg per day, in combination with proportionately lower doses of MPA[26–28]. These trials have already indicated therapeutic efficacy even in early-postmenopausal women, with associated favorable changes in cardiovascular risk factors and in bone density. Such lower-dose preparations therefore require proper assessment of the benefit/risk ratio where it might be expected that long-term risks may be less, particularly the risk of an increase in cardiovascular events in the first few months after initiating therapy. No such early increase has been reported in the lower-dose hormone trials. Lower dose transdermal therapy has also been evaluated, and some reports have indicated that, at such low doses, endometrial protection may not be necessary[29].

METHODS OF ADMINISTRATION

Because of the very extensive literature documenting the overall safety and efficacy of orally administered estrogen and progestogen, oral therapy is likely to remain a widely used option in the future. Much fewer data exist concerning long-term benefits and risks of transdermal preparations, although these may be viewed as being more physiological in their avoidance of hepatic first-pass effects. Oral estrogen preparations result in up to ten-fold higher levels of circulating estrone sulfate than with transdermally administered estradiol at comparable or even higher doses[30,31]. Estrogen-sensitive target tissues such as the breast and endometrium have a high capacity to metabolize estrone sulfate through to estradiol. This may be a mechanism by which concentrations of estrone and estradiol in breast cancer tissue are several-fold greater than circulating levels[32]. Thus, research into whether the benefits and risks of non-oral PHT are the same as those reported for oral regimens is urgently needed.

Orally administered estrogen therapy also increases sex hormone binding globulin (SHBG) to a greater extent than non-orally administered estrogens[33,34], and this may result in a clinically significant reduction in bio-available testosterone. Thus, it would seem that the prescription of oral estrogen therapy should be at the lowest available dose to mini-mize effects on circulating estrone sulfate and SHBG. Consistent with this, lower-dose combinations of micronized estradiol and norethisterone acetate are associated with equivalent symptom relief to that with higher-dose combinations, but with lower rates of mastalgia and vaginal bleeding[35].

Transdermal preparations are, and will almost certainly remain, the treatments of choice for women with a past history of venous thromboembolism, or those with malabsorption syndromes including the fairly common irritable bowel syndrome. Whether transdermal therapy will be more commonly indicated for women with hypertension and diabetes awaits the results of larger trials. The recently introduced intranasal estradiol spray has provided initially favorable results as far as patient acceptability and efficacy are concerned, but again requires more detailed evaluation. Buccal administration has not been studied extensively.

MODIFIED HORMONE THERAPIES

The future of modified therapies again remains uncertain. Tibolone has been used extensively in Europe for more than 10 years, but has been introduced only recently onto the Australian market and is not yet available in the USA. Tibolone has theoretical advantages in providing an estrogen, a progestogen and an androgen in a single tablet, the various activities resulting from tissue-specific metabolism[36]. Efficacy for relief of symptoms, for preservation of bone density and for enhancement of fibrinolysis has been demonstrated. No significant increase in breast density has been reported, and it therefore seems possible that tibolone will have no adverse effect on breast cancer incidence. Nevertheless, no data are currently available on cardiovascular event rates, fractures or breast cancer occurrence, and the more widespread adoption of tibolone therefore awaits adequately powered randomized controlled trials. Selective estrogen receptor modulators (SERMs) such as raloxifene are being used extensively for prevention of osteoporosis, or treatment of established osteoporosis. The reduction in breast cancer risk observed with raloxifene[15] makes it an attractive option for long-term osteoporosis management. The recent observation that women at significantly increased risk of cardiovascular disease had a 40% reduction in cardiovascular events with 4 years of raloxifene administration has also aroused interest[16]. Large prospective randomized trials are currently under way, comparing raloxifene with tamoxifen for reduction in breast cancer occurrence and for evaluation of the effects of raloxifene on the cardiovascular system. The future of raloxifene use in clinical practice will certainly be influenced significantly by the outcome of these studies. A number of companies are also developing newer SERMs, but there are insufficient data on any of these at the time of writing to make predictions about their likely applicability in the future of hormone therapy. Under evaluation also are combinations of SERMs with estradiol itself, with the aim of relieving symptoms of the menopause that are unaffected or exacerbated by currently available SERMs. Selective androgen receptor modulators are also in development, but insufficient data exist to make future predictions.

NEW METHODS

A recent report of an antiapoptotic effect of sex steroids on bone and other cell types, mediated by the region of the classical steroid hormone receptor distinct from that responsible for the genotropic actions of such steroids, has led to the possibility of developing function-specific as opposed to tissue-selective compounds. Such effects were demonstrated to be different from classic actions of estrogen or androgen, and the authors have suggested that this may lead to the development 'of an advantageous class of pharmacotherapeutic agents (true anabolic as opposed to anti-resorptive) and gender neutral for the management of osteopenic states'[37].

ANDROGEN THERAPY

The existence of a female androgen-deficiency syndrome has long been suspected, and a recent consensus conference developed guidelines for the clinical and biochemical diagnosis of such a deficiency[38]. More widespread application of such guidelines will depend on wider recognition of the syndrome, and the availability of testosterone assays of suitable sensitivity for measurements in the female range and below it. The therapeutic use of androgens in the future will require the development of gender-specific androgen preparations, such as a testosterone patch currently under intensive evaluation. Long-term randomized trials will be necessary to determine whether DHEA is an androgen of the future. Nevertheless, the future of hormone therapy may well lie in the development of combined preparations of estrogen, progestogen and androgen for many women.

References

1. Writing Group for the Women's Health Initiative Investigators. Risks and benefits of estrogen plus progestin in healthy postmenopausal women. Principal results from the Women's Health Initiative randomized controlled trial. *J Am Med Assoc* 2002;288:321–368

2. Hulley S, Grady D, Bush T, *et al.* Randomized trial of estrogen plus progestin for secondary prevention of coronary heart disease in postmenopausal women. *J Am Med Assoc* 1998;280:605–13

3. Greene JG, Cooke DJ. Life stress and symptoms at the climacterium. *Br J Psychiatry* 1980;136: 486–91

4. Avis NE, McKinlay SM. A longitudinal analysis of women's attitudes towards the menopause: results from the Massachusetts Women's Health Study. *Maturitas* 1991;13:65–79

5. Collaborative Group on Hormonal Factors in Breast Cancer. Breast cancer and hormone replacement therapy: collaborative reanalysis of data from 51 epidemiological studies of 52 705 women with breast cancer and 108 411 women without breast cancer. *Lancet* 1997; 350:1047–59

6. Mendelsohn ME, Karas RH. Mechanisms of disease: the protective effects of estrogen on the cardiovascular system. *N Engl J Med* 1999;340: 1801–11

7. Davis SR, Goldstat R, Newman A, *et al.* Differing effects of low dose estrogen–progestin therapy and pravastatin in postmenopausal hyper-cholesterolemic women. *Climacteric* 2002;5: 341–50

8. Adams MR, Kaplan JR, Manuck SB, *et al.* Inhibition of coronary artery atherosclerosis by 17β-estradiol in ovariectomized monkeys. Lack of an effect of added progesterone. *Arteriosclerosis* 1990;10:1051–7

9. Mikkola TS, Clarkson TB. Estrogen replacement therapy, atherosclerosis, and vascular function. *Cardiovasc Res* 2002;53:605–19

10. Stampfer MJ, Colditz GA, Willett WC, *et al.* Postmenopausal estrogen therapy and cardio-vascular disease: ten year follow-up from the Nurses' Health Study. *N Engl J Med* 1991; 325:756–62

11. Grodstein F, Stampfer MJ, Colditz GA, *et al.* Postmenopausal hormone therapy and mortality. *N Engl J Med* 1997;336:1769–75

12. Sullivan JM, El-Zeky F, Vander Zwaag R, Ramanathan KB. Effect on survival of estrogen replacement therapy after coronary artery bypass grafting. *Am J Cardiol* 1997;79:847–50

13. Hu FB, Stampfer MJ, Manson JE, *et al.* Trends in the incidence of coronary heart disease and changes in diet and lifestyle in women. *N Engl J Med* 2000;343:530–7

14. Ettinger B, Black D, Mitlak B, *et al.* Reduction of vertebral fracture risk of postmenopausal women with osteoporosis treated with raloxifene. *J Am Med Assoc* 1999; 282:637–45

15. Cummins SR, Eckert S, Krueger KA, *et al.* The effect of raloxifene on risk of breast cancer in postmenopausal women. *J Am Med Assoc* 1999;281:2189–97

16. Barrett-Connor E, Grady D, Sashegyi A, *et al.* Raloxifene and cardiovascular events in osteo-porotic postmenopausal women. Four-year results from the MORE (Mutliple Outcomes of Raloxifene Evaluation) randomised trial. *J Am Med Assoc* 2002;287:847–57

17. Yaffe K, Sawaya G, Leiderburg I, Grady D. Estro-gen therapy in postmenopausal women: effects on cognitive function and dementia. *J Am Med Assoc* 1998;279:688–95

18. Le Blanc E, Janowsky J, Chan B, Nelson T. HRT and cognition – systemic review and meta-analysis. *N Engl J Med* 2001;285:1489–99

19. Santen R, Pritchard K, Burger HG. The consen-sus conference on treatment of estrogen deficiency symptoms in women surviving breast cancer. *Obstet Gynecol Surv* 1998;53 (Suppl): S1–83

20. Loprinzi CL, Kugler JW, Sloan JA, *et al.* Venlafaxine in management of hot flashes in survivors of breast cancer: a randomised controlled trial. *Lancet* 2000;356:2059–64

21. O'Meara ES, Rossing MA, Daling JR, *et al.* Hormone replacement therapy after a diagnosis of breast cancer in relation to recurrence and mortality. *J Natl Cancer Inst* 2001;93:754–62

22. The Writing Group for the PEPI Trial. Effects of estrogen or estrogen/progestin regimens on heart disease risk factors in postmenopausal women. The Postmenopausal Estrogen/Progestin Interventions (PEPI) Trial. *J Am Med Assoc* 1995;273:199–208

23. Godsland IF. Effects of postmenopausal hor-mone replacement therapy on lipid, lipoprotein and apolipoprotein (a) concentrations: analysis of studies published from 1974–2000. *Fertil Steril* 2001;75:898–915

24. Sitruk-Ware R. Progestogens in hormonal replacement therapy: new molecules, risks and benefits. *Menopause* 2002;9:6–15

25. Stomati M, Monteleone P, Casarosa E, *et al.* Six-month oral dehydroepiandrosterone supple-mentation in early and late postmenopause. *Gynecol Endocrinol* 2000;14:342–63

26. Utian WH, Shoupe D, Bachmann G, *et al.* Relief of vasomotor symptoms and vaginal atrophy with lower doses of conugatged equine estrogens and medroxyprogesterone acetate. *Fertil Steril* 2001;75:1065–79

27. Lobo RA, Bush T, Carr BR, Pickar JH. Effects of lower doses of conjugated equine estrogens and medroxyprogesterone acetate on plasma lipids and lipoproteins, coagulation factors and carbohydrate metabolism. *Fertil Steril* 2001; 76:13–24

28. Gambacciani M, Ciaponi M, Cappagli B, Genazzani AR. Effects of low-dose continuous combined conjugated estrogens and medroxy-progesterone acetate on menopausal symptoms, body weight, bone density and metabolism in postmenopausal women. *Am J Obstet Gynecol* 2001;185:1180–5

29. Ettinger B. Personal perspective on low-dosage estrogen therapy for postmenopausal women. *Menopause* 1999;6:273–6

30. Slater C, Hodis H, Mack W, *et al.* Markedly elevated levels of estrone sulfate after long term oral, but not transdermal, administration of estradiol in postmenopausal women. *Menopause* 2001;8:200–203

31. Nachtigall L, Raju U, Banerjee S, *et al.* Serum estradiol binding profiles in postmenopausal women undergoing three common estrogen replacement therapies. *Menopause* 2000;7:243–50

32. Pasqualini JR, Chetrite G, Blacker C, *et al.* Concentrations of estrone, estradiol and estrone sulfate and evaluation of sulfatase and aromatase activities in pre- and postmenopausal breast cancer patients. *J Clin Endocrinol Metab* 1996; 81:1360–464

33. Raisz LG, Witta B, Artis A, *et al.* Comparison of the effects of estrogen alone and estrogen plus androgen on biochemical markers of bone formation and resorption in postmenopausal women. *J Clin Endocrinol Metab* 1995;81:37–43

34. Slowinska-Srzednicka J, Zgliczynski S, Jeske S, *et al.* A transdermal 17β-estradiol combined with oral progestogen increases plasma levels of insulin-like growth factor-I in postmenopausal women. *J Endocrinol Invest* 1992;15:533–8

35. Stradberg E, Mattsson L-A, Uvebrant M. 17β-Estradiol and norethisterone acetate in low doses as continuous combined hormone replacement therapy. *Maturitas* 1996;23:31–9

36. Modelska K, Cummings S. Tibolone for postmenopausal women: systematic review of randomized trials. *J Clin Endocrinol Metab* 2002; 87:16–23

37. Kousteni S, Bellido T, Plotkin LI, *et al.* Nongenotropic, sex-nonspecific signalling through the estrogen and androgen receptors: dissociation from transcriptional activity. *Cell* 2001;104: 719–30

38. Bachmann GA, Bancroft J, Braunstein G, *et al.* Female androgen insufficiency: The Princeton Consensus Statement on definition, classification and assessment. *Fertil Steril* 2002;77:660–5

2

National Osteoporosis Society statement, February 2003: hormone replacement therapy and the Women's Health Initiative study

D. Barlow

The premature termination of one component of the US Women's Health Initiative (WHI) study of the effects of hormone replacement therapy (HRT), in July 2002, has led to extensive debate in the field and in the public media[1]. This statement by the National Osteoporosis Society (NOS) seeks to clarify the view of the NOS Council members.

The WHI study was set up to examine the effect of HRT in a large group of 'healthy' American women aged 50–79 years. The women agreed to be randomly allocated a placebo or the appropriate HRT for their status. Those women who had undergone a hysterectomy received HRT involving only continuous daily oral estrogen (conjugated equine estrogens 0.625 mg); the rest received continuous combined daily oral estrogen and progestogen (conjugated equine estrogens 0.625 mg and 2.5 mg medroxyprogesterone acetate). The trial of hysterectomized women on estrogen or placebo continues. The premature trial termination relates only to the part of the study involving estrogen and progestogen. The declared reason for stopping this arm of the trial was that the statistic for overall hazard, combined with an increase in breast cancer risk, became sufficient in that group to necessitate cessation at an average duration of just over 5 years instead of the planned 8 years.

The overall results of the terminated WHI estrogen/progestogen study were published with minimal delay but more detailed publication of the trial data is required for a full assessment. At present the results for each condition relate to the 30-year age range as a whole. However, the absolute risk of each condition occurring changes greatly as women pass from 50 to 79 years of age. Thus, it is difficult to use the figures to advise a woman of a particular age about the balance of benefit and risk as it applies to her as an individual.

The study was a large, long duration, randomized controlled trial in a large number of postmenopausal women (more than 16 000) who took either placebo or estrogen/progestogen. This type of study is recognized to be more robust than the observational studies, which have provided the substantial information so far on the benefits and risks of HRT. The observational studies examined the effects of HRT in individuals who had been given HRT compared with those who had not used HRT. Such studies are recognized to be more subject to potential biases due to the fact that those who used the treatment may differ in many ways from those who did not. Thus randomized controlled studies are thought to give a more accurate estimate of the effects of treatments so long as there is a clear understanding of the questions tested by the randomized study. These questions can usually be summarized as:

(1) What was the specific intervention tested?

(2) What was the group of patients in whom it was used?

(3) What outcomes was the study designed to examine?

The observational studies reported over the past 20 years provided estimates of the expected benefits and risks of HRT when used by post-menopausal women over long periods. In order to test these expectations in a randomized controlled trial a very large, long duration trial was necessary.

Overall, most of the findings reported from the WHI trial have confirmed the expectations that were based on the previous observational studies. The important difference has been the failure to confirm the expected benefit in terms of coronary heart disease (CHD) and, in contrast, the demonstration of a small increase in the risk of CHD and stroke across the group as a whole.

Considering the benefits that were expected, there is confirmation of benefit in two important disease areas. Firstly, the trial demonstrated a significant 24% reduction in the risk of osteoporotic fractures as a whole and specifically a 34% reduction in the risk of hip fracture and a 34% reduction in the risk of spinal fracture. Secondly, the trial reported a significant 37% reduction in the risk of colorectal cancer, which is one of the most common cancers. These positive outcomes had been predicted by the observational studies but the new evidence strengthens our knowledge in those fields[2,3].

The trial confirmed certain risks that had been predicted by the previous observational studies. There was a 26% increase in the risk of breast cancer, which had been predicted by the previous meta-analysis of breast cancer studies that was published in the *Lancet* in 1997[4]. There was a 110% increase in the risk of venous thromboembolism. This doubling of risk is in keeping with previous reports[5]. With these breast cancer and thromboembolism findings there should be no necessity for any change in the advice being given to women so long as the previous advice made women aware of what was known about those risks in HRT users.

The trial reported a significant 41% increase in the risk of stroke. This had not been predicted by observational studies, which had mostly suggested either some reduction in stroke risk or no effect[6]. The level of absolute risk this involves for an HRT user will be very much influenced by age since stroke is rare at the younger end of the age spectrum of the study. Over the whole age spectrum (50–79 years) this translates annually into three stroke events per 1000 HRT users and two stroke events per 1000 women not using HRT. Concerning fatal stroke, the difference in the number of events was not statistically significant in a study of this size. The annualized figures are four fatal strokes per 10 000 HRT users and three fatal strokes in 10 000 women not using HRT.

The trial did not demonstrate the expected reduction in CHD[7,8] but instead reported a significant 26% increase in risk. In 1998 the Heart and Estrogen/progestogen Replacement Study (HERS) reported an increased risk of coronary events in women who already had heart disease when started on HRT[9] but there remained an expectation that HRT would have a protective effect in a 'healthy' group of women. The effect seen in the WHI trial is equivalent annually to four coronary events in 1000 HRT users across the age spectrum of the study (50–79) compared with three coronary events in 1000 women not using HRT. As with stroke, the difference in fatal coronary events was not statistically significant in a study of this size. The annualized figures are seven fatal coronary events per 10 000 HRT users and six fatal coronary events in 10 000 women not using HRT.

A meta-analysis that places the WHI findings in the context of other relevant randomized trial evidence has subsequently been published[10]. The conclusion from that analysis is confirmation that HRT does not reduce the risk of coronary artery disease, but that the overall effect of estrogen/progestogen HRT on coronary artery disease is neutral. In that analysis the slight increased risk of stroke reported in the WHI trial remained a significant increase and was recorded as a 27% increase in risk. In terms of how an individual woman might view this information, it does not take into account the difference in the absolute risk in the younger and older age groups who might use HRT, the absolute risk of stroke being expected to be relatively low in the younger age groups and higher in the older age groups.

There has been, and continues to be, discussion about the implications of these findings and to what extent they can be extrapolated to HRT formulations that differ from that used in the WHI. It is not possible to provide a definitive answer to the question of how other HRT formulations might have performed in this trial, since the question has not been tested. However, it is known that the greatest difference in effect between different HRT regimens has been on the metabolic and functional aspects of the cardiovascular system – the system in which the greatest adverse effect was noted. Another area of ongoing discussion is whether it is possible that HRT might reduce the risk of CHD in women who do not yet have deterioration of coronary arteries, but may not be effective in this if there is already significant coronary deterioration, which could have been the case for many of the 'healthy' women in the WHI trial. Such a suggestion would be in keeping with the animal research in this field but it remains unresolved in relation to the WHI study.

In advising women wishing to use HRT for the relief of menopausal symptoms or the management of osteoporosis risk – the two commonest reasons for using HRT – they can take from the WHI trial a continuing reassurance that solid trial evidence concerning fracture prevention has been added to the already solid evidence on the relief of menopausal symptoms and the preservation of bone density in HRT users. Women have not generally used HRT for the prevention of colorectal cancer but they can take reassurance from the reduction in risk demonstrated by the

trial. When deciding whether to use HRT women have already had to face the advice that treatment involves small but significant increases in the risks of breast cancer and venous thromboembolism. Up until recently, women have been able to be advised that HRT use may confer a benefit in terms of the risk of CHD. But now that cannot be advised, and they may have to consider that there could be a small increase in the risk of CHD or stroke which will be lowest, in absolute terms, in women between 50 and 60 years and greatest, in absolute terms, in women between 70 and 79 years.

Those women using estrogen without progestogen because they have had a hysterectomy should be reminded that the WHI study of their form of HRT continues because the analysis of global risk was lower than for estrogen/progestogen. They should gain reassurance from that information and await the final report of their aspect of the trial in a few years' time.

The UK Medical Research Council (MRC) has funded an equivalent study to the US WHI named the WISDOM study. This has a similar trial design to the US study but was commenced relatively recently. Following the publication of the estrogen/progestogen results of the WHI study, the Steering Committee of WISDOM recommended continuation of the trial but a review of the trial by an independent international committee was set up. On 23 October 2002 the MRC announced that after the review by the independent international committee there had been a decision to discontinue the WISDOM trial. The grounds for discontinuation were that in the light of the new evidence and the slow recruitment to date, WISDOM was considered unlikely to provide substantial evidence to influence clinical practice in the next 10 years. The MRC stressed that there were no safety concerns for the 5700 women involved in the study.

This statement is published by kind permission of the National Osteoporosis Society, PO Box 10, Radstock, Bath BA3 3YB, UK.

References

1. Writing Group for the Women's Health Initiative Investigators. Risks and benefits of estrogen plus progestin in healthy postmenopausal women. *J Am Med Assoc* 2002;288:321–33

2. RCP guidelines on the prevention and treatment of osteoporosis, 1999. London: RCP, 1999

3. Grodstein F, Newcombe PA, Stampfer MJ, *et al*. Postmenopausal hormone therapy and the risk of colorectal cancer: a review and meta-analysis. *Am J Med* 1999;106:574–82

4. Collaborative Group on Hormonal Factors in Breast Cancer. Breast cancer and hormone replacement therapy: collaborative reanalysis of data from 51 epidemiological studies of 52 705 women with breast cancer and 108 411 women without breast cancer. *Lancet* 1997;350:1047

5. Daly E, Vessey MP, Hawkins MM, *et al*. Risk of venous thromboembolism in users of hormone replacement therapy. *Lancet* 1996;348:977–80

6. Paganini-Hill A. Hormone replacement therapy and stroke: risk, protection or no effect? *Maturitas* 2001;38:243–61

7. Stampfer MJ, Coldity GA. Estrogen replacement therapy and coronary heart disease: a quantitative assessment of the epidemiologic evidence. *Prev Med* 1991;20:47–63

8. Grodstein F, Manson JE, Coldity GA, *et al*. A prospective, observational study of postmenopausal hormone therapy and primary prevention of cardiovascular disease. *Ann Intern Med* 2000;133:933–41

9. Heart and Estrogen/progestin Replacement Study (HERS) Research Group, Hulley S, Good D, *et al*. Randomized trial of estrogen plus progestin for secondary prevention of coronary heart disease in postmenopausal women. *J Am Med Assoc* 1998;280:605–13

10. Beral V, Banks E, Reeves G. Evidence from randomised controlled trials on the long-term effects of hormone replacement therapy. *Lancet* 2002;360:942–4

3

Estrogen therapy for cardiovascular disease

G. Samsioe

INTRODUCTION

Coronary heart disease (CHD) is the most common cause of morbidity and mortality in both women and men. At younger ages, men are at a significantly greater risk of developing CHD, but as women age, the female risk for CHD approaches that of men. The prevalence of CHD in women aged between 45 and 64 years is 1 in 7. Over the age of 65 it is 1 in 3. A significant number of women have atherosclerotic lesions even if they have no clinical signs of CHD. Mortality rises by age in both genders. The male/female excess is 5 : 1 for those aged 35–44 years, but only 1. 5 : 1 for those over 75 years. One in four women of age 60 and older will eventually die of CHD. A 50-year-old woman has a 46% risk of developing CHD and a 31% risk of death due to CHD[1]. Women hospitalized with myocardial infarction (MI) have a mortality rate twice that of men. The high risk of death emphasizes the need for better understanding of heart disease in women. Only 50% of cases are related to predictable risk factors, suggesting the need for a different approach to risk factors in women. Despite the fact that CHD incidence increases at the time of the menopause, the change is gradual rather than abrupt.

Although CHD overall represents a greater risk of morbidity and mortality, cancer remains a woman's greatest fear, even among university graduates who are normally better informed of CHD risks.

Women have a different clinical presentation of an acute ischemic event, compared with men. Women have unstable angina more frequently than men, while men have acute ischemic syndromes more frequently. Women have a worse outcome after acute MI, in part because they receive slower medical attention, with a greater delay in receiving care, and later and less thrombolysis. In addition, they present more risk factors and higher rates of complications, owing to their different pathophysiology or other yet unknown reasons.

The highest mortality rates from ischemic heart disease in Europe are found in Northern European countries, while Central and Eastern Europe have intermediate rates. The risk differs in different countries in different parts of the world, in relation to ethnic group, diet and life-style. Populations characterized by different patterns of mortality may have different hormone replacement therapy (HRT) risk–benefit balances with regard to morbidity as well as mortality. Such epidemiological differences should be considered in evaluation of the HRT risk–benefit profile.

CARDIOVASCULAR DISEASE RISK FACTORS IN WOMEN

Women share several cardiovascular disease (CVD) risk factors with men, such as family history, diet, obesity, smoking, unfavorable lipid profile, high homocystine levels, high fibrinogen, low physical activity, diabetes mellitus and hypertension. In addition, women have one unique risk factor: the menopause. Women have a greater relative risk than men if they are diabetic, have raised triglyceride levels, or low levels of high-density lipoprotein (HDL), or if they are smokers. CHD is more common in countries with high-saturated-fat diets and high cholesterol levels. In addition, hypercholesterolemic patients are prone to early CHD, while cholesterol-lowering reduces CHD. For CHD in middle-aged women, high triglyceride levels are more important than high low-density lipoprotein (LDL) and low HDL cholesterol levels. Nevertheless, CHD prevention trials using statins have demonstrated that women benefit from LDL cholesterol reduction as much as men do. Recent studies have revealed that intensive multiple interventions such as life-style modifications including diet, weight reduction, smoking cessation and exercise, may reduce the risk of CHD and can result in fewer cases of heart disease in a very cost-effective manner. Aspirin, beta-blockers and cholesterol-lowering drugs are also beneficial in women with documented CVD.

MENOPAUSE AND CARDIOVASCULAR DISEASE

Presumably because of the protective effects of estrogen, women tend to develop CHD about 10 years later than do men. Being male and above 45 years of age is a risk factor for CHD, whereas females are not considered at risk until they reach 55 years of age. This '10-year advantage' can be lost, however, if a woman starts the menopause prematurely or if she has other risk factors, such as smoking or diabetes mellitus.

Although a few, well-designed longitudinal studies have reported some conflicting results, large cross-sectional studies indicate that, in addition to the effect of aging, the menopause *per se* is associated with lipid modifications, such as an increase in total cholesterol, LDL cholesterol and triglycerides that can cause an increased risk of developing CVD. This increase in total cholesterol results from increases in levels of LDL cholesterol, and increases in very-low-density lipoprotein (VLDL) and lipoprotein(a). The oxidation of LDL cholesterol is also enhanced. HDL cholesterol levels may decrease over time, but these changes are small

and insignificant relative to the increases in LDL cholesterol and triglycerides. The coagulation balance is not altered significantly with the menopause because a counterbalance of changes occurs: some procoagulation factors increase (factor VII, fibrinogen), but so do certain fibrinolytic factors such as antithrombin III and plasminogen. In addition, at the time of the menopause, changes in vascular reactivity take place: prostacyclin production decreases, endothelin levels increase and endothelium-dependent vasodilatation is impaired. At the same time, increases in blood pressure and body weight and changes in body fat distribution, plus alterations in insulin sensitivity and glucose metabolism, have been reported; in healthy, non-obese, postmenopausal women, carbohydrate tolerance decreases as a result of an increase in insulin resistance.

Prior to publication of the Heart and Estrogen/progestin Replacement Study (HERS)[2] in 1998, primary and especially secondary prevention of heart disease by HRT was regarded as almost established medicine. Admittedly, cardiac prevention was never an established official indication, but more or less all available data pointed to this possibility. Apart from beneficial effects on several surrogate markers for CVD, observational studies and experimental data were in agreement. Several observational studies with hard end-points as well as angiographic data on the extent of coronary arteriosclerosis strongly suggested a cardioprotective effect. These data were also backed up by animal experiments, and results for the cynomolgus monkey were considered pivotal. These concepts formed the rationale for the HERS and Women's Health Initiative (WHI)[3] trials, which, surprisingly, could not verify the hypothesis. Despite well-founded criticism of the HERS, an era of negativism regarding CVD and HRT commenced. None the less, estrogens and estrogen–progestin combinations have repeatedly been shown positively to influence several factors of pivotal importance for subsequent CVD.

In most Western countries, women suffer more cardiovascular events than do men. In addition, female mortality is higher, particularly when occurring in women with coexisting diabetes. An MI occurs as a result of preceding vascular disease, usually in the form of arteriosclerosis which, in turn, has developed over decades.

Several studies have also produced compelling evidence that CVD increases after oophorectomy at premenopausal ages, and CVD is also more common in women with a premature menopause.

In conclusion, nature suggests that premature loss of ovarian function is associated with a higher incidence of CVD.

Given the perceived benefit of female gonadal hormones on CVD, several studies have been undertaken to underline this benefit further. These include a variety of experimental studies in both animals and women. An immense database on various surrogate markers exists, which in essence demonstrates beneficial effects on a huge variety of surrogate markers ranging from intima–media thickness and smooth muscle cell proliferation, to markers of inflammation, coagulation, fibrinolysis and carbohydrate metabolism. An overwhelming amount of data also exist on various HRT regimens and their effects on serum lipids and lipoproteins.

An extensive review of HRT and lipids, covering data reported between 1974 and 2000, was recently published by Godsland[4]. In this review, 248 studies provided information on the effects of 42 different HRT regimens. All estrogen-alone preparations increased HDL cholesterol and lowered total and LDL cholesterol. Oral estrogens raised triglycerides, while transdermal estradiol lowered them. Added progestogens had little effect on estrogen-induced reductions in LDL, but attenuated estrogen-induced increases in triglycerides and HDL. Apart from dose, the magnitude of this attenuation was dependent on the type of progestogen. In order of least to greatest effects, the progestogens were: dydrogesterone, medrogestone, progesterone, cyproterone, medroxyprogesterone, norgestrel and norethisterone. It should be pointed out that this included both HDL- and triglyceride-lowering, and whether a great or small effect is more advantageous from the aspect of cardiovascular risk is not known to date. In addition, apolipoprotein A was generally lowered by HRT.

DATA FROM HERS AND WHI

Post hoc analyses of the HERS data showed a statistically significant time trend, with more coronary events in the hormone group than in the placebo group during the first year of treatment, and fewer in years 3–5. Further analyses of subgroups did not add much new information[5].

The HERS II[6] was a follow-up study including women enrolled in the HERS. In HERS II, treatment assignment was unblinded in 1998. Subsequent use of HRT was based on decisions made by women and their physicians. Of the 2763 women enrolled in the HERS, 2510 were alive at the time of enrolment in HERS II (1260 in the placebo group and 1250 in the hormone group). Of these, 2321 (93%) agreed to enrol in HERS II (1165 in the placebo group and 1156 in the hormone group). At the end of HERS II, close-out telephone contacts were completed for 99% of surviving women in both placebo and hormone groups. The results were published after an average additional follow-up of 2.7 years. Among women randomly assigned to hormone treatment in the HERS, the proportion reporting 80% or more adherence to hormones was 81% during year 1 and declined to 45% during year 6 of follow-up in HERS II. The results showed no differences between women originally assigned to the hormone and the placebo groups in rates of coronary events during the HERS. As the study lost over half of its participants and was open, it is hardly possible to draw any well-founded conclusions from the extension part.

Less than 1 week after publication of HERS II, the HRT arm of the WHI was stopped. This part of the WHI was a randomized trial of a continuous estrogen–progestin regimen versus placebo in healthy postmenopausal women. However, increased incidences of breast cancer and an overall index measure suggested that the harms outweighed the benefits. In brief, the WHI trial setting included participants who were randomized to a continuous combined combination of 0.625 mg/day of conjugated equine estrogens (CEE) and 2.5 mg/day of medroxyprogesterone acetate (MPA), or placebo.

It is of interest that the WHI used exactly the same preparation as the HERS, despite that this particular preparation was never used in trials on heart disease, and cardioprotection has never been suggested for any continuous combined regimen. Data to date has related to estrogen monotherapy and sequential estrogen–progestin combinations.

The WHI was the first randomized trial to address directly whether oral continuous combined estrogen plus a progestin had a favorable effect on CHD incidence and on overall risks and benefits in predominantly healthy women, since only 7.7% of participating women reported having prior CVD. However, a substantial proportion were hypertensive and had a body mass index (BMI) greater than 28 kg/m^2, suggesting that the participants were at increased risk of CVD compared with a normal population, at least by European standards. In the WHI, 8506 women were randomized to placebo and 8106 received the active treatment. Demographic data prior to commencement of the study were similar for the groups of women. It should be remembered that the recruitment strategy was such that one-third of the participants were aged between 50 and 59 and two-thirds between 60 and 79 years. Hence, the mean age was 66.3, which is similar to that in the HERS. The trial was stopped early, based on health risks that exceeded health benefits over an average follow-up of 5.2 years. However, the

estrogen-alone arm in women with a hysterectomy is continuing, and the planned termination of this arm is March 2005, by which time the average follow-up will be about 8.5 years.

The major difference between the estrogen-only arm and the continuous combined arm was the higher incidence of breast cancer in the latter. However, it was subsequently reported that this increased risk of breast cancer was confined to those women who had been using combined HRT prior to study entry, and had only a 3-month wash-out period before entry. In this subset, the hazards ratio (HR) for breast cancer was around 2, whereas in new acceptors it was 1.06, the difference between which was not statistically significant.

The principal results from a trial of combined estrogen and progestin in women with a uterus were reported[2]. Several outcomes suggested no benefit and possibly harm, including increased coronary heart disease (HR 1.29; 95% confidence interval (CI) 1.02–1.63), stroke (HR 1.41; 95% CI 1.07–1.85) and pulmonary embolism (HR 2.13; 95% CI 1.39–3.25) (Table 1). Beneficial results included decreases in colorectal cancer (HR 0.63; 95% CI 0.43–0.92) and hip fracture (HR 0.66; 95% CI 0.45–0.98). Most adverse outcomes began appearing within 1–2 years, but the increased breast cancer risk did not begin until 3 years after the start of the study. These findings are more or less in agreement with findings from major observational studies in terms of seven of the eight outcomes, the exception being CHD. This would suggest that the type of study does

Table 1 Hazards ratio (HR) risks for important diseases and benefits for other important events from the Women's Health Intitiative. 95% confidence interval is given in parentheses. Adapted with permission from Writing Group for the Women's Health Initiative Investigators. Risks and benefits of estrogen plus progestin in healthy postmenopausal women. *J Am Med Assoc* 2002;288:321–33[3]

Risks	HR	Benefits	HR
CHD	1.29 (1.02–1.63)	colorectal cancer	0.63 (0.43–0.62)
Breast cancer	1.26 (1.00–1.59)		
Stroke	1.41 (1.07–1.85)	endometrial cancer	0.83 (0.47–1.47)
PE	2.13 (1.39–3.25)		
Total CVD	1.22 (1.09–1.36)	hip fracture	0.66 (0.45–0.98)

CHD, coronary heart disease; PE, pulmonary embolism; CVD, cardiovascular disease

not, to any major extent, influence the outcome, and that specific attention must be paid to the effects on CHD. The findings in the WHI for stroke are consistent with those from the HERS, as is the pattern in the WHI related to the occurrence of venous thromboembolism, which is a well-known complication of postmenopausal hormone therapy.

In the WHI report, the magnitude of the relative risks is fairly impressive. However, absolute risks are small. At the end of 5.2 years, 7968 women remained in the treated group and 7608 in the placebo group, with an additional eight strokes, seven heart attacks and eight cases of breast cancer per 2000 women treated for 5 years.

Combining all outcomes monitored, women taking estrogen plus a progestin might expect 19 more events per year per 10 000 women than women taking placebo. These figures underline the need to present also the data related to harm and not merely relative risks, to prevent public scare and confusion among users. Indeed, when applying the adjusted figures the risks were even smaller, and only those for venous thromboembolism and fracture prevention reached statistical significance.

One obvious limitation of the WHI study is that the trial tested just one specific drug regimen, the oral administration of CEE 0.625 mg/day plus MPA 2.5 mg/day. The results do not necessarily apply to lower dosages, to other formulations of oral estrogens and progestins or to estrogens and progestins administered via non-oral routes.

The WHI finding that CEE plus continuous administration of the progestin MPA does not confer benefit for preventing CHD among women with a uterus concurs with the HERS and its extension study, HERS II.

Over the years, several meta-analyses have been published. However, it is questionable whether they add anything more to our knowledge than a summary of existing data. The problem with meta-analyses is that, if a bias or confounder exists in observational studies, this cannot be corrected. The simple meta-analysis does not control for size, duration or quality of the studies included. Grading by quality is often done by the authors prior to performing the statistics leading to the results of the meta-analysis. This procedure is subjective and, hence, subject to bias.

One recent meta-analysis[7] attempted to minimize such bias by using established criteria on study quality issued by an independent body, in this case the US Preventive Services Task Force criteria. From the literature comprising 3035 papers evaluating primary prevention and published between 1966 and 2000, only 24 cohort studies, 18 case–control studies and one randomized clinical trial were found to meet the criteria of the US Task Force. Whether it is justifiable to disregard 98.5% of the published literature could well be debated.

The meta-analysis by Humphrey and colleagues[7] also differs from previous work by evaluating potential explanatory variables of the relationship between HRT and CVD. The results revealed a reduction of incidence and mortality in coronary artery disease in current users, and decreased mortality among current users of HRT in total cardiovascular disease. There were no statistically significant effects in past-, ever- or any-users of HRT (Table 2).

Numerous attempts have been made to mimic the natural hormonal situation in women by producing a huge variety of HRT regimens. As CVD is a major killer, the effect of HRT on cardiovascular morbidity and mortality has been meticulously studied. Given the enormous variation among HRT regimens, however, only a few of these have been studied to produce

Table 2 Hormone replacement therapy (HRT) and coronary heart disease: principal results from a recent meta-analysis. Reproduced with permission from Humphrey L, Chan B, Sox H. Postmenopausal hormone replacement therapy and the primary prevention of cardiovascular disease. *Ann Intern Med* 2002;137:273–84[7]

HRT use	Mortality	Incidence
Current	0.62*	0.80*
Past	0.76	0.89
Ever	0.81	0.91
Any	0.74	0.88

*Significant difference compared with non-users

results relating to treatment or prevention of CVD. Concerning hard end-points, there are limited data on types and doses of estrogens other than oral CEE at 0.625 or 1.25 mg/day.

There are almost no data on transdermal administration, but in a recent UK publication[8] involving a fairly small number of patients, no benefit, but no harm either, was encountered after use of a transdermal patch. As in many other recent studies of HRT and CVD, doses used were high, in this case 80 µg/day, compared with the standard dose of 50 µg daily which is commonly used to treat menopausal symptoms.

In the limited number of studies using combined HRT, data only relate to oral MPA at doses of 2.5–10 mg daily. In other words, the term HRT must be interpreted with care, as it refers to a very limited number from the huge family of HRT preparations. In addition, the majority of data on cardiovascular events are from North America, with only few European studies and no data from Asia, Africa or Latin America. Generalization of conclusions is therefore not justifiable.

CVD is multifactorial, and the risk of a cardiovascular event depends largely on the occurrence of one or more risk factors. Some of these, such as male gender, age and family history, are not possible to change, whereas others, such as perturbations of the lipid and carbohydrate metabolisms, obesity, hypertension and (oxidative) stress, are clearly modifiable. Also, a healthy diet, smoking cessation and increased physical activity impact heavily upon future risk.

The WHI has an observational arm that recently produced data on exercise and cardiovascular events in postmenopausal women belonging to the WHI poulation. This study[9] compared, prospectively, walking and vigorous exercise for the prevention of cardiovascular events among 73 743 postmenopausal women aged 50–79. Increasing physical activity had a strong inverse association with the risk of both coronary events and total CVD. Both walking and vigorous exercise were associated with similar risk reductions provided that they produced similar energy expenditure. Expressed in quintiles from lowest to highest energy expend-

iture, the relative risks were 1.00, 0.73, 0.69, 0.68 and 0.47, the trend being highly statistically significant.

Again, compelling evidence suggests that the reduction of one or several established risk factors by pharmacological or non-pharmacological means reduces subsequent cardiovascular events.

In line with nature's own experiments as outlined above, almost all experimental data for animals as well as humans suggest a reduction of surrogate markers for atherosclerosis, as well as the extent of atherosclerotic plaques, by estrogens and commonly also by combinations of estrogens and progestogens.

Recently, long-term studies includng tens of thousands of women, leading to more than 100 000 woman-years, have been pushed aside by shorter-term and smaller-scale studies with superior methodology, i.e. double-blind, placebo-controlled and randomized. By mid-2002, already several such studies have shown that it is not advisable to start HRT solely for cardioprevention, because of an increase in the incidence of cardiovascular events. The HERS trial did not show any benefit of HRT. It also did not show any benefit of statins, or any detrimental effect of hypertension or smoking.

While shortcomings and interpretation problems with surrogate end-point studies and observational data are well recognized, the magnitude and diversity of these studies are such that the overall results should carry considerable weight in our understanding of the relationship between HRT and CVD. Randomized clinical trials (RCTs) are not problem free, and are subject to bias[10] as exemplified by the following:

(1) Inclusion and exclusion criteria for RCTs are much more rigid than those for observational studies, and many of them have implications for CVD such as hypertension, high BMI, lipid abnormalities and impaired hepatic or renal function, leading to recruitment of a lower-than-average-risk population. Hence, results are valid only for those women who meet these inclusion and exclusion criteria.

(2) According to the Helsinki declaration, information to RCT participants must be such that they understand the current scientific knowledge on which the hypothesis of the RCT is based, recognizing that there is a 50% chance to be on placebo for a considerable time. This is likely to recruit a population at lower-than-average risk into RCTs, which seems to be the case for both the HERS and the WHI.

(3) Subjects are new starters, but whether they have never used HRT, or used HRT for a considerable time prior to the trial, is not without importance for the development of CVD. Of particular relevance for primary prevention is the possibility that women void of climacteric symptoms, and with previously higher endogenous estrogens, are recruited into RCTs.

(4) RCTs use one preparation at one given dose and mode of administration. Interpretation of the results should be limited to this and to the target group of the RCT, and not generalized to include all populations and all HRT preparations regardless of their composition, dose and mode of administration. In addition, the composition of the target population regarding age and concomitant medication must be considered, as this may impact upon steroid pharmacology.

(5) RCTs are usually short-term, and are at present limited to some 5 years' observation time.

In summary, both RCTs and observational studies are subject to bias but such biases are likely to differ between the two study types. Another important difference is that an RCT will bear weight for the initial phase of a chronic treatment, whereas cohort studies are poor captors of this phase. RCTs are extremely poor at giving data on effects beyond 5 years of treatment, whereas observational data readily supply this.

Time seems to be crucial in several studies, and in many observational studies a clear reduction cannot be seen until 4–5 years of HRT. (However, this time effect could well be influenced by study dropouts.)

It could also be a potential explanatory factor as to why the WHI agrees with observational data in seven of eight outcome measures, the exception being CHD. It is known today that an MI occurs after thrombotization of a ruptured unstable atherosclerotic plaque which in turn showed signs of inflammation. In the initial phase of HRT the risk of thromboembolic episodes is likely to be captured by an RCT, but not by a cohort study.

As evident from the observational arm of the WHI[11], almost all MIs occurred in women with high C-reactive protein (CRP) levels, irrespective of HRT use. At least initially, continuous combined oral CEE + MPA elevates CRP and possibly other markers of inflammation. This could be the reason why the maximum difference in stroke was demonstrated in years 2–4 in the WHI, suggestive of enhanced inflammation and an increased tendency for plaque rupture.

A recent publication from the Multiple Outcomes of Raloxifene Evaluation (MORE) trial[12] indicates that raloxifene does not impose an increased risk of CVD, and, in the subset of 1035 women with risk factors for CVD, even induced protection with a relative risk of 0.60 (95% CI 0.38–0.95). This occurred despite that raloxifene in earlier reports was shown to cause a similar increased risk of venous thromboembolism to that with estrogens. One possibility to explain this finding is that raloxifene may not induce an inflammatory response, as suggested by the reduction also in stroke. The increase of CRP could be indicative of such an induction by oral estrogens, which in turn may promote rupture of unstable atherosclerotic plaques and thereby induce cardiovascular events.

FUTURE DEVELOPMENT

Hence, in the aftermath of the HERS and the WHI, it is essential to revisit the current situation and provide ideas for the future role of HRT regarding its effects on CVD.

CVD is multifactorial and can be influenced by life-style. For both primary and secondary prevention of CVD, much could be gained by modifying life-style factors, for example stopping smoking, comsuming a well-balanced low-fat diet and exercising regularly. Modification of these very important risk factors is non-controversial, and this should be emphasized to all women as well as men.

Incidence and mortality can also be modified by the use of pharmacological agents other than HRT. There is evidence that antifibrinolytic drugs, beta-blockers, angiotensin-converting enzyme (ACE) inhibitors and statins all can lower risk, in both primary and especially secondary prevention settings. Despite their proven benefits, it should be remembered that all these agents are not natural compounds for humans. Widespread long-term use of such compounds may lead to other untoward effects, as exemplified by the recent withdrawal of a marketed statin owing to side-effects.

As mentioned above, the consumption of a healthy diet should be encouraged. Such a diet should be low in saturated fat but should have a high content of polyunsaturated fatty acids (PUFAs), especially from the so-called omega-3 series, i.e. n-3 fatty acids. Such a diet should also be rich in fibers and contain relevant amounts of vitamins, antioxidants and trace elements.

The antioxidative properties of vitamins C and E are well documented, as they are for several estrogens, and antioxidation is believed to be cardioprotective. Port and red wine contain antioxidants and could hence be included in the diet, but not more than 1–2 glasses per day.

Seafood is a rich source of PUFAs, particularly salmon and other fish with a high fat content. It is a long-standing observation that Inuits have lower risk of thromboembolism and longer bleeding time than, for example, Caucasians. This phenomenon is attributed to the high content of PUFAs in their diet. In addition, it is possible to reduce blood coagulability by intake of cod liver oil. Another important quality of PUFAs is to reduce triglycerides and particularly to stabilize cardiac rhythm. The latter was demonstrated clearly in GISSI 3, an Italian study[13] of secondary prevention.

Administration of PUFAs from the n-3 seires was associated with an increased survival rate after MI, attributed to this antiarrhythmic effect.

Given the results of the HERS and the follow-up HERS II as well as the WHI, it is intriguing to suggest a combination of estrogens and a healthy diet. This could also be complemented by low-dose administration of aspirin to reduce the risk of early thrombosis, particularly prudent in secondary prevention trials.

CLINICAL IMPLICATIONS

The incidence of harmful effects in the WHI study was really very small in terms of individual health. There is no reason to avoid postmenopausal hormonal medication in women with climacteric symptoms.

It should be stressed that the main aim of all health-care should be improvement of women's health, and not just by means of hormonal therapies. In the Nurses' Health Study[14], between 1980 and 1994 there was a 31% reduction in CHD. Better nutrition, smoking cessation and hormonal treatments in the menopause were responsible for 18, 13 and 9% of the reduction, respectively.

The main goal should remain the maintenance of health as well as primary and secondary prevention of disabling diseases, in particular those that are more prevalent after the age of 50.

The WHI is an important study. However, it does not necessarily introduce new rules into good clinical practice. Based on recent developments the European Menopause and Andropause Society have issued a policy document[15] outlining guidelines to prescribers:

(1) To recommend the use of any HRT to women with climacteric symptoms likely to impact upon quality of life and to re-emphasize that topical low-dose vaginal estrogens can be used by any woman bearing an indication for such therapy.

(2) To reassess the need for continuous combined oral HRT after 4–5 years of therapy and not recommend HRT for the sole

purpose of preventing chronic disease, such as CVD or osteoporosis, as other alternatives are available.

(3) To promote the use of additional and alternative non-hormonal strategies for the maintenance of health and prevention of disease in symptom-free women of middle age and beyond.

CONCLUSIONS

Until we have further evidence, it seems prudent not to include CVD prevention as a sole indication for HRT. However, there is little evidence to support withdrawal of HRT in long-term users, should a CVD event occur. There is also no good evidence to deny HRT to women with increased CVD risk, including those with established CVD. The 'grey zone' in between must be considered on an individual basis. So far most studies have been performed with CEE alone or combined with MPA. Indeed, one randomized trial[16] using estradiol showed less progression of intima–media thickness, compared with controls, suggesting that composition of the HRT may well have the greatest influence. However, it must be pointed out that, owing to the low number of participants, this study warrants confirmation. Hence, firm recommendations cannot be made until further studies of a variety of HRT preparations and regimens inclusive of different delivery systems, doses and components have been performed, and these are obviously urgently required.

Data based almost exclusively on CEE suggest that HRT in doses used to treat climacteric symptoms increases the incidence of venous thrombembolism, but only during the first 1–3 years of usage[17]. The reason for this remains obscure. Our current insufficient understanding of HRT administration and surveillance should encourage further research, especially into the effects of lower doses and non-oral approaches. It should not impact upon the overall concept, which is that estrogens may well be beneficial for the heart.

References

1. Hu FB, Grodstein F. Postmenopausal hormone therapy and the risk of cardiovascular disease: the epidemiologic evidence. *Am J Cardiol* 2002; 90(Suppl 1):F26–9
2. Hulley S, Grady D, Bush T, *et al.* Randomized trial of estrogen plus progestin for secondary prevention of coronary artery disease in post menopausal women. *J Am Med Assoc* 1998;280: 605–13
3. Writing Group for the Women's Health Initiative Investigators. Risks and benefits of estrogen plus progestin in healthy postmenopausal women. *J Am Med Assoc* 2002;288:321–33
4. Godsland IF. Effects of postmenopausal hormone replacement therapy on lipid, lipoprotein, and apolipoprotein(a) concentrations: analysis of studies published from 1974–2000. *Fertil Steril* 2001;75:898–915
5. Furberg CD, Vittinghoff E, Davidson M, *et al.* Subgroup interactions in the Heart and Estrogen/progestin Replacement Study. *Circulation* 2002;105:917–22
6. Grady D, Herrington D, Bitner V, *et al.* Cardiovascular disease outcomes during 6.8 years of hormone therapy. Heart and Estrogen/progestin Replacement Study follow-up (HERS II). *J Am Med Assoc* 2002;288:49–57
7. Humphrey L, Chan B, Sox H. Postmenopausal hormone replacement therapy and the primary prevention of cardiovascular disease. *Ann Intern Med* 2002;137:273–84
8. Clarke SC, Kelleher J, Lloyd-Jones H, Slack M, Schofield PM. A study of hormone replacement therapy in postmenopausal women with ischaemic heart disease: the Papworth HRT Atherosclerosis Study. *Br J Obstet Gynaecol* 2002; 109:1056–62
9. Manson JE, Greenland P, Lacroix AZ, *et al* Walking compared with vigorous exercise for the

prevention of cardiovascular events in women. *N Engl J Med* 2002;347:755–6

10. Samsioe G, Neves-e-Castro M, Pines A, *et al.* Critical comments. *Maturitas* 2001;40:5–15

11. Ridker PM, Rifai N, Rose L, Buring JE, Cook NR. Comparison of C-reactive protein and low density lipoprotein cholesterol levels in the prediction of first cardiovascular events. *N Engl J Med* 2002;347:1557–65.

12. Barrett-Connor E, Grady D, Sashegyi A, *et al* Raloxifene and cardiovascular events in osteoporotic postmenopausal women. *J Am Med Assoc* 2002;287:847–57

13. GISSI Investigators. Dietary supplementation with n-3 polyunsaturated fatty acids and vitamin E after myocardial infarction: results of the GISSI-Prevenzione trial. Gruppo Italiano per lo Studio della Sopravivenza nell'Infarto miocardico. *Lancet* 1999;354:447–55

14. Stampfer MJ, Hu FB, Manson JE, *et al.* Primary prevention of coronary heart disease in women through diet and lifestyle. *N Engl J Med* 2000; 343:16–22

15. Neves-e-Castro M, Doren M, Samsioe G, Skouby S. Results from WHI and HERS-II. Implications for women and the prescriber of HRT. *Maturitas* 2002;9:255

16. Hodis HN, Mack WJ, Lobo RA, *et al.* Estrogen in the prevention of atherosclerosis. A randomised double-blind, placebo-controlled trial. *Ann Intern Med* 2001;135:939–53

17. Perez-Gutthann SP, Rodríguez LG, Castellsague J, Oliart AD. Hormone replacement therapy and risk of venous thromboembolism: population based case–control study. *Br Med J* 1997;314: 796–800.

4

Urogenital atrophy

D. Robinson and L. Cardozo

INTRODUCTION

Urogenital atrophy is a manifestation of estrogen withdrawal following the menopause and symptoms may appear for the first time more than 10 years after the last menstrual period[1]. The female genital and lower urinary tract share a common embryological origin from the urogenital sinus and both are sensitive to the effects of female sex steroid hormones. Estrogen is known to have an important role in the function of the lower urinary tract throughout adult life and estrogen and progesterone receptors have been demonstrated in the vagina, urethra, bladder and pelvic floor musculature[2-5]. Estrogen deficiency occurring following the menopause is known to cause atrophic changes within the urogenital tract[6] and is associated with urinary symptoms, such as frequency, urgency, nocturia, incontinence and recurrent infection. These may co-exist with symptoms of vaginal atrophy, such as dyspareunia, itching, burning and dryness. The role of estrogen replacement in the treatment of these symptoms of urogenital atrophy has still not been clearly defined despite several randomized trials and widespread clinical use. This review presents an overview of the pathogenesis and management of urogenital atrophy.

EPIDEMIOLOGY

Increasing life expectancy has led to an increasingly elderly population and it is now common for women to spend a third of their lives in the estrogen-deficient postmenopausal state[7].

The average age of the menopause is 50 years although there is some cultural and geographical variation[8]. World-wide in 1990 there were approximately 467 million women aged 50 years or over and this is expected to increase to 1200 million over the next 30 years[9]. Furthermore, postmenopausal women comprise 15% of the population in industrialized countries, with a predicted growth rate of 1.5% over the next 20 years. Overall, in the developed world 8% of the total population have been estimated to have urogenital symptoms[10], this representing 200 million women in the United States alone.

UROGENITAL ATROPHY

The prevalence of symptomatic urogenital atrophy is difficult to estimate since many women accept the changes as being an inevitable consequence of the aging process and thus do not seek help. It has been estimated that 10–40% of all postmenopausal women are symptomatic[11] although only 25% are thought to seek medical help. In addition, vaginal symptoms associated with urogenital atrophy are reported by two out of three women by the age of 75 years[12].

More recently, a study assessing the prevalence of urogenital symptoms in 2157 Dutch women has been reported[13]. Overall 27% of women complained of vaginal dryness, soreness and dyspareunia, whilst the prevalence of urinary symptoms such as leakage and recurrent

27

infections was 36%. When considering severity, almost 50% reported moderate to severe discomfort although only one-third had received medical intervention. Interestingly, women who had previously had a hysterectomy reported moderate to severe complaints more often than those who had not.

The prevalence of urogenital atrophy and urogenital prolapse has also been examined in a population of 285 women attending a menopause clinic[14]. Overall, 51% of women were found to have anterior vaginal wall prolapse, 27% posterior vaginal prolapse and 20% apical prolapse. In addition, 34% of women were noted to have urogenital atrophy, and 40% complaining of dyspareunia; whilst urogenital atrophy and symptoms of dyspareunia were related to menopausal age, the prevalence of prolapse showed no association.

Whilst urogenital atrophy is an inevitable consequence of the menopause, women may not always be symptomatic. In a recent study of 69 women attending a gynecology clinic, they women were asked to fill out a symptom questionnaire prior to examination and undergoing vaginal cytology[15]. Urogenital symptoms were found to be relatively low and were poorly correlated with age and physical examination findings, although not with vaginal cytological maturation index. Women who were taking estrogen replacement therapy had higher symptom scores and physical examination scores. In conclusion, it would appear that urogenital atrophy is a universal consequence of the menopause, although often elderly women may be minimally symptomatic and hence treatment should not be the only indication for replacement therapy.

URINARY INCONTINENCE

The prevalence of urinary incontinence is known to increase with age, affecting 15–35% of community-dwelling women over the age of 60 years[16], with other studies reporting a prevalence of 49% in women over 65 years[17]. In addition, rates of 50% have been reported in elderly nursing-home residents[18]. Little work has been done to examine the incidence of urinary incontinence, although a study in New Zealand of women over the age of 65 years found 10% of the originally continent developed urinary incontinence in the 3-year study period[19].

ECONOMIC CONSIDERATIONS

The economic cost of urogenital atrophy is difficult to estimate due to under-reporting and also since some of the cost is borne by the patients themselves without involving the health services. The price of incontinence is slightly easier to estimate although it is still affected by under-reporting. It is comprised of the 'direct' costs of treatment, supplies and provision of medical staff whilst 'indirect' costs relate to loss of earnings and productivity. A study performed in 1994 in Scotland estimated that the cost of pad supplies alone in the UK may be in the region of £57.3 million per year whilst the cost of incontinence has been estimated at $16 billion a year in the USA. More recent data from the UK have shown the annual expenditure on incontinence to be £163 million with appliances and containment accounting for £59 million and £69 million respectively and the cost of drugs and surgery being £23 million and £12 million (Department of Health figures, 2001).

ESTROGEN RECEPTORS, HORMONAL FACTORS AND THEIR EFFECTS

The effects of the steroid hormone 17β-estradiol are mediated by ligand-activated transcription factors known as estrogen receptors which are glycoproteins sharing common features with androgen and progesterone receptors. The classic estrogen receptor (ERα) was first discovered by Elwood Jensen in 1958 and was cloned from uterine tissue in 1986[20]. It was not until 1996, however, that the second estrogen receptor (ERβ) was identified[21].

Estrogen receptors have been demonstrated throughout the lower urinary tract and are expressed in the squamous epithelium of the proximal and distal urethra, vagina and trigone of the bladder[3,22], although not in the dome of the bladder, reflecting its different embryological origin. The pubococcygeus and the musculature of the pelvic floor have also been shown to be estrogen sensitive[23,24], although estrogen receptors have not yet been identified in the levator ani muscles[25].

More recently, the distribution of estrogen receptors throughout the urogenital tract has been studied, with both α and β receptors being found in the vaginal walls and uterosacral ligaments of premenopausal women, although the latter was absent in the vaginal walls of postmenopausal women[26]. In addition, α receptors are localized in the urethral sphincter and, when sensitized by estrogens, are thought to help maintain muscular tone[27].

In addition to estrogen receptors, both androgen and progesterone receptors are expressed in the lower urinary tract although their role is less clear. Progesterone receptors are expressed inconsistently and their presence may be dependent on estrogen status[5], whilst androgen receptors are present in both the bladder and urethra although their role has not been defined[28].

Lower urinary tract function

In order to maintain continence, the urethral pressure must remain higher than the intravesical pressure at all times, except during micturition[29]. Estrogens play an important role in the continence mechanism, with bladder and urethral function becoming less efficient with age[30].

Elderly women have been found to have a reduced flow rate, increased urinary residuals, higher filling pressures, reduced bladder capacity and lower maximum voiding pressures[31]. Estrogens may affect continence by increasing urethral resistance, raising the sensory threshold of the bladder or by increasing α-adrenoreceptor sensitivity in the urethral smooth muscle[32,33]. In addition, exogenous estrogens have been shown to increase the number of intermediate and superficial cells in the vagina of postmenopausal women[34] and these changes have also been demonstrated in the bladder and urethra[35].

Bladder function

Estrogen receptors, although absent in the transitional epithelium of the bladder, are present in the areas of the trigone which have undergone squamous metaplasia[23]. Estrogen is known to have a direct effect on detrusor function through modifications in muscarinic receptors[36,37] and by inhibition of movement of extracellular calcium ions into muscle cells[38]. Consequently, estradiol has been shown to reduce the amplitude and frequency of spontaneous rhythmic detrusor contractions[39] and there is also evidence that it may increase the sensory threshold of the bladder in some women[40].

Neurological control

Sex hormones are known to influence the central neurological control of micturition, although their exact role in the micturition pathway has yet to be elucidated. Estrogen receptors have been demonstrated in the cerebral cortex, limbic system, hippocampus and cerebellum[41,42], whilst androgen receptors have been demonstrated in the pontine micturition centre and the pre-optic area of the hypothalamus[43].

Urethra

Estrogen receptors have been demonstrated in the squamous epithelium of both the proximal and distal urethra[22] and estrogen has been shown to improve the maturation index of urethral squamous epithelium[44]. It has been suggested that estrogen increases urethral closure pressure and improves pressure transmission to the proximal urethra, both promoting continence[45–48]. Estrogens have been shown to cause vasodilatation in the systemic and cerebral circulation and these changes are also seen in the urethra[49–51]. The vascular pulsations seen on urethral pressure profilometry secondary to blood flow in the urethral submucosa and urethral sphincter have been shown to increase in size following estrogen administration[52], whilst the effect is lost following estrogen withdrawal at the menopause.

Collagen

Estrogens are known to have an effect on collagen synthesis and they have been shown to have a direct effect on collagen metabolism in the lower genital tract[53]. Changes found in women with urogenital atrophy may represent an alteration in systemic collagenase activity[54] and urodynamic stress incontinence and urogenital prolapse have been associated with a reduction in both vaginal and periurethral collagen[55–57]. There is a reduction in skin collagen content following the menopause[58] and rectus muscle fascia has been shown to become less elastic with increasing age, resulting in a lower energy requirement to cause irreversible damage[59]. Changes in collagen content have also been identified, the hydroxyproline content in connective tissue from women with stress incontinence being 40% lower than in continent controls[60].

Urogenital atrophy

Withdrawal of endogenous estrogen at the menopause results in well-documented climacteric symptoms, such as hot flushes and night sweats, in addition to the less commonly reported symptoms of urogenital atrophy. Symptoms do not usually develop until several years following the menopause when levels of endogenous estrogens fall below the level required to promote endometrial growth[61]. This temporal relationship would suggest estrogen withdrawal as the cause.

Vaginal dryness is commonly the first reported symptom and is caused by a reduction in mucus production within the vaginal glands. Atrophy within the vaginal epithelium leads to thinning and an increased susceptibility to infection and mechanical trauma. Glycogen depletion within the vaginal mucosa following the menopause leads to a decrease in lactic acid formation by Doderlein's lactobacillus and a consequent rise in vaginal pH from around 4 to between 6 and 7. This allows bacterial overgrowth and colonization with Gram-negative bacilli, compounding the effects of vaginal atrophy and leading to symptoms of vaginitis, such as pruritis, dyspareunia and discharge.

Lower urinary tract symptoms

Epidemiological studies have implicated estrogen deficiency in the etiology of lower urinary tract symptoms, with 70% of women relating the onset of urinary incontinence to their final menstrual period[6]. Lower urinary tract symptoms have been shown to be common in postmenopausal women attending a menopause clinic, with 20% complaining of severe urgency and almost 50% complaining of stress incontinence[62]. Urge incontinence in particular is more prevalent following the menopause and the prevalence would appear to rise with increasing years of estrogen deficiency[63]. There is, however, conflicting evidence regarding the role of estrogen withdrawal at the time of the menopause. Some studies have shown a peak incidence in perimenopausal women[64,65], whilst other evidence suggests that many women develop incontinence at least 10 years prior to the cessation of menstruation, with significantly more premenopausal women than postmenopausal women being affected[61,66].

Cyclical variations in the levels of both estrogen and progesterone during the menstrual cycle have also been shown to lead to changes in urodynamic variables and lower urinary tract symptoms, with 37% of women noticing a deterioration in symptoms prior to menstruation[67]. Measurement of the urethral pressure profile in nulliparous premenopausal women shows that there is an increase in functional urethral length midcycle and early in the luteal phase corresponding to an increase in plasma estradiol[68]. Furthermore, progestogens have been associated with an increase in irritating bladder symptoms[69,70] and urinary incontinence in those women taking combined hormone replacement therapy[71]. The incidence of detrusor overactivity in the luteal phase of the menstrual cycle may be associated with raised plasma progesterone following ovulation, and progesterone has been shown to antagonize the inhibitory effect of estradiol on rat detrusor contractions[72]. This may help to explain the increased prevalence of detrusor overactivity found in pregnancy[73].

Urinary tract infection is also a common cause of urinary symptoms in women of all ages. This is a particular problem in the elderly, with a reported incidence of 20% in the community and over 50% in institutionalized patients[74,75]. Pathophysiological changes, such as impairment of bladder emptying, poor perineal hygiene and both fecal and urinary incontinence, may partly account for the high prevalence observed. In addition, as previously described, changes in the vaginal flora due to estrogen depletion lead to colonization with Gram-negative bacilli, which in addition to causing local symptoms of irritation also act as uropathogens. These microbiological changes may be reversed with estrogen replacement following the menopause which offer a rationale for treatment and prophylaxis.

ESTROGENS IN THE MANAGEMENT OF INCONTINENCE

Estrogen preparations have been used for many years in the treatment of urinary incontinence[76,77], although their precise role remains controversial. Many of the studies performed have been uncontrolled observational series examining the use of a wide range of different preparations, doses and routes of administration. The inconsistent use of progestogens to provide endometrial protection is a further confounding factor making interpretation of the results difficult.

In order to clarify the situation, a meta-analysis from the Hormones and Urogenital Therapy (HUT) Committee has been reported[78]. Of 166 articles identified which were published in English between 1969 and 1992 only six were controlled trials and 17 were uncontrolled series. Meta-analysis found an overall significant effect of estrogen therapy on subjective improvement in all subjects and for subjects with urodynamic stress incontinence alone. Subjective improvement rates with estrogen therapy in randomized controlled trials ranged from 64% to 75%, although placebo groups also reported an improvement of 10% to 56%. In uncontrolled series subjective improvement rates were 8–89%, with subjects with urodynamic stress incontinence showing improvement of 34–73%. However, when assessing objective fluid loss there was no significant effect. Maximum urethral closure pressure was found to increase significantly with estrogen therapy although this outcome was influenced by a single study showing a large effect[79].

ESTROGENS IN THE MANAGEMENT OF STRESS INCONTINENCE

In addition to the studies included in the HUT meta-analysis several authors have also investigated the role of estrogen therapy in the management of urodynamic stress incontinence only (Table 1). Oral estrogens have been reported to increase the maximum urethral pressures and lead to symptomatic

Table 1 Summary of randomized controlled trials assessing the use of estrogens in the management of urinary incontinence

Study	Year	Type of incontinence	Estrogen	Route
Henalla et al.[79]	1989	stress incontinence	conjugated estrogen	vaginal
Hilton et al.[88]	1990	stress incontinence	conjugated estrogen	vaginal
Beisland et al.[87]	1984	stress incontinence	estriol	vaginal
Judge[109]	1969	mixed incontinence	quinestradol	oral
Kinn and Lindskog[110]	1988	stress incontinence	estriol	oral
Samsioe et al.[89]	1985	mixed incontinence	estriol	oral
Walter et al.[83]	1978	urge incontinence	estradiol and estriol	oral
Walter et al.[111]	1990	stress incontinence	estriol	oral
Wilson et al.[82]	1987	stress incontinence	piperazine estrone sulphate	oral

improvement in 65–70% of women[80,81], although other work has not confirmed this[82,83]. More recently, two placebo-controlled studies have been performed examining the use of oral estrogens in the treatment of urodynamic stress incontinence in postmenopausal women. Neither conjugated equine estrogens and medroxyprogesterone[84], or unopposed estradiol valerate[85] showed a significant difference in either subjective or objective outcomes. Furthermore, a review of eight controlled and 14 uncontrolled prospective trials concluded that estrogen therapy was not an efficacious treatment for stress incontinence but may be useful for symptoms of urgency and frequency[86].

From the available evidence estrogen does not appear to be an effective treatment for stress incontinence although it may have a synergistic role in combination therapy. Two placebo-controlled studies have examined the use of oral and vaginal estrogens with the α-adrenergic agonist, phenylpropanolamine, used separately and in combination. Both studies found that combination therapy was superior to either drug given alone, although whilst there was subjective improvement in all groups[87], there was only objective improvement in the combination therapy group[88]. This may offer an alternative conservative treatment for women who have mild urodynamic stress incontinence.

ESTROGENS IN THE MANAGEMENT OF URGE INCONTINENCE

Estrogens have been used in the treatment of urinary urgency and urge incontinence for many years although there have been few controlled trials to confirm their efficacy (Table 1). A double-blind, placebo-controlled crossover study using oral estriol in 34 postmenopausal women produced subjective improvement in eight women with mixed incontinence and 12 with urge incontinence[89]. However, a double-blind multicenter study of the use of estriol (3 mg/day) in postmenopausal women complaining of urgency has failed to confirm these findings[90], showing both subjective and objective improvements but not significantly better than placebo. Estriol is a naturally occurring, weak estrogen which has little effect on the endometrium and does not prevent osteoporosis, although it has been used in the treatment of urogenital atrophy. Consequently it is possible that the dosage or route of administration in this study was not appropriate for the treatment of urinary symptoms and higher systemic levels may be required.

The use of sustained release 17β-estradiol vaginal tablets (Vagifem®) has also been examined in postmenopausal women with urgency and urge incontinence or a urodynamic diagnosis of sensory urgency or detrusor overactivity. These vaginal tablets have been shown to be well absorbed from the vagina and to induce maturation of the vaginal epithelium within 14 days[91]. However, following a 6-month course of treatment the only significant difference between active and placebo groups was an improvement in the symptom of urgency in those women with a urodynamic diagnosis of sensory urgency[92]. A further double-blind, randomized, placebo-controlled trial of 17β-estradiol vaginal tablets has shown lower urinary tract symptoms of frequency, urgency, urge and stress incontinence to be significantly improved, although there was no objective urodynamic assessment performed[93]. In both of these studies the subjective improvement in symptoms may simply represent local estrogenic effects reversing urogenital atrophy rather than a direct effect on bladder function.

To try and clarify the role of estrogen therapy in the management of women with urge incontinence a meta-analysis of the use of estrogen in women with symptoms of 'overactive bladder' has been reported by the HUT Committee (unpublished results). In a review of ten randomized, placebo-controlled trials, estrogen was found to be superior to placebo when considering symptoms of urge incontinence, frequency and nocturia, although vaginal estrogen administration was found to be superior for symptoms of urgency. In those taking estrogens there was also a significant increase in first sensation and bladder capacity as compared to placebo.

ESTROGENS IN THE MANAGEMENT OF RECURRENT URINARY TRACT INFECTION

Estrogen therapy has been shown to increase vaginal pH and reverse the microbiological changes that occur in the vagina following the menopause[94]. Initial small uncontrolled studies using oral or vaginal estrogens in the treatment of recurrent urinary tract infection appeared to give promising results[95,96], although unfortunately this has not been supported by larger randomized trials. Several studies have been performed examining the use of oral and vaginal estrogens, although these have had mixed results (Table 2).

Kjaergaard and colleagues[97] compared vaginal estriol tablets with placebo in 21 postmenopausal women over a 5-month period and found no significant difference between the two groups. However, a subsequent randomized, double-blind, placebo-controlled study assessing the use of estriol vaginal cream in 93

Table 2 Summary of randomized controlled trials assessing the use of estrogens in the management of recurrent lower urinary tract infection (UTI)

Study	Study group	Type of estrogen	Route of delivery	Duration of therapy	Results
Kjaergaard et al. 1990[97]	21 postmenopausal women with recurrent cystitis (10 active group 11 placebo)	estradiol	vaginal tablets	5 months	Number of positive cultures not statistically different between the two groups.
Kirkengen et al. 1992[99]	40 postmenopausal women with recurrent UTIs (20 active group 20 placebo)	estriol	oral	12 weeks	Both estriol and placebo significantly reduced the incidence of UTIs ($p < 0.05$). After 12 weeks estriol was significantly more effective than placebo ($p < 0.05$).
Raz and Stamm 1993[98]	93 postmenopausal women with recurrent UTIs (50 active group 43 placebo)	estriol	vaginal cream	8 months	Significant reduction in the incidence of UTIs in the group given estriol compared to placebo ($p < 0.001$).
Cardozo et al. 1998[100]	72 postmenopausal women with recurrent UTIs (36 active group 36 placebo)	estriol	oral	6-month treatment period with a further 6 months follow-up	Reduction in urinary symptoms and incidence of UTIs in both groups. Estriol no better than placebo.
Eriksen 1999[101]	108 women with recurrent UTIs (53 active group 55 no treatment)	estradiol	Estring	36 weeks for the active group 36 weeks or until first recurrence for the controls	Cumulative likelihood of remaining free of infection was 45% in active group and 20% in control group ($p = 0.008$)

postmenopausal women during an 8-month period did reveal a significant effect[98].

Kirkengen and colleagues randomized 40 postmenopausal women to receive either placebo or oral estriol and found that although initially both groups had a significantly decreased incidence of recurrent infections, after 12 weeks estriol was shown to be significantly more effective[99]. These findings, however, were not confirmed subsequently in a trial of 72 postmenopausal women with recurrent urinary tract infections randomized to oral estriol or placebo. Following a 6-month treatment period and a further 6-month follow-up, estriol was found to be no more effective than placebo[100].

More recently a randomized, open, parallel-group study assessing the use of an estradiol-releasing silicone vaginal ring (Estring®) in postmenopausal women with recurrent infections has been performed which showed that the cumulative likelihood of remaining infection free was 45% in the active group and 20% in the placebo group[101]. Estring was also shown to decrease the number of recurrences per year and to prolong the interval between infection episodes.

ESTROGENS IN THE MANAGEMENT OF UROGENITAL ATROPHY

Symptoms of urogenital atrophy do not occur until the levels of endogenous estrogen are lower than that required to promote endometrial proliferation[61]. Consequently it is possible to use a low-dose estrogen replacement therapy in order to alleviate urogenital symptoms whilst avoiding the risk of endometrial proliferation and removing the necessity of providing endometrial protection with progestogens[102]. The dose of estradiol commonly used in systemic estrogen replacement is usually 25–100 μg, although studies investigating the use of estrogens in the management of urogenital symptoms have shown that 8–10 μg of vaginal estradiol is effective[103]. Thus, only 10–30% of the dose used to treat vasomotor symptoms may be effective in the management of urogenital symptoms. Since 10–25% of women receiving systemic hormone replacement therapy still experience the symptoms of urogenital atrophy[104], low-dose local preparations may have an additional beneficial effect.

A recent review of estrogen therapy in the management of urogenital atrophy has been performed by the Hormones and Urogenital Therapy Committee[105]. Ten randomized trials and 54 uncontrolled series were examined from 1969 to 1995, assessing 24 different treatment regimens. Meta-analysis of ten placebo-controlled trials confirmed the significant effect of estrogens in the management of urogenital atrophy (Table 3).

The route of administration was assessed and oral, vaginal and parenteral (transcutaneous patches and subcutaneous implants) were compared. Overall, the vaginal route of administration was found to correlate with better symptom relief, greater improvement in cytological findings, and higher serum estradiol levels.

Table 3 Summary of randomized controlled trials assessing the use of estrogens in urogenital atrophy

Study	Year	Estrogen	Route
Bellatoni et al.[112]	1991	estradiol	transdermal
Campbell et al.[113]	1977	conjugated estrogen	oral
Erikson and Ramussen[93]	1992	estradiol	pessary
Felding et al.[114]	1992	estradiol	pessary
Foidart et al.[115]	1991	estriol	vaginal cream
Laufer et al.[116]	1983	estradiol	transdermal
Mettler and Olsen[102]	1991	estradiol	pessary
Molander et al.[117]	1990	estriol	oral
Raz and Stamm[98]	1993	estriol	vaginal cream
Van der Linden et al.[118]	1993	estriol	oral

With regard to the type of estrogen preparation, estradiol was found to be most effective in reducing patient symptoms, although conjugated estrogens produced the most cytological change and the greatest increase in serum levels of estradiol and estrone.

Finally the effect of different dosages was examined. Low-dose vaginal estradiol was found to be the most efficacious according to symptom relief, although oral estriol was also effective. Estriol had no effect on the serum levels of estradiol or estrone, whilst vaginal estriol had minimal effect. Vaginal estradiol was found to have a small effect on serum estrogen although not as great as systemic preparations. In conclusion it would appear that estrogen is efficacious in the treatment of urogenital atrophy and low-dose vaginal preparations are as effective as systemic therapy.

More recently the use of Estring®, which releases estradiol at 5–10 µg/24 hr, has been investigated in postmenopausal women with symptomatic urogenital atrophy[101]. There was a significant effect on symptoms of vaginal dryness, pruritis vulvae, dyspareunia and urinary urgency, with improvement being reported in over 90% of women in an uncontrolled study. The maturation of vaginal epithelium was also significantly improved. The patient acceptability was high and whilst the maturation of vaginal epithelium was significantly improved there was no effect on endometrial proliferation.

These findings were supported by a 1-year multicenter study of Estring® in postmenopausal women with urogenital atrophy which found subjective and objective improvement in 90% of patients up to 1 year. However, there was a 20% withdrawal rate, with 7% of women reporting vaginal irritation, two having vaginal ulceration, and three complaining of vaginal bleeding although there were no cases of endometrial proliferation[106]. Long-term safety has been confirmed by a 10-year review of the use of the estradiol ring delivery system, which has found its safety, efficacy and acceptability to be comparable to other forms of vaginal administration[107]. A comparative study of safety and efficacy of Estring® with conjugated equine estrogen vaginal cream in 194 postmenopausal women complaining of urogenital atrophy found no significant difference in vaginal dryness, dyspareunia and resolution of atrophic signs between the two treatment groups. Furthermore, there was a similar improvement in the vaginal mucosal maturation index and a reduction in pH in both groups with the vaginal ring being found to be preferable to the cream[108].

CONCLUSIONS

Estrogens are known to have an important physiological effect on the female lower genital tract throughout adult life, leading to symptomatic, histological and functional changes. Urogenital atrophy is the manifestation of estrogen withdrawal following the menopause, presenting with vaginal and/or urinary symptoms. The use of estrogen replacement therapy has been examined in the management of lower urinary tract symptoms as well as in the treatment of urogenital atrophy although only recently has it been subjected to randomized, placebo-controlled trials and meta-analysis.

Estrogen therapy alone has been shown to have little effect in the management of urodynamic stress incontinence, although when used in combination with an α-adrenergic agonists it may lead to an improvement in urinary leakage. When considering the irritative symptoms of urinary urgency, frequency and urge incontinence, estrogen therapy may be of benefit, although this may simply represent reversal of urogenital atrophy rather than a direct effect on the lower urinary tract. The role of estrogen replacement therapy in the management of women with recurrent lower urinary tract infection remains to be determined although there is now some evidence that vaginal administration may be efficacious. Finally, low-dose vaginal estrogens have been shown to have a role in the treatment of urogenital atrophy in postmenopausal women and would appear to be as effective as systemic preparations.

References

1. Iosif CS. Effects of protracted administration of oestriol on the lower genitourinary tract in postmenopausal women. *Acta Obstet Gynecol Scand* 1992;251:115–20

2. Cardozo LD. Role of oestrogens in the treatment of female urinary incontinence. *J Am Geriatr Soc* 1990;38:326–8

3. Iosif S, Batra S, Ek A, Astedt B. Oestrogen receptors in the human female lower urinary tract. *Am J Obstet Gynecol* 1981;141:817–20

4. Batra SC, Fossil CS. Female urethra, a target for oestrogen action. *J Urol* 1983;129:418–20

5. Batra SC, Iosif LS. Progesterone receptors in the female urinary tract. *J Urol* 1987;138:130–4

6. Iosif C, Bekassy Z. Prevalence of genitourinary symptoms in the late menopause. *Acta Obstet Gynecol Scand* 1984;63:257–60

7. American National Institute of Health Population Figures. Washington DC: US Treasury Department. NIH, 1991

8. WHO Research on the menopause in the 1990s. Report of a WHO Scientific Group. In: *WHO Technical Report Series* 866 Geneva: WHO, 1994.

9. Hill K. The demography of the menopause. *Maturitas* 1996;23:113–27

10. Barlow D, Samsioe G, van Geelan H. Prevalence of urinary problems in European countries. *Maturitas* 1997;27:239–48

11. Greendale GA, Judd JL. The menopause: health implications and clinical management. *J Am Geriatr Soc* 1993;41:426–36

12. Samsioe G, Jansson I, Mellstrom D, Svanborg A. The occurrence, nature and treatment of urinary incontinence in a 70 year old population. *Maturitas* 1985;7:335–43

13. Van Geelen JM, Van de Weijer PH, Arnolds HT. Urogenital symptoms and resulting discomfort in non-institutionalised Dutch women aged 50–75 years. *Int Urogynecol J Pelvic Floor Dysfunct* 2000;11:9–14

14. Versi E, Harvey MA, Cardozo L, *et al.* Urogenital prolapse and atrophy at menopause: a prevalence study. *Int Urogynecol J Pelvic Dysfunct* 2001;12:107–10

15. Davila GW, Karapanagiotou I, Woodhouse S, *et al.* Are women with urogenital atrophy symptomatic? *Obstet Gynecol* 2001;97(4 Suppl 1): S48

16. Diokno AC, Brook BM, Brown MB. Prevalence of urinary incontinence and other urological symptoms in the non-institutionalised elderly. *J Urol* 1986;136:1022

17. Yarnell J, Voyle G, Richards C, Stephenson T. The prevalence and severity of urinary incontinence in women. *J Epidemiol Community Health* 1981;35:71–4

18. Ouslander JG. Urinary incontinence in nursing homes. *J Am Geriatr Soc* 1990;38:289–91

19. Kok AL, Voorhorst FJ, Burger CW, *et al.* Urinary and faecal incontinence in community residing elderly women. *Age Ageing* 1992;21:211

20. Green S, Walter P, Kumar V, *et al.* Human oestrogen receptor cDNA: sequence, expression and homology to v-erbA. *Nature* 1986; 320:134–9

21. Kuiper G, Enmark E, Pelto-Huikko M, *et al.* Cloning of a novel oestrogen receptor expressed in rat prostate and ovary. *Proc Natl Acad Sci USA* 1996;93:5925–30

22. Blakeman PJ, Hilton P, Bulmer JN. Mapping oestrogen and progesterone receptors throughout the female lower urinary tract. *Neurourol Urodyn* 1996;15:324–5

23. Ingelman-Sundberg A, Rosen J, Gustafsson SA. Cytosol oestrogen receptors in urogenital tissues in stress incontinent women. *Acta Obstet Gynecol Scand* 1981;60:585–6

24. Smith P. Oestrogens and the urogenital tract. *Acta Obstet Gynecol Scand* 1993;72:1–26

25. Bernstein IT. The pelvic floor muscles: muscle thickness in healthy and urinary-incontinent women measured by perineal ultrasonography with reference to the effect of pelvic floor training. Oestrogen receptor studies. *Neurourol Urodyn* 1997;16:237–75

26. Chen GD, Oliver RH, Leung BS, *et al.* Oestrogen receptor α and β expression in the vaginal walls and uterosacral ligaments of premenopausal and postmenopausal women. *Fertil Steril* 1999;71:1099–102

27. Screiter F, Fuchs P, Stockamp K. Oestrogenic sensitivity of α receptors in the urethral musculature. *Urol Int* 1976;31:13–19

28. Blakeman PJ, Hilton P, Bulmer JN. Androgen receptors in the female lower urinary tract. *Int Urogynecol J* 1997;8:S54

29. Abrams P, Blaivas JG, Stanton SL, *et al.* The standardisation of terminology of lower urinary tract dysfunction. *Br J Obstet Gynaecol* 1990; 97:1–16

30. Rud T, Anderson KE, Asmussen M, *et al.* Factors maintaining the urethral pressure in women. *Invest Urol* 1980;17:343–7

31. Malone-Lee J. Urodynamic measurement and urinary incontinence in the elderly. In Brocklehurst JC, ed. *Managing and Measuring Incontinence. Proceedings of the Geriatric Workshop on Incontinence,* July 1988. (Geriatric Medicine). London: Churchill Livingstone,1988

32. Versi E, Cardozo LD. Oestrogens and lower urinary tract function. In Studd JWW,

Whitehead MI, eds. *The Menopause*. Oxford: Blackwell Scientific Publications, 1988:76–84

33. Kinn AC, Lindskog M. Oestrogens and phenyl-propanolamine in combination for stress incontinence. *Urology* 1988;32:273–80

34. Smith PJB. The effect of oestrogens on bladder function in the female. In Campbell S, ed. *The Management of the Menopause and Postmenopausal Years*. Carnforth: MTP, 1976:291–8

35. Samsioe G, Jansson I, Mellstrom D, Svandborg A. Occurrence, nature and treatment of urinary incontinence in a 70 year old female population. *Maturitas* 1985;7:335–42

36. Shapiro E. Effect of oestrogens on the weight and muscarinic receptor density of the rabbit bladder and urethra. *J Urol* 1986;135:1084–7

37. Batra S, Anderson KE. Oestrogen induced changes in muscarinic receptor density and contractile responses in the female rat urinary bladder. *Acta Physiol Scand* 1989;137: 135–141

38. Elliott RA, Castleden CM, Miodrag A, Kirwan P. The direct effects of diethylstilboestrol and nifedipine on the contractile responses of isolated human and rat detrusor muscles. *Eur J Clin Pharmacol* 1992;43:149–55

39. Shenfield OZ, Blackmore PF, Morgan CW, *et al.* Rapid effects of oestriol and progesterone on tone and spontaneous rhythmic contractions of the rabbit bladder. *Neurourol Urodyn* 1998;17: 408–9

40. Fantl JA, Wyman JF, Anderson RL, *et al.* Post menopausal urinary incontinence: comparison between non-oestrogen and oestrogen supplemented women. *Obstet Gynecol* 1988;71:823–8

41. Maggi A, Perez J. Role of female gonadal hormones in the CNS. *Life Sci* 1985;37:893–906

42. Smith SS, Berg G, Hammar M. (eds.) The modern management of the menopause. Hormones, mood and neurobiology – a summary. Carnforth, UK: Parthenon Publishing, 1993:204

43. Blok EFM, Holstege G. Androgen receptor immunoreactive neurones in the hypothalamic preoptic area project to the pontine micturition centre in the male cat. *Neurourol Urodyn* 1998; 17:404–5

44. Bergman A, Karram MM, Bhatia NN. Changes in urethral cytology following oestrogen administration. *Gynecol Obstet Invest* 1990;29:211–13

45. Rud T. The effects of oestrogens and gestogens on the urethral pressure profile in urinary continent and stress incontinent women. *Acta Obstet Gynecol Scand* 1980;59:365–70

46. Hilton P, Stanton SL. The use of intravaginal oestrogen cream in genuine stress incontinence. *Br J Obstet Gynaecol* 1983;90:940–4

47. Bhatia NN, Bergman A, Karram MM, *et al.* Effects of oestrogen on urethral function in

women with urinary incontinence. *Am J Obstet Gynecol* 1989;160:176–80

48. Karram MM, Yeko TR, Sauer MV, *et al.* Urodynamic changes following hormone replacement therapy in women with premature ovarian failure. *Obstet Gynecol* 1989;74:208–11

49. Ganger KF, Vyas S, Whitehead RW, *et al.* Pulsitility index in the internal carotid artery in relation to transdermal oestradiol and time since the menopause. *Lancet* 1991;338:839–42

50. Jackson S, Vyas S. A double blind, placebo controlled study of postmenopausal oestrogen replacement therapy and carotid artery pulsatility index. *Br J Obstet Gynaecol* 1998;105:408–12

51. Penotti M, Farina M, Sironi L, *et al.* Long term effects of postmenopausal hormone replacement therapy on pulsatility index of the internal carotid and middle cerebral arteries. *Menopause* 1997;4:101–4

52. Versi E, Cardozo LD. Urethral instability: diagnosis based on variations in the maximum urethral pressure in normal climacteric women. *Neurourol Urodyn* 1986;5:535–41

53. Falconer C, Ekman-Ordeberg G, Ulmsten U, *et al.* Changes in paraurethral connective tissue at menopause are counteracted by oestrogen. *Maturitas* 1996;24:197–204

54. Kushner L, Chen Y, Desautel M, *et al.* Collagenase activity is elevated in conditioned media from fibroblasts of women with pelvic floor weakening. *Int Urogynecol* 1999;10(S1):34

55. Jackson S, Avery N, Shephered A, *et al.* The effect of oestradiol on vaginal collagen in postmenopausal women with stress urinary incontinence. *Neurourol Urodyn* 1996;15:327–8

56. James M, Avery N, Jackson S, *et al.* The pathophysiological changes of vaginal skin tissue in women with stress urinary incontinence: A controlled trial. *Int Urogynecol* 1999;10(S1):35

57. James M, Avery N, Jackson S, *et al.* The biochemical profile of vaginal tissue in women with genitourinary prolapse: a controlled trial. *Neurourol Urodyn* 1999;18:284–5

58. Brincat M, Moniz CF, Studd JWW. Long term effects of the menopause and sex hormones on skin thickness. *Br J Obstet Gynaecol* 1985; 92:256–9

59. Landon CR, Smith ARB, Crofts CE, Trowbridge EA. Biochemical properties of connective tissue in women with stress incontinence of urine. *Neurourol Urodyn* 1989;8:369–70

60. Ulmsten U, Ekman G, Giertz G. Different biochemical composition of connective tissue in continent and stress incontinent women. *Acta Obstet Gynecol Scand* 1987;66:455

61. Samicoe G. Urogenital ageing – a hidden problem. *Am J Obstet Gynecol* 1998;178:S245–9

62. Cardozo LD, Tapp A, Versi E, *et al.*, eds. The lower urinary tract in peri- and postmenopausal

women. In *The Urogenital Defiency Syndrome*. Bagsverd, Denmark: Novo Industri AS, 1987: 10–17

63. Kondo A, Kato K, Saito M, *et al.* Prevalence of hand washing incontinence in females in comparison with stress and urge incontinence. *Neurourol Urodyn* 1990;9:330–1

64. Thomas TM, Plymat KR, Blannin J, *et al.* Prevalence of urinary incontinence. *Br Med J* 1980;281:1243–5

65. Jolleys JV. Reported prevalence of urinary incontinence in a general practice. *Br Med J* 1988;296:1300–2

66. Burgio KL, Matthews KA, Engel B. Prevalence, incidence and correlates of urinary incontinence in healthy, middle aged women. *J Urol* 1991;146:1255–9

67. Hextall A, Bidmead J, Cardozo L, Hooper R. Hormonal influences on the human female lower urinary tract: a prospective evaluation of the effects of the menstrual cycle on symptomatology and the results of urodynamic investigation. *Neurourol Urodyn* 1999;18:282–3

68. Van Geelen JM, Doesburg WH, Thomas CMG. Urodynamic studies in the normal menstrual cycle: the relationship between hormonal changes during the menstrual cycle and the urethral pressure profile. *Am J Obstet Gynecol* 1981;141:384–92

69. Burton G, Cardozo LD, Abdalla H, *et al.* The hormonal effects on the lower urinary tract in 282 women with premature ovarian failure. *Neurourol Urodyn* 1992;10:318–19

70. Cutner A, Burton G, Cardozo LD, *et al.* Does progesterone cause an irritable bladder? *Int Urogynecol J* 1993;4:259–61

71. Benness C, Gangar K, Cardozo LD, Cutner A. Do progestogens exacerbate urinary incontinence in women on HRT? *Neurourol Urodyn* 1991;10:316–18

72. Elliot RA, Castleden CM. Effect of progestagens and oestrogens on the contractile response of rat detrusor muscle to electrical field stimulation. *Clin Sci* 1994;87:342

73. Cutner A. *The urinary tract in pregnancy*. MD Thesis. 1993. University of London

74. Sandford JP. Urinary tract symptoms and infection. *Annu Rev Med* 1975;26:485–505

75. Boscia JA, Kaye D. Asymptomatic bacteria in the elderly. *Infect Dis Clin North Am* 1987;1: 893–903

76. Salmon UL, Walter RI, Gast SH. The use of oestrogen in the treatment of dysuria and incontinence in postmenopausal women. *Am J Obstet Gynecol* 1941;14:23–31

77. Youngblood VH, Tomlin EM, Davis JB. Senile urethritis in women. *J Urol* 1957;78:150–2

78. Fantl JA, Cardozo LD, McClish DK and the Hormones and Urogenital Therapy Com-

mittee. Oestrogen therapy in the management of incontinence in postmenopausal women: a meta-analysis. First report of the Hormones and Urogenital Therapy Committee. *Obstet Gynecol* 1994;83:12–18

79. Henalla SM, Hutchins CJ, Robinson P, Macivar J. Non-operative methods in the treatment of female genuine stress incontinence of urine. *Br J Obstet Gynaecol* 1989;9:222–225

80. Caine M, Raz S. The role of female hormones in stress incontinence. In *Proceedings of the 16th Congress of the International Society of Urology, Amsterdam, the Netherlands.*

81. Rud T. The effects of oestrogens and gestagens on the urethral pressure profile in urinary continent and stress incontinent women. *Acta Obstet Gynecol Scand* 1980;59:265–70

82. Wilson PD, Faragher B, Butler B, *et al.* Treatment with oral piperazine oestrone sulphate for genuine stress incontinence in postmenopausal women. *Br J Obstet Gynaecol* 1987;94:568–74

83. Walter S, Wolf H, Barlebo H, Jansen H. Urinary incontinence in postmenopausal women treated with oestrogens: a double-blind clinical trial. *J Urol* 1978;33:135–43

84. Fantl JA, Bump RC, Robinson D, *et al.* Efficacy of oestrogen supplementation in the treatment of urinary incontinence. *Obstet Gynecol* 1996;88:745–9

85. Jackson S, Shepherd A, Brookes S, Abrams P. The effect of oestrogen supplementation on post-menopausal urinary stress incontinence: a double-blind, placebo controlled trial. *Br J Obstet Gynaecol* 1999;106:711–18

86. Sultana CJ, Walters MD. Oestrogen and urinary incontinence in women. *Maturitas* 1995;20: 129–38

87. Beisland HO, Fossberg E, Moer A, *et al.* Urethral insufficiency in post-menopausal females: treatment with phenylpropanolamine and oestriol separately and in combination. *Urol Int* 1984;39:211–16

88. Hilton P, Tweddel AL, Mayne C. Oral and intravaginal oestrogens alone and in combination with alpha adrenergic stimulation in genuine stress incontinence. *Int Urogynecol J* 1990;12:80–6

89. Samsioe G, Jansson I, Mellstrom D, Svanberg A. Urinary incontinence in 75 year old women. Effects of oestriol. *Acta Obstet Gynecol Scand* 1985;93:57

90. Cardozo LD, Rekers H, Tapp A, *et al.* Oestriol in the treatment of postmenopausal urgency: a multicentre study. *Maturitas* 1993;18:47–53

91. Nilsson K, Heimer G. Low dose oestradiol in the treatment of urogenital oestrogen deficiency – a pharmacokinetic and pharmacodynamic study. *Maturitas* 1992;15:121–7

92. Benness C, Wise BG, Cutner A, Cardozo LD. Does low dose vaginal oestradiol improve frequency and urgency in postmenopausal women. *Int Urogynaecol J* 1992;3:281

93. Eriksen PS, Rasmussen H. Low dose 17β-oestradiol vaginal tablets in the treatment of atrophic vaginitis: a double-blind placebo controlled study. *Eur J Obstet Gynecol Reprod Biol* 1992;44:137–44

94. Brandberg A, Mellstrom D, Samsioe G. Low dose oral oestriol treatment in elderly women with urogenital infections. *Acta Obstet Gynecol Scand* 1987;140:33–8

95. Parsons CL, Schmidt JD. Control of recurrent urinary tract infections in postmenopausal women. *J Urol* 1982;128:1224–6

96. Privette M, Cade R, Peterson J, *et al.* Prevention of recurrent urinary tract infections in postmenopausal women. *Nephron* 1988;50:24–7

97. Kjaergaard B, Walter S, Knudsen A, *et al.* Treatment with low dose vaginal oestradiol in postmenopausal women. A double blind controlled trial. *Ugeskr Laeger* 1990;152:658–9

98. Raz R, Stamm WE. A controlled trial of intravaginal oestriol in postmenopausal women with recurrent urinary tract infections. *N Engl J Med* 1993;329:753–6

99. Kirkengen AL, Anderson P, Gjersoe E, *et al.* Oestriol in the prophylactic treatment of recurrent urinary tract infections in postmenopausal women. *Scand J Prim Health Care* 1992;10:142

100. Cardozo LD, Benness C, Abbott D. Low dose oestrogen prophylaxis for recurrent urinary tract infections in elderly women. *Br J Obstet Gynaecol* 1998;105:403–7

101. Eriksen B. A randomised, open, parallel-group study on the preventive effect of an oestradiol-releasing vaginal ring (Estring) on recurrent urinary tract infections in postmenopausal women. *Am J Obstet Gynecol* 1999;180:1072–9

102. Mettler L, Olsen PG. Long term treatment of atrophic vaginitis with low dose oestradiol vaginal tablets. *Maturitas* 1991;14:23–31

103. Smith P, Heimer G, Lindskog M, Ulmsten U. Oestradiol-releasing vaginal ring for treatment of postmenopausal urogenital atrophy. *Maturitas* 1993; 16:145–54

104. Smith RJN, Studd JWW. Recent advances in hormone replacement therapy. *Br J Hosp Med* 1993;49:799–809

105. Cardozo LD, Bachmann G, McClish D, *et al.* Meta-analysis of oestrogen therapy in the management of urogenital atrophy in postmenopausal women: Second report of the Hormones and Urogenital Therapy Committee. *Obstet Gynecol* 1998;92: 722–7

106. Henriksson L, Stjernquist M, Boquist L, *et al.* A one-year multicentre study of efficacy and safety of a continuous, low dose, oestradiol-releasing vaginal ring (Estring) in postmenopausal women with symptoms and signs of urogenital aging. *Am J Obstet Gynecol* 1996;174:85–92

107. Bachmann G. Oestradiol-releasing vaginal ring delivery system for urogenital atrophy. Experience over the last decade. *J Reprod Med* 1998;43:991–8

108. Ayton RA, Darling GM, Murkies AL, *et al.* A comparative study of safety and efficacy of low dose oestradiol released from a vaginal ring compared with conjugated equine oestrogen vaginal cream in the treatment of postmenopausal vaginal atrophy. *Br J Obstet Gynaecol* 1996;103:351–8

109. Judge TG. The use of quinestradol in elderly incontinent women: a preliminary report. *Gerontol Clin* 1969;11:159–64

110. Kinn AC, Lindskog M. Oestrogens and phenylpropanolamine in combination for stress incontinence in postmenopausal women. *Urology* 1988;32:273–80

111. Walter S, Kjaergaard B, Lose G, *et al.* Stress urinary incontinence in postmenopausal women treated with oral oestrogen (oestriol) and an α-adrenoceptor stimulating agent (phenylpropanolamine): A randomised double-blind placebo-controlled study. *Int Urogynecol J* 1990; 1:74–9

112. Bellatoni MF, Harman SM, Cullins VE, *et al.* Transdermal oestradiol with oral progestin: biological and clinical effects in younger and older postmenopausal women. *J Gerontol* 1991; 46:M216–22

113. Campbell S, Whitehead M. Oestrogen therapy and the menopausal syndrome. *Clin Obstet Gynecol* 1977;4:31–47

114. Felding C, Mikkelse AL, Chausen HV, *et al.* Preoperative treatment with oestradiol in women scheduled for vaginal operations for genital prolapse. A randomised double blind trial. *Maturitas* 1992;15:241–9

115. Foidart JM, Vervliet J, Buytaert P. Efficacy of sustained release vaginal formulation of oestriol in alleviating urogenital and systemic climacteric complaints. *Maturitas* 1991;13: 99–107

116. Laufer LR, Defazio JL, Lu JKH. Oestrogen replacement therapy by transdermal oestradiol administration. *Am J Obstet Gynecol* 1983;146: 533–40

117. Molander U, Milson I, Ekelund P, Mellstrom D. An epidemiological study of urinary incontinence and related urogenital symptoms in elderly women. *Maturitas* 1990;12:51–60

118. Van der Linden MCGJ, Gerretsen G, Brandhurst MS, *et al.* The effects of oestriol on the cytology of urethra and vagina in postmenopausal women with genitourinary symptoms. *Eur J Obstet Gynecol Reprod Biol* 1993;51:29–33

5

Urogenital collagen turnover and hormone replacement therapy

C. Falconer

INTRODUCTION

Like all other structures in the human body, those of the urogenital system also undergo aging. This degenerative process may induce a variety of dysfunctions in the organs and structures, which in turn lead to various symptoms. It remains unclear whether this is due to the hormonal changes associated with the menopause, or is just part of the aging process. Lack of estrogen may be related to some of these changes, but the effects of estrogen replacement on these conditions have not been demonstrated conclusively. However, several factors suggest that some lower urinary tract changes are related to loss of estrogen stimulation. The urethra and vagina share a common derivation from the urogenital sinus, and the mucosa of the urethra undergoes cyclic variation during menses. With the arrival of the menopause, there is regression of the thick squamous epithelium that is found during the reproductive period. Estrogen affects collagen content and metabolism differently depending on site and function of the involved tissue.

Our knowledge of connective tissue changes in the genitourinary tract is limited. Since paraurethral connective tissue is crucial for the mechanical properties of the genitourinary region, it is important to characterize the biochemical nature of this tissue and to record possible changes related to estrogen status.

ULTRASTRUCTURE OF FIBROUS CONNECTIVE TISSUE

Connective tissue is analogous to a fiber-reinforced composite, including fibrous elements (collagen and elastic fibers) and a viscoelastic matrix containing proteoglycans. The relationship between the fibers and the other matrix components is important for the physical properties of the tissue. The cells in the connective tissues, making up about 20% of the tissue volume, are embedded in the extracellular matrix (ECM). All the matrix proteins and polysaccharides are secreted locally by cells in contact with the matrix, and they can be ordered by close association with the exterior surface of the plasma membrane. Because the structure and orientation of the matrix, in turn, influence the orientation of the cells it contains, an order is likely to be propagated from cell to cell through the matrix[1–3].

A model of the organization of fibrous connective tissue components is presented in Figure 1. The biomechanical properties of a soft tissue are determined by the structure and distribution of the various ECM components.

Collagens

Collagen is the most abundant protein in the human body and the dominating structure of the connective tissue. The collagen fibers, mainly types I and III, are responsible for the tensile strength of the tissue. Other collagens,

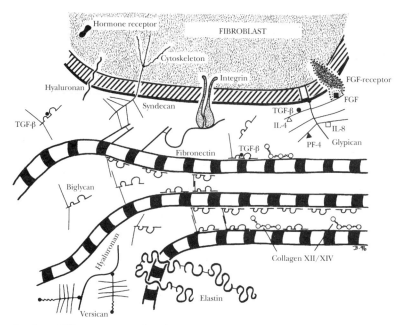

Figure 1 Organization of fibrous connective tissue components

present in smaller quantities in tissues, serve as connecting elements between the major structures and other tissue components. The fibril-associated collagens types IX, XII and XIV (FACIT collagens) appear to connect collagen fibrils to other matrix elements. Collagen IX is found along fibers of collagen II in cartilage, whereas collagens XII and XIV are found primarily in non-cartilage tissue and, therefore, mostly along fibers of the dominating collagen I (Figure 1)[4].

Collagen fibrils, constituting the fibers, are made up of tropocollagen molecules staggered in a special way, resulting in the cross-striation typical of the collagen fibrils seen with electron microscopy (Figure 2). This arrangement presumably maximizes the tensile strength of the aggregate. However, it is still not certain how these staggered molecules are packed in the three dimensions of a cylindrical fibril[4]. Each tropocollagen molecule consists of three polypeptide chains of about 1000 amino acids each, twisted into a triple helix. A proper helix formation requires the presence of glycine in every third position. Collagen is also rich in two other amino acids, hydroxyproline, which stabi-

lizes the helical structure, and hydroxylysine, involved in the covalent cross-links holding the tropocollagen together. These intermolecular as well as intramolecular cross-links are responsible for the tensile properties of the collagen molecule[5]. The extracellular enzyme lysyl oxidase converts certain lysine and hydroxylysine residues into reactive aldehydes[6]. Although cross-linking is the last step in the biosynthesis of collagens, it is very important for fibrillar collagens, because it greatly increases the tensile strength of fibers, and therefore contributes significantly to tissue integrity.

Collagen fibrils are between 10 and 300 nm in diameter[7]. In general, the fibrils increase in diameter with increasing age, coupled with a marked dispersion of the size distribution. In extreme old age the fibrils grow thinner[8]. The FACITs are non-fibrillar collagens with several short triple-helical sequences interrupted by non-triple-helical domains. FACIT collagens are attached to the surfaces of pre-existing fibrils of the fibril-forming collagens, and thus influence the fibrillization process[6] (Figure 1). The exact nature of this interaction remains to be elucidated.

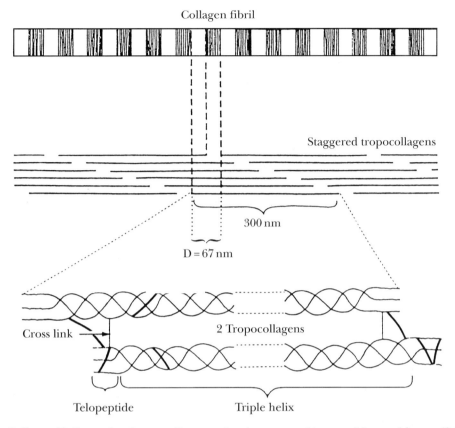

Figure 2 Collagen fibrils consist of tropocollagen molecules staggered in a special way, with gaps (0.6 D) and overlaps (0.4 D) resulting in the typical cross-striation of fibrillar collagens seen with electron miscroscopy

Proteoglycans

Proteoglycans (PGs) have the potential for almost limitless heterogeneity. Proteoglycans are special types of glycoproteins consisting of a protein core with one or several covalently bound glycosaminoglycans (GAGs) and a number of oligosaccharides[9,10]. They are called glycosaminoglycans because one of the two sugar residues in the repeating disaccharide is always an aminosugar. In most cases this aminosugar is sulfated and the second sugar is a uronic acid. Because of the sulfate or carboxyl groups on most of their sugar residues, GAGs are highly negatively charged, causing the attraction of large quantities of water. Four main groups of GAGs have been distinguished by their sugar residues, the type of linkage

between these residues and the number and location of sulfate groups: hyaluronic acid; chondroitin sulfate and dermatan sulfate; heparan sulfate and heparin; and keratan sulfate. The PGs can differ markedly in protein content, molecular size and number and types of GAG chains per molecule[1]. Of the many divergent functions associated with the PGs, some are connected with the core proteins, some with the GAG chains and others with the whole molecules[11]. The PGs are essential for organization of the collagen fibrils and the cells, as well as for hydration and resilience of the tissue molecules[1,11,12].

Proteoglycans substituted with heparan sulfate are found mainly on cell surfaces, where they are of importance for cell adhesion and proliferation, and in basement membranes, where they interact with other molecules such as collagen type IV and laminin[1,13]. Chondroitin sulfate proteoglycans on the other hand appear to act as a lubricant, allowing collagen fibrils to slide by each other[10]. Some PGs can bind growth factors, modulating their activity and serving as reservoirs for them in the tissue[2,10,12,13].

Three small PGs with homologous core proteins have been identified in most fibrous connective tissues: decorin and biglycan with protein cores of 40–45 kDa and fibromodulin with a protein core of 59 kDa. Both decorin and fibromodulin bind to collagen types I and II and influence fibrillogenesis[14–17]. Decorin may, by specific side-chain reactions, organize the collagen fibrils[14]. Biglycan and larger aggregating PGs might instead split up the collagen fibers[16] (Figure 1).

Other connective tissue components of importance are the following.

Elastin

Elastin is the major component of elastic fibers, which form a network of thin fibers[7]. The elastin molecules in tissues are in the form of an insoluble protein and, as such, very difficult to isolate.

Fibronectin

Fibronectin is a multifunctional molecule which can bind to collagen, to heparin and to specific receptors of various types of cells. In this way it contributes to the organization of the matrix and helps cells attach to it[7].

Hyaluronan

Hyaluronan can aggregate with the core proteins of versican and has a great capacity for binding water, contributing to swelling pressure between the collagen fibrils[7] (Figure 1).

Integrins

The integrins are a family of glycoproteins which, via specific receptors, bind the cell surface to the ECM and transmit information from the cytoplasmic domain to the extra-cellular domain[3].

ASPECTS OF CONNECTIVE TISSUE METABOLISM

Several factors, such as age, mechanical stress, hormones, enzymes and their inhibitors, growth factors and cytokines, are involved in the regulation of connective tissue metabolism[18]. Collagen turnover becomes slower with increasing age[19], but little is known about the impact of age on urogenital connective tissue. The simultaneous progressive formation of stable collagen molecule networks through the continous increase in stable cross-link content may further slow down protein turnover, with possible deleterious consequences for the aging organism. Mechanical load (compression) changes PG metabolism depending on whether it is dynamic or static[20]. Hormones also influence fibroblast PG metabolism differently in different tissues, for example glucocorticoids decrease PG synthesis in skin fibroblasts whereas they increase it in lung fibroblasts[21]. This also means that changes in connective tissue properties at one location in the human body do not necessarily reflect changes in other parts[22].

A family of proteolytic enzymes known as matrix metalloproteinases (MMPs) is mainly responsible for degradation of the ECM components[23]. The synthesis of MMPs is regulated by cytokines and growth factors such as interleukin-1 (IL-1), tumor necrosis factor (TNF), epidermal growth factor, platlet-derived growth factor (PDGF) and transforming growth factor-β (TGF-β)[24,25].

Hence, the ECM is a very dynamic tissue. Variations in the relative amounts of the various types of matrix molecules and the way they are organized in the ECM give rise to a diversity of forms, each highly adapted to the functional requirements of the particular tissue. It is clear that the matrix plays an active and complex role in regulating proliferation, shape and metabolic functions. The matrix is also under the continual influence of factors such as physical stress, hormones, biological aging and various diseases.

PARAURETHRAL COLLAGEN, THE MENOPAUSE AND HORMONE REPLACEMENT THERAPY

The changes occurring at the menopause seem to generate a paraurethral connective tissue with higher collagen concentration and different properties due to lower extractability by pepsin, indicating the presence of more cross-links[26] (Figure 3). These changes, in connection with a decrease in the proteoglycan/collagen ratio, suggest a tissue with an increase in load-bearing ability, but a decrease in elasticity[27]. Studies have not revealed any change in mRNA levels, either for collagens or proteoglycans, indicating a decrease in degradation (Figure 4). This in turn might explain the changes in ECM composition found after the menopause. Estrogen treatment after the menopause seems to induce an increase in mRNA levels for both collagens I and III and also a decrease in total collagen concentration (Figures 3 and 4). These findings indicate an increase in collagen turnover[26,28]. The data are supported by a simultaneous decrease in non-extractable collagen as a measure of the number of cross-links. In contrast, neither the concentration nor the mRNA levels for the proteoglycans seem to be affected, resulting in reversal of the proteoglycan/collagen ratio to almost premenopausal levels (Figure 5). Consequently, estrogen treatment after the menopause seems to reverse connective tissue properties towards the premenopausal status[26].

An interesting observation is that women of fertile age suffering from stress urinary incontinence (SUI) are more similar to post-menopausal women regarding paraurethral connective tissue status. They seem to have a higher concentration of less elastic and thus less supportive collagen[29]. After the menopause no such difference between women with and without SUI is to be found. Also, there is a significant difference in collagen ultrastructure between women of fertile age with SUI and healthy controls. This difference is not found in

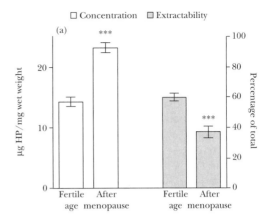

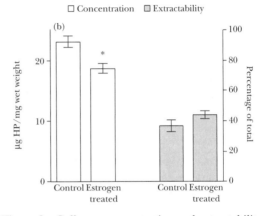

Figure 3 Collagen concentration and extractability. Collagen was determined as hydroxyproline (HP) concentration after extraction with acetic acid and digestion with pepsin. Non-extractable collagen is given as hydroxyproline concentration in collagen not extracted by pepsin digestion; (a) menopausal changes; (b) effect of estrogen treatment after menopause; *significance

comparison of incontinent women and controls after the menopause (Figure 6)[29,30].

The discrepancy in paraurethral connective tissue biochemistry and ultrastructure between SUI women before and after the menopause gives rise to some speculations. In SUI women of fertile age, it is possible that the biochemical and ultrastructural changes found are due to a constitutional divergency, causing weakness of the tissue and early onset of SUI. It is possible that the abnormal fibrillization process registered in SUI women of fertile age can be

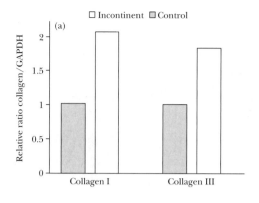

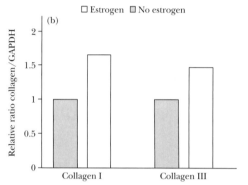

Figure 4 Intensity of Northern blot hybridization for collagens I and III in biopsies from stress incontinent women and controls using a Fuji 2000 Bio Imaging System™; (a) collagen mRNA in incontinent women and controls at fertile age; (b) effects of estrogen treatment on collagen mRNA in controls after menopause

related to a genetic disturbance of collagen synthesis, as described in many other human disorders affecting collagen fibril formation[6,31]. As a consequence, fibrillization might be disturbed, resulting in the increase in fibril diameter found. After the menopause, no differences in ECM composition between continent and incontinent women can be detected. It is possible, however, that urogenital connective tissue after the menopause reacts differently to estrogen replacement therapy in SUI women, compared with continent controls. In clinical practice, estrogen as monotherapy also seems to be insufficient in the restoration of continence, even if the steroid hormone

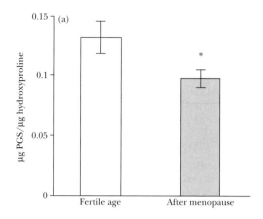

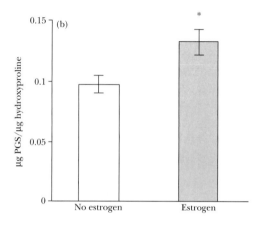

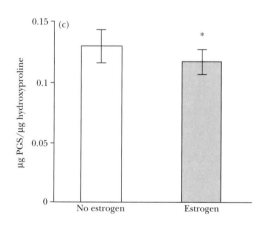

Figure 5 Ratio of proteoglycan/collagen in biopsies from stress incontinent women and controls; (a) menopausal changes in controls; (b) effects of estrogen treatment on controls after menopause; (c) effects of estrogen treatment on incontinent women after menopause; *significant

receptors found in pelvic muscles and ligaments make an influence possible[32,33]. Also, a higher proteoglycan/collagen ratio in continent controls taking estrogen replacement therapy compared with the untreated group has been observed, but not between SUI women with and without estrogen[26,30]. This may reflect a change in responsiveness to hormone replacement therapy in SUI women, compared with healthy controls.

There are also data supporting changes in urogenital connective tissue in other manifestations of pelvic floor insufficiency such as genitourinary prolapse[34,35]. Also, differences in collagen content between pre- and postmenopausal women suffering from genitourinary prolapse have been recorded, suggesting different etiologies at work[36].

CONCLUSIONS

The menopause causes changes of the urogenital connective tissue metabolism, resulting in a tissue with impaired elastic qualities. Estrogen replacement therapy appears to reverse these findings. If this is true, it should be of importance for the understanding and treatment of disorders such as urogenital prolapse and stress urinary incontinence. Recent studies indicate that stress urinary incontinence and urogenital prolapse can, at least in part, be defined as connective tissue diseases. It is possible that the pathophysiology of stress urinary incontinence and urogenital prolapse in women is different in those of fertile age and those after the menopause. Also, there are data indicating the amount of fresh 'elastic' collagen rather than the total concentration to be of crucial importance. Estrogen replacement therapy tends to restore the elastic properties of the urogenital connective tissue, even if the effect on symptoms of pelvic floor insufficiency has not been demonstrated conclusively. The elucidation of tentative defects in urogenital connective tissue and related structures involves new surgical thinking whereby reconstruction of tissue defects needs permanent support of foreign mesh material to minimize the risk of relapse.

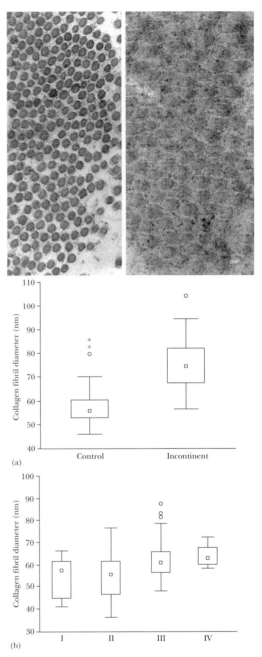

Figure 6 Collagen ultrastructure examined with transmission electron microscopy. Cross-section of collagen fibrils in paraurethral biopsies from stress incontinent women (right) and controls of fertile age, magnification ×55; (a) difference in collagen fibril diameter (nm) between the two groups, expressed as D_{min}; (b) difference in collagen fibril diameter (nm) expressed as D_{min}, between controls with or without estrogen after menopause (I, II) and stress urinary incontinent women with or without estrogen after menopause (III, IV)

References

1. Fransson L-Å. Structure and function of cell-associated proteoglycans. *Trends Biochem Sci* 1987;12:406–11
2. Ruoslahti E. Proteoglycans in cell regulations. *J Biol Chem* 1989;264:13369–72
3. Schwartz MA, Schaller MD, Ginsberg MH. Integrins: emerging paradigms of signal transduction. *Annu Rev Cell Dev Biol* 1995;II:549–99
4. Van der Rest M, Garrone R. Collagen family of proteins. *FASEB J* 1991;5:2814–23
5. Ricard-Blum S, Ville G. Collagen cross-linking. *Int J Biochem* 1989;21:1185–9
6. Prockop DJ, Kivirikko KI. Heritable diseases of collagen. *N Engl J Med* 1984;311:376–86
7. In: Alberts B, Dennis B, Lewis J, *et al*, eds. *Molecular Biology of The Cell*. New York: Garland Publishing, 1994:971–99
8. Hall D. *The Ageing of Connective Tissue*. London: Academic Press, 1976:70
9. Ruoslahti E. Structure and biology of proteoglycans. *Annu Rev Cell Biol* 1988;4:229–55
10. Kjellén L, Lindahl U. Proteoglycans structure and interactions. *Annu Rev Biochem* 1991;60:443–75
11. Iozzo RV, Murdoch AD. Proteoglycans and the extracellular environment: clues from the gene and protein side offer novel perspectives in molecular diversity and function. *FASEB J* 1996;10:598–614
12. Yamaguchi Y, Mann DM, Ruoslahti E. Negative regulation of transforming growth factor-β by the proteoglycan decorin. *Nature (London)* 1990;346:281–4
13. Bernfield M, Kokenyesi R, Kato M, *et al*. Biology of the syndecans: a family of transmembrane heparan sulfate proteoglycans. *Annu Rev Cell Biol* 1992;8:366–93
14. Vogel KG, Paulsson M, Heinegård D. Specific inhibition of type I and type II collagen fibrillogenesis by the small proteoglycan of tendon. *Biochem J* 1984;223:587–97
15. Uldbjerg N, Danielsson CC. A study of the interaction *in vitro* between type I collagen and a small dermatan sulphate proteoglycan. *Biochem J* 1988;251:643–8
16. Hedbom E, Heinegård D. Binding of fibromodulin and decorin to separate sites on fibrillar collagens. *J Biol Chem* 1993;268:27307–12
17. Oldberg Å, Antonsson P, Lindblom K, Heinegård D. A collagen-binding 59-kd protein (fibromodulin) is structurally related to the small interstitial proteoglycans PG-S1 and PG-S2 (decorin). *EMBO J* 1989;8:2601–4
18. Kovacs EJ, DiPietro LA. Fibrogenic cytokines and connective tissue production. *FASEB J* 1994;8:854–61
19. Mays PK, McAnulty RJ, Campa JS, Laurent GJ. Age-related changes in collagen synthesis and degradation in rat tissues. Importance of degradation of newly synthesized collagen in regulating collagen production. *Biochem J* 1991;276:307–13
20. Larsson T, Aspden RM, Heinegård D. Effects of mechanical load on cartilage matrix biosynthesis *in vitro*. *Matrix* 1991;11:388–94
21. Särnstrand B, Brattsand R, Malmström A. Effect of glucocorticoids on glycosaminoglycan metabolism in cultured human skin fibroblasts. *J Invest Dermatol* 1982;79:412–17
22. Buckwalter JA, Goldberg VM, Woo SL-Y. *Musculoskeletal Soft-Tissue Aging: Impact on Mobility*. Rosemont, IL: American Academy of Orthopedic Surgeons, 1993
23. Nagase H. Matrix metalloproteinases 1, 2 and 3: substrate specificities and activation mechanisms. In Leppert PC, Woessner JF, eds. *The Extracellular Matrix of the Uterus, Cervix and Fetal Membranes: Synthesis, Degradation and Hormonal Regulation*. New York: Perinatal Press, 1991:28–44
24. Alexander CM, Werb Z. Proteinases and extracellular matrix remodelling. *Curr Opin Cell Biol* 1989;1:974–82
25. Woessner JF Jr. Matrix metalloproteinases and their inhibitors in connective tissue remodelling. *FASEB J* 1991;5:2145–54
26. Falconer C, Ekman-Ordeberg G, Ulmsten U, *et al*. Changes in paraurethral connective tissue at menopause are counteracted by estrogen. *Maturitas* 1996;24:197–204
27. Peacock EE. Structure, synthesis and interaction of fibrous protein and matrix. In *Wound Repair*, 3rd edn. Philadelphia: WB Saunders, 1984:56–101
28. Jackson S, James M, Abrams P. The effect of oestradiol on vaginal collagen metabolism in postmenopausal women with genuine stress incontinence. *Br J Obstet Gynaecol* 2002;109:339–44
29. Falconer C, Blomgren B, Johansson O, *et al*. Different organization of collagen fibrils in stress incontinent women of fertile age. *Acta Obstet Gynecol Scand* 1998;77:87–94
30. Falconer C, Ekman-Ordeberg G, Blomgren B, *et al*. Paraurethral connective tissue in stress incontinent women after menopause. *Acta Obstet Gynecol Scand* 1998;77:95–100

31. Holmes GB Jr, Mann RA. Possible epidemiological factors associated with rupture of the posterior tibial tendon. *Foot Ankle* 1992;13: 70–9

32. Cardozo L, Versi E. Estrogens and the lower urinary tract. In Asch RH, Studd JWW, eds. *Annual Progress in Reproductive Medicine.* Carnforth, UK: Parthenon Publishing, 1993: 311–25

33. Smith P, Heimer G, Norgren A, Ulmsten U. Steroid hormone receptors in pelvic muscles and ligaments in women. *Gynecol Obstet Invest* 1990; 30:27–30

34. Söderberg MW, Falconer C, Byström B, *et al.* Young women with genital prolapse have a lower collagen concentration. *Int Urogynecol J* 2002; 13(Suppl 1):S40

35. Adams EJ, Richmond DH, Avery N, *et al.* Biomechanical alterations in prolapse. *Int Urogynecol J* 2002;13(Suppl 1):S81

36. Bezerra LRPS, Junior PCFM, Kati LM, *et al.* Quantitative and qualitative analysis of glycosaminoglycans in the paraurethral connective tissue of women with and without genuine stress incontinence. *Int Urogynecol J* 2002;13(Suppl 1): S15

6

Progestins in premenopausal women

A. E. Schindler

INTRODUCTION

For clinical use there are various groups of progestins available; these are classified in Table 1. The progestins include compounds with different partial effects, as shown in Table 2[1]. The different biological effects of the various progestins are shown in Table 3 using ovulation inhibition and endometrial transformation as parameters[1]. The progestins can be administered in various forms: tablet, depot, patch, gel and vaginal suppository. The routes of application are: oral, parenteral, transdermal and vaginal.

There are a number of benefits of progestins in symptomatic premenopausal women:

(1) Bleeding disorder;

(2) Premenstrual syndrome, dysmenorrhea;

(3) Vasomotor symptoms;

(4) Benign breast disease;

(5) Endometrial hyperplasia;

(6) Endometriosis;

(7) Contraception;

(8) Bone;

(9) Endometrial, ovarian and breast cancer;

(10) Signs of androgenization.

As suggested by Prior[2], premenopausal women pass through several phases (phases A to D) before amenorrhea occurs (phase E). During these phases, bleeding pattern, cycle-related symptoms, vasomotor symptoms and hormonal levels undergo various changes, all of which must be considered when treatment is indicated.

Table 1 Classification of progestins

Progestin	Example
Natural progesterone	
Progesterone derivatives	medrogestone
Retroprogesterone derivatives	dydrogesterone
17-Hydroxyprogesterone derivatives	medroxyprogesterone acetate, megestrol acetate, chlormadinone acetate, cyproterone acetate
19-Norprogesterone derivatives	demegestone, promegestone
17-Hydroxy-19-norprogesterone derivatives	nomegestrol acetate
Testosterone derivatives	ethisterone
19-Nortestosterone derivatives	norethisterone acetate, lynestrenol, levonorgestrel, gestodene, desogestrel, norgestimate, dienogest

Table 2 Mechanism of action of progestins (modified according to Neumann and Düsterberg[1])

Progestins	Endo-metrium effect	Anti-gonadotropic effect	Anti-estrogenic effect	Estrogenic effect	Anabolic effect	Anti-androgenic effect	Gluco-corticoid effect	Anti-mineralo-corticoid effect
Progesterone	+	+	+	−	−	±	+	+
Dydrogesterone	+	−	+	−	−	±	−	±
Medrogestone	+	+	+	−	−	±	−	−
17-Hydroxyprogesterone derivatives								
Chlormadinone acetate	+	+	+	−	−	+	−	−
Cyproterone acetate	+	+	+	−	−	++	+	−
Megestrol acetate	+	+	+	−	−	+	−	−
Medroxyprogesterone acetate	+	+	+	−	±	−	+	−
19-Norprogesterone derivatives								
Nomegestrol acetate	+	+	+	−	−	+	−	−
Promegestone	+	+	+	−	−	−	−	−
Trimegestone	+	+	+	−	−	±	−	±
Spironolactone derivative								
Drospirenone	+	+	+	−	−	+	−	+
19-Nortestosterone derivatives								
Norethisterone	+	+	+	+	+	−	−	−
Lynestrenol	+	+	+	+	+	−	−	−
Norethinodrel	±	+	±	+	±	−	−	−
Levonorgestrel	+	+	+	−	+	−	−	−
Norgestimate	+	+	+	−	+	−	−	−
3-Keto-desogestrel	+	+	+	−	+	−	?	−
Gestodene	+	+	+	−	+	−	+	+
Dienogest	+	+	−	−	−	+	−	−

+, effective; ±, weakly effective; −, not effective

BLEEDING DISTURBANCES

Menstrual bleeding disorders are one of the most disturbing symptoms in premenopausal women[3]. The prevalence of menorrhagia is 45% in early premenopausal women and 48% in late premenopausal women[4]. Appropriate therapy can be realized by progestins when used in the following ways: orally cyclic; orally continuous; as depot, as intrauterine devices (IUDs) containing progestins and as implants.

Effective therapy for menorrhagia or metromenorrhagia can be provided by cyclic progestin administration (10 to 15 days per cycle). This leads to a counterbalance regarding high endogenous estrogen levels or high non-protein-bound estradiol concentrations[5].

Studies have been performed with either 5 mg of norethisterone acetate three times per day from day 15 to 24 of the cycle, or 100 mg progesterone three times per day. The results have documented a regression of hyperplastic changes with both preparations. However, the carry-over effect is short: 3 months after discontinuation, proliferation of hyperplastic changes occurred in 24% and 10% of patients, respectively[6]. Continuous administration of progestins may be more effective in treating uterine bleeding disorders than cyclic doses. Amenorrhea is the goal in all continuous systemic progestin applications.

A significant decrease of blood loss has been demonstrated in a number of publications[7,8].

Table 3 Biological effects of progesterone and progestins (modified according to Neumann and Düsterberg[1])

Progestin	Dose of ovulation inhibition (mg/day p.o.)	Transformation dose (mg/cycle p.o.)
Progesterone	> 100	200 (i.m.)
Medrogestone	10	60
Dydrogesterone	> 30	140
Norethisterone	0.5	100–150
Norethisterone acetate	0.5	30–60
Lynestrenol	2	70
Norgestimate	0.2	7
Levonorgestrel	0.05	6
Desogestrel	0.06	2
Gestodene	0.03	3
Dienogest	1	6
Chlormadinone acetate	1.5–2	20–30
Cyproterone acetate	1	20
Medroxyprogesterone acetate	10	80
Drospirenone	2	40–80

p.o., *per os*; i.m., intramuscular

In recent years many clinical data have been gathered on the use of levonorgestrel-containing IUDs. Recurrent hypermenorrhea refractory to oral treatment can be effectively treated by the levonorgestrel-IUD[9]. This IUD treatment can replace approximately 75% of the endometrial ablations[10]. The clinical effect increases with time. A maximum appears to be reached after 12 months[11]. This positive effect seems to be achieved regardless of ethnicity. For example, Chinese women who had menorrhagia without organic cause and suffered from anemia had a 54%, 87%, and 95% reduction in menstrual blood loss at the first, third and sixth months of treatment. These reductions were statistically significant, with p values of 0.004, 0.03 and 0.008 respectively[12]. In a randomized comparative trial of a levonorgestrel IUD and norethisterone for treatment of idiopathic menorrhagia the levonorgestrel IUD reduced blood loss by 94% and oral norethisterone reduced blood loss by 87% when given as 5 mg three times a day from day 5 to day 26 for three cycles[8]. Both the levonorgestrel IUD and oral norethisterone are effective in menorrhagia in terms of reducing menstrual blood loss to within normal limits. The levonorgestrel IUD was associated with higher rates of satisfaction and continuation of treatment[8].

Therefore, the levonorgestrel IUD appears to be an effective non-surgical treatment modality for the management of both menorrhagia and dysmenorrhea. In addition, it should be noted that a marked and safe relief from adenomyosis-associated menorrhagia can be obtained with the use of the levonorgstrel IUD[13]. This was confirmed by others[14]. Similar control of uterine bleeding disorders can be obtained with progestin implants[15]. Recent studies have indicated a continuous induction of plasminogen activator inhibitor-1, which may contribute to the therapeutic effect on menorrhagia[16].

ENDOMETRIAL HYPERPLASIA

In premenopausal women, endometrial hyperplasia can become a relevant clinical feature. Progestins are ideal compounds for the treatment of this condition[7]. Different progestins, such as medroxyprogesterone acetate (MPA) and cyproterone acetate, are effective[17]. In order to choose the most effective dose the degree of endometrial hyperplasia has to be taken into account[18].

When endogenous progesterone secretion is diminished, endometrial cancer can develop[19]. However, the exogenously applied dose of progestins may be too low or the duration of use may be too short to prevent this[20]. Progestins act in different ways to prevent or to regress endometrial hyperplasia, e.g. by decreasing insulin-like growth factor-1 (IGF-1) action on the endometrium by increasing IGF-binding proteins[21], changing the activity of the 17β-hydroxysteroid dehydrogenase[21] or up-regulating the tumor suppressor gene[22].

Control of endometrial proliferation can be achieved using the scheme proposed by Druckmann[23]. In the case of estrogen dominance he suggests starting with progestins alone on day 5 of the cycle and adding estradiol or conjugated estrogens at the end. During the premenopause there can be a gradual shift in the levels of progestins and estrogens by extending the duration of estrogen application and shortening the progestin phase[23].

PREMENSTRUAL SYNDROME AND DYSMENORRHEA

Premenstrual syndrome and its symptoms occur when higher estradiol levels are present and there is a relative or absolute lack of progesterone or progestins[23,24]. Therefore, individually adapted progestin use is the therapy of choice. Cyclic progestin treatment for 10 or more days per cycle can be adequate.

VASOMOTOR SYMPTOMS

Vasomotor symptoms occur in 11–67% of menstruating premenopausal women[25]. Commonly, they start when estrogen levels are high and erratic in the premenopausal years and are often associated with a decrease of life quality, mainly caused by sleep disturbances[2]. It is clinically interesting that vasomotor symptoms are associated with an increased risk of osteoporosis[2]. It appears, however, that there is no correlation between the severity of vasomotor symptoms and the level of estradiol[26]. With the application of progestins, hot flushes can be reduced by 85%[27].

BENIGN BREAST DISEASE

Epidemiological data, clinical experience and endocrine studies show ample evidence of progesterone's role in benign breast disease[7,28,29]. Since an overwhelming number of publications have demonstrated that progesterone deficiency is a major link for the development of cystic breast disease, progestins are a medical treatment of choice. The relief of breast pain and, also, a decrease of nodularity have been obtained with progestins[30]. Data from our group have shown that cyclic treatment with 10 mg of medrogestone or dydrogesterone resulted in relief of mastodynia in 88% and 78%, respectively. Clinically, the nodularity decreased by 64% and 58%, respectively. Ultrasound findings showed improvements between 54% and 58%, with similar findings being reported by others[29]. In a large prospective study, a decrease in the breast cancer risk after the use of progestins was found[31]. A study of patients on hormonal replacement therapy has shown changes of breast density by mammography depending on the type of progestins used[32]. Similar data were recently presented by von Schoultz (personal communication). It has been demonstrated that norethisterone or norethisterone acetate are converted to ethinylestradiol in 0.4% to 1.0%. That means that an oral intake of 1 mg norethisterone per day leads to ethinylestradiol serum levels comparable with 5–10 μg orally administered ethinylestradiol per day[33]. Indeed, patients using hormonal replacement products containing norethisterone acetate showed a higher density of breast tissue in mammography[32]. Furthermore, a recently published study indicated an increased breast cancer risk with continuous combined use of nortestosterone derivatives and estrogens[34].

ENDOMETRIOSIS

In the case of symptoms due to endometriosis, which could be related to a preponderance of an estrogenic effect, progestins are suitable for controlling symptoms and the endometriosis itself. There are ample data to show a good endometriosis-associated pelvic pain response[35] and such treatments are comparable with the effects of other drugs[36]. With continuous long-term use of progestins, regression of the endometriotic lesions and elimination of clinical symptoms can be accomplished[37].

CONTRACEPTION

In premenopausal women progestins can be used effectively for contraception in four different modalities:

(1) Continuous low-dose ('mini-pill');

(2) Depot preparation;

(3) Intrauterine device containing progestin;

(4) Progestin implant.

Because of the very low Pearl Index and the reduced menstrual flow, and also amenorrhea with diminished pelvic pain, the new levonorgestrel IUD and the progestin implant are very suitable for premenopausal women[9,15].

BONE

During the transition from premenopause to menopause the prevalence of osteoporosis increases from 0.4 to 12.7% and the prevalence of osteopenia increases from 4.5 to 42.8%[38].

In premenopausal women the lack of consistent, normal ovulation is associated with accelerated bone loss[2]. In premenopausal women with cycle disturbances (i.e. corpus luteum insufficiency, anovulation), cyclic progestins, such as 10 mg MPA for 10 days, lead to a significant increase of bone density ($p < 0.0001$)[39]. Depot MPA over a period of 5–16 years does not markedly influence bone loss[40]. Levonorgestrel implants, however, have demonstrated positive effects on bone[41].

SIGNS OF ANDROGENIZATION

When signs of androgenization (acne, seborrhea, hirsutism) prevail, progestins with anti-androgenic activity should be considered. There are two compounds available, chlormadinone acetate and cyproterone acetate, the latter of these being the strongest anti-androgenic steroid so far available for clinical use.

ENDOMETRIAL CANCER, OVARIAN CANCER AND BREAST CANCER

Low-dose progestins can be used in patients with these malignant neoplasms without any restrictions (i.e. to alleviate menopausal symptoms)[27]. High doses of progestins are a medical treatment of choice in the adjuvant therapy of metastases of endometrial cancer. In ovarian cancer, in particular, if associated with cachexia, high-dose progestins are used. In breast cancer, high-dose progestins are generally considered as a third or fourth line endocrine therapy.

References

1. Neumann F, Düsterberg B. Entwicklung auf dem Gebiete der Gestagene. *Reproduktionsmedizin* 1998;14:257–64
2. Prior JC. Perimenopause: the complex endocrinology of the menopausal transition. *Endocr Rev* 1998;14:347–59
3. Kaufert PA. The perimenopausal woman and her use of the health service. *Maturitas* 1980; 2:191–205
4. Ballinger CB, Browning NC, Smith AHW. Hormonal profiles and psychological symptoms in perimenopausal women. *Maturitas* 1987; 9:235–51
5. Hirvonen E, Malkonen M, Mamninen V. Effects of different progestins on lipoproteins during postmenopausal therapy. *N Engl J Med* 1981; 304:560–3
6. Saarikoski S, Yliskoski M, Penttilä I. Sequential use of norethisterone and natural progesterone in premenopausal bleeding disorders. *Maturitas* 1990;12:89–97
7. Schindler AE. *Gutartige proliferative Erkrankungen der Frau. Bücherei des Frauenarztes*, Vol. 40. Stuttgart: Ende, 1991
8. Irwine GA, Cample-Brown NB, Lumbston MA, *et al.* Randomized comparative trial of the levonorgestrel intrauterine system and norethisterone for treatment of idiopathic menorrhagia. *Br J Obstet Gynaecol* 1998;105: 592–8

9. Munro M.G. Medical management of abnormal uterine bleeding. *Obstet Gynecol Clin North Am* 2000;27:287–304

10. Römer Th. Prospective comparison study of levonorgesterol IUD versus Roller-Ball endometrial ablation in the management of refractory recurrent hypermenorrhea. *Eur J Obstet Gynecol Reprod Biol* 2000;90:27–9

11. Andersson JK, Rybo G. Levonorgestrel releasing intrauterine device in the treatment of menorrhagia. *Br J Obstet Gynaecol* 1999;97:690–4

12. Tang GWK, Lo SST. Levonorgestrel intrauterine device in the treatment of menorrhagia in Chinese women: efficacy versus acceptability. *Contraception* 1995;51:231–5

13. Fedele L, Portuese A, Bianchi S, *et al.* Treatment of adenomyosis-associated menorrhagia with a levonorgestrel-releasing intrauterine device. *Fertil Steril* 1997; 68:426–9

14. Fong Y-F, Singh K. Medical treatment of a grossly enlarged adenomyotic uterus with the levonorgestrel-releasing intrauterine system. *Contraception* 1999;60:173–5

15. Affandi B. Eine integrierte Analyse des Vaginalblutungsverhaltens in klinischen Studien über Implanon®. *Contraception* 1998;58:99–107

16. Rutanen EM, Hurskainen R, Finne P, Nokelainen K. Induction of endometrial plasminogen activator-inhibitor 1: a possible mechanism contributing to the effect of intrauterine levonorgestrel in the treatment of menorrhagia. *Fertil Steril* 2000;73:1020–4

17. Orlandi C, Martinelli G, Marabini A. Treatment of endometrial hyperplasia with progestins. Comparison between medroxyprogesterone acetate and cyproterone acetate. *Gynecol Endocrinol* 1985;1:25–9

18. Dallenbach-Hellweg B, Czernobilski KY, Allemann J. Medroxyprogesteronancetat bei adenomatöser Hyperplasie des Korpusendometriums. *Geburtsh Frauenheilk* 1986;46:601–8

19. Modan B, Ron E, Lerner-Geva L, *et al.* Cancer incidence in a cohort of infertile women. *Am J Epidemiol* 1998;147:1038–42

20. McGonigle KF, Karlan BY, Barbuto DA, *et al.* Development of endometrial cancer in women on estrogen and progestin replacement therapy. *Gynecol Oncol* 1994;55:126–32

21. Schindler AE. Konservative Therapiemöglichkeiten bei glandulärer und adenomatöser Endometriumhyperplasie. *Zbl Gynäkol* 1996;118:359–69

22. Ace CI, Okulicz WC. A progesterone-induced endometrial homolog of a new candidate suppressor, DMBT1. *J Clin Endocrinol Metab* 1998;83:3569–73

23. Druckmann R. Die Prämenopause: Eine Zeit des Übergangs. *J Menopause* 1995;2:17–21

24. Wang M, Seippel L, Purdy RH, *et al.* Relationship between symptom severity and steroid variation in women with premenstrual syndrome: study on serum pregnenolone, pregnenolone sulfate, 5α-pregnane-3, 20-dione and 3α-hydroxy-5α-pregnan-20-one. *J Clin Endocrinol Metab* 1996;81:1076–82

25. Kronenberg F. Hot flashes: epidemiology and physiology. *Ann NY Acad Sci* 1990;592:52–86

26. Rannevik G, Jeppsson S, Johnell O, *et al.* A longitudinal study of the perimenopausal transition: altered profiles of steroid and pituitary hormones, SHBG and bone mineral density. *Maturitas* 1995;21:103–13

27. Loprinzi CL, Michalak JC, Quella SK, *et al.* Megestrol acetate for the prevention of hot flashes. *N Engl J Med* 1994;331:347–52

28. Schindler AE. Ätiologie und Epidemiologie gutartiger Veränderungen der Brust. *Der Gynäkologe* 1989;22:212–15

29. Schindler AE. Gestageneinwirkung an der Brust – protektiv oder proliferativ? *Zbl Gynäkol* 1997; 119:359–65

30. Goebel R, Junkermann H, von Fournier D. Danazoltherapie bei gutartigen Brusterkrankungen. *Der Gynäkologe* 1989;22:263–70

31. Plu-Bureau G, Li M, Sitruk-Ware R, *et al.* Progestins and the hormonal risk of breast cancer in a cohort of premenopausal women with benign breast cancer disease. *Br J Cancer* 1994;70:270–7

32. Persson I, Thurfjell E, Holmberg L. Effect of estrogen and estrogen-progestin replacement regimens on mammografic breast parenchymal density. *J Clin Oncol* 1997;15:3201–7

33. Kuhnz W, Heuner A, Hümpel M, *et al.* In vivo conversion of norethisterone and norethisterone acetate to ethinylestradiol in postmenopausal women. *Contraception* 1997;55:379–85

34. Magnusson C, Baron JA, Correia N, *et al.* Breast-cancer risk following long-term oestrogen and oestrogen-progestin replacement therapy. *Int J Cancer* 1999;55:339–44

35. Vercellini P, Cortesi I, Crosignani PG. Progestins for symptomatic endometriosis: a critical analysis of the evidence. *Fertil Steril* 1997;68:393–401

36. Schweppe KW. Die Bedeutung der Gestangene zur Behandlung der Endometriose. *Zbl Gynäkol* 1997;119:64–9

37. Schorer P, Schindler AE. Falldarstellung von zwei Endometrioselangzeit-Behandlungen mit Cyproteronazetat. *Zbl Gynäkol* 2001;123:1–4

38. Smeets-Goevaers CG, Lesusink GL, Papapouluos SE, *et al.* The prevalence of low bone mineral density in Dutch perimenopausal women: the Eindhoven perimenopausal osteoporosis study. *Osteoporosis Int* 1998;8:404–9

39. Prior JC, Vigna YM, Barr SI, *et al.* Cyclic medroxyprogesterone treatment increases bone

density: a controlled trial in active women with menstrual cycle disturbances. *Am J Med* 1994; 96:521–30

40. Gbolade B, Ellis S, Muby B, *et al.* Bone density in long term users of depot medroxyprogesterone acetate. *Br J Obstet Gynaecol* 1999;93(Suppl. 4): 25–39

41. Thijssen JHH, Druckmann R. Effect of progestins on bone: an up-date. *Gynecol Endocrinol* 1999;93 (Suppl.4):25–39

7

Effects of progestogen on the breast

E. Lundström and B. von Schoultz

INTRODUCTION

There is strong evidence that reproductive factors and endogenous sex hormones are important in the etiology of breast cancer. As for many other malignancies the incidence of breast cancer shows a continuous increase with age, until around 50 years. Thereafter when the average woman enters a postmenopausal state there is a decline in the incidence[1]. The number of ovulatory menstrual cycles during the reproductive period of a woman's life has a positive correlation with breast cancer risk[2]. Women with an early menarche and late menopause have an increase in relative risk of around 1.5–2, whereas an early menopause has a protective effect[3]. Early childbirth, multiple pregnancies and lactation have been associated with a reduced risk of breast cancer, while the increased incidence following childbirth after the age of 30 implies an age-dependent increase in risk[4]. The risk of breast cancer seems to rise in parallel with an increase of endogenous estradiol levels[5]. Young women with obesity have a lower breast cancer risk, whereas obesity after the menopause has been connected with an increase in breast cancer. This could relate to hormonal factors, since obese young women often have anovulatory cycles, and obese elderly woman with more fatty tissue may have an enhanced local production of estrogens by peripheral aromatization of androgen precursors[6]. In fact, endogenous estrogen levels may be the key factor for a variety of associations reported, such as body mass, bone mass, reproductive history, menarche, menopause, and dietary habits. This concept is also supported by the fact that an early menopause or oophorectomy is strongly protective and also increases survival in young breast-cancer patients[1,7].

HORMONAL TREATMENTS

Numerous women are currently treated with different combinations of estrogen and progestogen for hormonal contraception and for replacement after the menopause. While there are also contradictory findings, epidemiologic data overall indicate an increase in the risk of breast cancer during such hormonal treatment. When treatment is discontinued the excess risk is normalized within 5–10 years[8,9]. According to large meta- and re-analyses of epidemiological data, the relative risk for breast cancer during long-term HRT, i.e. for more than 5 years, is in the order of 1.5–2.5. The pathophysiologic mechanisms behind this association are incompletely understood. Furthermore, many different therapeutic regimens are used for hormonal replacement in clinical practice. It is well known that different therapeutic principles, such as estrogen alone, estrogen in cyclic combination with progestogen and estrogen in continuous combination with progestogen, have quite different effects in many target organs such as the endometrium. Long-term treatment with estrogen alone is known to increase the risk for endometrial cancer but this increase is abolished when progestogens are added to the treatment[10]. At present there is limited information about the effects of different treatment regimens on the normal breast, but it seems clear that progestogen addition has no protective effect. On the contrary, a number of recent studies suggest that combined estrogen–progestogen treatment may carry a risk for breast cancer beyond that of estrogen alone[11–15]. This notion is also supported by prospective clinical treatment data from the Women's Health Initiative (WHI)[16]. After a mean follow-up of 5.2 years, there was an increase in breast cancer among women on continuous combined estrogen–progestogen treatment. Therefore the continuous combined treatment arm of the WHI project was closed early. Apparently, no such increase has so far been observed during estrogen only treatment and this part of the WHI project, after monitoring of safety, was allowed to continue.

The interpretation of available data is complicated by a remarkable lack of basic understanding of how hormones work in the normal breast. Furthermore, hormone replacement therapy (HRT) is not a uniform concept. A wide range of different estrogens and progestogens are available on the market and they are used at different doses, combinations and by different routes of administration. It may well be, but has not yet been demonstrated, that different compounds, for example progestogens, have specific differences with respect to their influence on the breast.

HORMONES AND THE BREAST

The breast is a hormonal target organ, and proliferation of both the normal and the malignant epithelium is influenced by sex steroids, peptide hormones and growth factors[17]. During the menstrual cycle, the breast epithelium undergoes proliferation followed by apoptosis[18]. However, in contrast to the endometrium, the proliferative rate in breast epithelium is low under the influence of estrogen only, in the follicular phase of the cycle. In the breast, the highest proliferation occurs during the luteal phase under the combined influence of both estrogen and progesterone[18–20]. During the

increased proliferation of the luteal phase, there is also a down-regulation of estrogen receptors while the expression of progesterone receptors is maintained[21,22]. The same pattern, with the most pronounced proliferation during the luteal phase, has also been observed in tissue samples from premenopausal women with breast cancer[23].

Estrogen is a well-known mitogen in human breast epithelium but the action of progestogen is complex and incompletely understood. In particular, there is remarkable confusion about the mitogenic effects of progestogen. Over the years, numerous studies in cell lines[24,25], animal models[26,27] and in women[28,29] have reported either a proliferative or an antiproliferative effect of progestogen. High doses of progestogen, for example medroxyprogesterone acetate (MPA), are used in breast cancer treatment. The mechanism for the therapeutic action is unclear but may be mediated via down-regulation of gonadotropins or estrogen receptors or by a direct cytotoxic effect[30]. Clearly the effects of different progestogens could be dependent on type, dose, route of administration and the estrogenic environment[31]. Native progesterone is extensively metabolized by the liver and therefore oral preparations in general have a low effectiveness. Synthetic progestogens completely devoid of estrogenic or androgenic action have been difficult to synthesize. The 19-nor steroids, like norethindrone, levonorgestrel, lynestrenol and desogestrel are derived from testosterone whereas the 17-hydroxyprogesterone compounds like medroxyprogesterone are more similar to natural progesterone. The many different progestogens may also have quite different effects on sex steroid receptor expression and breast cell proliferation[32]. The progesterone receptor (PR) is expressed in two protein isoforms, PRA and PRB. They seem to have a dual role and studies indicate that PRA has a repressive function on PRB action[33]. In the endometrium, the different PRs display estrogen-dependent variations during the menstrual cycle[34]. To what extent the PRA and B levels undergo similar changes in the breast is unknown.

ASSESSMENT OF BREAST CELL PROLIFERATION

The basis of breast cancer risk associated with hormonal therapies may lie in the regulation of cell proliferation[35]. A better knowledge of the proliferative response induced by different treatment regimens is of crucial importance for the interpretation of epidemiologic data and to evaluate the potential risks of different treatments.

Carefully conducted *in vitro* studies of both normal and transformed breast cells in culture have produced a wealth of information about the hormonal regulation of breast epithelium[24]. However, cultured breast epithelial cells lack the normal complement of blood vessels, fat tissues, stroma and myoepithelial cells. These components are known to exert considerable paracrine and hormonal influence *in vivo*[36]. In fact, the results from many proliferation analyses in cell cultures of the effects of progestogen are quite opposite to the findings obtained under *in vivo* conditions[19,24]. While many cell-culture experiments indicate an inhibitory effect of progestogen on estrogen induced proliferation, the majority of *in vivo* studies show an enhanced proliferative activity.

Many experiments with normal human breast tissue have been performed on tissue sections either from reduction mammoplasties or from 'normal' breast tissue near a benign or malignant lesion. Clearly studies on excisional biopsies also have inherent limitations since the tissue may not be entirely normal and analysis is possible only at one single occasion. However, in a recent study of such breast tissue, Hofseth and co-workers[29] demonstrated that combined estrogen–progestogen treatment increased the rate of cell proliferation compared with treatment with estrogen alone.

The fine needle aspiration (FNA) biopsy technique was developed at the Karolinska Hospital and has become an established tool for the preoperative diagnosis of palpable tumors in the breast[37]. Over the years, numerous studies have shown a high concordance between cytological findings obtained by FNA and the histopathologic assessment after surgery[38].

Using a 0.6 mm needle, the procedure is simple, fast and causes very little inconvenience for the patient. The development of monoclonal antibodies has made it possible to assess hormone receptor expression, as well as proliferative activity in cytologic breast cell samples. FNA biopsies can be used for monitoring and can easily be repeated during the course of different treatments.

Using this method we demonstrated an increased proliferative activity in normal breast epithelium from young women during the luteal phase of the menstrual cycle and also a significant correlation with blood levels of progesterone[20]. Likewise, in women using combined oral contraceptives we found increased breast epithelial proliferation and also a marked interindividual variation in the response to treatment. Proliferation during oral contraceptive use showed a positive correlation with circulating levels of the progestogen levonorgestrel and a negative correlation with levels of free testosterone[39]. We have recently shown that it is possible to assess breast epithelial proliferation also in postmenopausal women, who have a lower cellularity in the breast, by using cytologic samples obtained with the FNA biopsy technique[40]. During 6 months of HRT with continuous combined estrogen–progestogen treatment, we found a three- to four-fold increase in proliferating cells as recorded by staining for the marker Ki-67/Mib-1[41]. The results were quite similar for two different combinations of estradiol and progestogen.

For obvious reasons, studies on long-term hormonal treatment can be difficult to perform in women. Thus, there is a need for relevant animal models. Raafat and co-workers[42,43] studied the hormonal influence on the normal postmenopausal mammary gland in a murine model. They found an association between combined estrogen–progesterone therapy and epithelial breast cell proliferation in this model. The cynomolgus macaque (*Maccaca fascicularis*) is a primate. Macaques have well-documented similarities to women in terms of reproductive physiology and anatomy, mammary gland development, peripheral steroid hormone metabolism and sex steroid receptor expression[44]. The breast epithelial cells also share a characteristic cytokeratin immunophenotype, which reflects the close phylogenetic relationship with the human species[45]. In general, experimental findings in macaques have been predictive of outcome in human reproductive studies. Data from this experimental *in vivo* model, where surgically postmenopausal macaques were given HRT, also suggest a proliferative action of progestogen. The proliferative response after combined treatment with conjugated equine estrogens plus MPA was much more pronounced than for treatment with estrogen alone[27,46].

MAMMOGRAPHIC BREAST DENSITY

Mammography is a valuable tool for the early detection of breast cancer. It has been clearly shown that mammographic mass screening programs reduce breast cancer mortality rates in women over 50 years of age[47]. Currently, all women receiving HRT are also recommended to attend regular mammographic screening. The mammographic picture of the breast varies between women according to the relative amount of fat, connective and epithelial tissues. Fat is radiologically lucent and appears dark on the image whereas connective and epithelial tissues are more dense and appear white. High amounts of connective and epithelial cells yield an increased density in the mammogram. Variations in mammographic density are apparently associated with ovarian function: density is increased in women with an early menarche and during the luteal phase of the menstrual cycle[48]. Breast parenchymal density in individual women has also been found to vary with age, menopausal status, parity, height, and body weight. Possible associations with nutritional status, exercise, alcohol intake, and family history of breast cancer have also been reported[48]. The histologic correlates to the increase in mammographic density are not fully clear. It may tentatively be caused by epithelial proliferation but also by vasodilatation, fibrosis and edema.

Irrespective of its cause, mammographic breast density may be an important surrogate marker for the development of breast cancer. In several epidemiological studies breast density has been established as a strong and independent risk factor. Odds ratios and relative risks in different studies range between 2 and 6, which is higher than for many other risk factors like age at menarche, menopause, parity, and body-weight[48]. In fact, density seems to be more important than all other risk factors currently identified except for female sex, age and genetic predisposition. It has even been suggested that high mammographic density may account for as much as 30% of all breast cancer cases. This impact would be of the same importance as for circulating lipid patterns in coronary heart disease. However, at present there is no consensus about the interpretation of these data. There are also reports that mammographic screening sensitivity may be reduced by increased density which may hamper the diagnosis of clinically occult tumors.

Many different methods have been used to classify and quantify mammographic breast density including visual parenchymal methods, estimations of the percentage of the breast area that is dense, measurement by planimetry of the area of density and measurement of density in digitized images with computer assisted methods[48]. The classic Wolfe scale[49,50] is a visual parenchymal method classified into four categories: N1, essentially normal breast with parenchyma composed primarily of fat with at most a few fibrous connective tissue strands; P1, a prominent ductal pattern in up to one quarter of the volume; P2, a prominent ductal pattern in more than one quarter of the breast volume; and DY, an extremely dense parenchyma, which usually denotes connective tissue hyperplasia.

During recent years there have been numerous reports that breast density is increased in a significant proportion of women using HRT (Figure 1). There is also clear evidence that different regimens have a different impact in this respect[51–53]. We have used information from ongoing mass-screening programs where treatment data on HRT, including type of estrogen and progestogen, have been available. Overall data from such material and the results

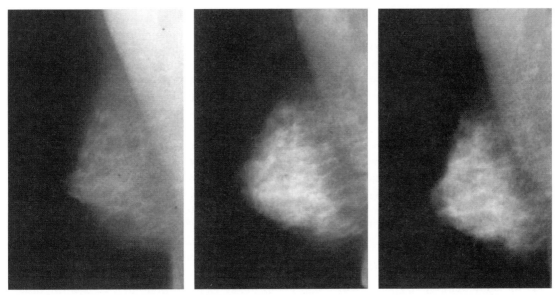

Figure 1 Change in mammographic breast density in a postmenopausal woman during hormone replacement therapy (HRT). The left mammogram was obtained at the age of 50 and before any hormonal treatment. The picture in the middle was taken 6 months after starting continuous combined HRT. The apparent increase in breast density is unchanged also after 2 years (right) on the same HRT regimen

from prospective clinical trials show that an increase in breast density is much more frequent among women on combined estrogen/progestogen treatment than in those receiving estrogen alone[52,53]. Similar findings regarding progestogen addition to estrogen treatment have been reported from the ongoing Postmenopausal Estrogen/Progestin Interventions (PEPI) trial[54]. During treatment with common continuous combined regimens, such as conjugated equine estrogens (CEE) 0.625 mg + MPA 5 mg and estradiol 2 mg + norethisterone acetate 1 mg, about 40–50% of women respond with an increase in mammographic density that fulfils the criteria for an up-grading according to the Wolfe classification[52]. In contrast, during treatment with different forms of unopposed estrogen, for example a patch releasing estradiol 50 µg every 24 hours or orally administered tablets of estradiol 2 mg or CEE 0.625 mg, only a few percent of women react with an increased density[53]. In a randomized prospective study we also found tibolone, a compound with partly estrogenic, progestogenic and also androgenic properties, to have little effect on breast density[55]. The number of women

reacting with an increase was roughly the same as for unopposed estrogen treatment.

Mammographic breast density may be of particular importance since it is to date the only known risk factor that is present in the very organ that will eventually develop the disease. The increase in mammographic density, when it occurs, seems to be an early event during HRT. In our studies where all women continued on the same regimen, we observed little change in mammographic status after the first 6 months of treatment[52,53]. There are also data to indicate that breast density during HRT is dynamic, increasing with initiation and decreasing with discontinuation and change of therapy[51]. It may also be that an increase in mammographic density is associated with subjective symptoms of breast discomfort and pain[55]. While an effect of the estrogen dosage during combined treatment could be important, the marked differences observed between treatment regimens are most likely to be associated with the addition of progestogen. So far there seems to be little difference between the effects of a 19-nor steroid like norethisterone and a 17-hydroxyprogesterone compound like MPA in this respect. The effects of different doses, routes of administration and types of estrogen and progestogen should be further explored. Information regarding breast density may be an important part of future clinical management in women receiving HRT.

SUMMARY

At present there is no consensus on the proliferative effects of progestogen addition to estrogen treatment. However, during the past few years, accumulating data from animal, clinical and observational studies strongly suggest a proliferative effect of progestogen in human breast tissue. Findings in surrogate markers like breast density and proliferation add to epidemiologic reports and clearly suggest that continuous combined HRT may carry a higher risk of breast cancer than treatment with estrogen alone. All these data are also consistent with the findings from the WHI randomized controlled trial. Whether the results are valid for all progestogens as a group or if there are indeed alternative progestogen compounds without stimulatory effects on the breast remains to be elucidated. It should also be recalled that the absolute risk for an individual women to develop breast cancer during treatment is low.

From a clinical perspective increased breast epithelial proliferation and mammographic density during hormonal treatment should be regarded as an unwanted and potentially hazardous side effect. Efforts should be made to identify those women who are most sensitive and react with excessive proliferation during treatment. Still, in many women no apparent increase in proliferation or density will be detected. Not all women respond in the same way to the same treatment and the biologic basis for the marked individual variation has to be clarified. Further knowledge about the role of growth factors like insulin-like growth factor-I (IGF-I) and of the balance between the different sex steroid receptor isoforms is important in this respect. There is an apparent need to develop clinical and non-invasive methods for monitoring breast response during hormonal treatment in order to identify women at risk for breast cancer. Our present knowledge on the impact of hormonal treatments on the breast is based largely on epidemiologic observations and experimental data. Prospective randomized clinical studies are needed to further explore the effects of different HRT regimens on the normal breast.

ACKNOWLEDGEMENTS

This work was supported by grants from the Swedish Research Council (05982), the Swedish Cancer Society and funds from the Karolinska Institute.

References

1. Spicer DV, Pike MC. Breast cancer prevention through modulation of endogenous hormones. *Breast Cancer Res Treat* 1993;28:179–93
2. Henderson BE, Ross RK, Judd HL, *et al.* Do regular ovulatory cycles increase breast cancer risk? *Cancer* 1985;56:1206–8
3. Clavel-Chapelon F, the E3N-EPIC Group. Differential effects of reproductive factors on the risk of pre- and postmenopausal breast cancer. Results from a large cohort of French women. *Br J Cancer* 2002;86:723–7
4. Spratt JS, Donegan WL, Sigdestad CP. Epidemiology and etiology. In: Harris JR, Lippman ME, Morrow M, Hellman S, eds. *Diseases of The Breast.* Lipincott-Raven Publishers: Philadelphia, 1996: 116–41
5. Cauley JA, Lucas FL, Kuller LH, *et al.* Elevated serum estradiol and testosterone concentrations are associated with a high risk for breast cancer. Study of Osteoporotic Fractures Research Group. *Ann Intern Med* 1999;130:270–77

6. Clemons M, Goss P. Estrogen and the risk of breast cancer. *N Engl J Med* 2001;344:276–85

7. Henderson BE, Ross R, Bernstein L. Estrogens as a cause of human cancer. *Cancer Res* 1988;48: 246–53

8. Early Breast Cancer Trialists' Collaborative Group. Ovarian ablation in early breast cancer: overview of the randomized trials. *Lancet* 1996;348:1189–96

9. Collaborative group on hormonal factors in breast cancer. Breast cancer and hormonal contraceptives: collaborative reanalysis of individual data on 53 297 women with breast cancer and 100 239 women without breast cancer; data from 54 epidemiological studies. *Lancet* 1996; 347:1713–27

10. Collaborative group on hormonal factors in breast cancer. Breast cancer and hormone replacement therapy: collaborative reanalysis of data from 51 epidemiological studies of 52 705 women with breast cancer and 108 411 women without breast cancer. *Lancet* 1997;350:1047–59

11. Persson I, Weiderpass E, Bergkvist L, *et al.* Risks of breast and endometrial cancer after estrogen and estrogen–progestin replacement. *Cancer Caus Contr* 1999;10:253–60

12. Magnusson C, Baron JA, Correia N, *et al.* Breast cancer risk following long-term oestrogen and oestrogen–progestin replacement therapy. *Int J Cancer* 1999;38:325–34

13. Ross RK, Paganini-Hill A, Wan PC, *et al.* Effect of hormone replacement therapy on breast cancer risk: estrogen versus estrogen plus progestin. *J Natl Cancer Inst* 2000;93:328–32

14. Schairer C, Lubin J, Troisi R, *et al.* Estrogen–progestin replacement and risk of breast cancer. *J Am Med Assoc* 2000;284:691–4

15. Santen RJ, Pinkerton J, McCartney C, *et al.* Risk of breast cancer with progestins in combination with estrogen as hormone replacement therapy. *J Clin Endocrinol Metab* 2001;86:16–23

16. Writing group for the Women's Health Initiative Investigators. Risks and benefits of estrogen plus progestin in healthy postmenopausal women. *J Am Med Assoc* 2002;288:321–33

17. Reid SE, Murthy MS, Kaufman M, *et al.* Endocrine and paracrine hormones in the promotion, progression and recurrence of breast cancer. *Br J Surg* 1996;83:1037–46

18. Potten CS, Watson RJ, Williams GT, *et al.* The effect of age and menstrual cycle upon proliferative activity of the normal human breast. *Br J Cancer* 1988;58:163–70

19. Longacre TA, Bartow SA. A correlative morphologic study of human breast and endometrium in the menstrual cycle. *Am J Surg Pathol* 1986;10:382–93

20. Söderqvist G, von Schoultz B, Tani E, *et al.* Estrogen and progesterone receptor content in breast epithelial cells from healthy women during the menstrual cycle. *Am J Obstet Gynecol* 1993;168:874–9

21. Battersby S, Robertson BJ, Anderson TJ, *et al.* Influence of menstrual cycle, parity and oral contraceptive use on steroid hormone receptors in normal breast. *Br J Cancer* 1992;65:601–7

22. Söderqvist G, Isaksson E, von Schoultz B, *et al.* Proliferation of breast epithelial cells in healthy women during the menstrual cycle. *Am J Obstet Gynecol* 1997;176:123–8

23. Pujol P, Daures J-P, Thezenas S, *et al.* Changing estrogen and progesterone receptor patterns in breast carcinoma during the menstrual cycle and menopause. *Cancer* 1998;83:698–705

24. Gompel A, Malet C, Spritzer P, *et al.* Progestin effect on cell proliferation and 17-β-hydroxysteroid dehydrogenase activity in normal human breast cells in culture. *J Clin Endocrinol Metab* 1986;63:1174–80

25. Dran G, Luthy IA, Molinolo AA, *et al.* Effects of medroxyprogesterone acetate (MPA) and serum factors on cell proliferation in primary cultures of an MPA-induced mammary adenocarcinoma. *Breast Cancer Res Treat* 1995;35:173–86

26. Haslam SZ. Progesterone effects on deoxyribonucleic acid synthesis in normal mouse mammary glands. *Endocrinology* 1988;122:464–70

27. Cline JM, Söderqvist G, von Schoultz B, *et al.* Effects of hormone replacement therapy on the mammary gland of surgically postmenopausal macaques. *Am J Obstet Gynecol* 1996;174:93–100

28. Hargreaves DF, Knox F, Swindell R, *et al.* Epithelial proliferation and hormone receptor status in the normal post-menopausal breast and the effects of hormone replacement therapy. *Br J Cancer* 1998;78:945–49

29. Hofseth LJ, Raafat AM, Osuch JR, *et al.* Hormone replacement therapy with estrogen or estrogen plus medroxyprogesterone acetate is associated with increased epithelial proliferation in the normal postmenopausal breast. *J Clin Endocrinol Metab* 1999;184:4559–65

30. Della Cuna R. Progestins. In Cvitkovic E, Droz JP, Armand JP, Khoury S, eds. *Handbook of Chemotherapy in Clinical Oncology.* Jersey: Scientific Communication International, 1993:371–3

31. Miller WR, Langdon SP. Steroid hormones and cancer. II Lessons from experimental systems. *Eur J Surg Oncol* 1997;23:163–83

32. Rabe T, Bohlmann MK, Rehberger-Schneider S, Profto S. Induction of estrogen receptor-α and -β activities by synthetic progestins. *Gynecol Endocrinol* 2000;14:118–26

33. Conneely OM, Lydon JP, De Mayo F, *et al.* Reproductive functions of the progesterone receptor. *J Soc Gynecol Invest* 2000;7:25–32

34. Mangal RK, Wiehle RD, Poindexter AN III, *et al.* Differential expression of uterine progesterone

receptor forms A and B during the menstrual cycle. *J Steroid Biochem Mol Biol* 1996;56:93–6

35. Preston-Martin S, Pike MC, Ross RK, *et al.* Increased cell division as a cause of human cancer. *Cancer Res* 1990;50:7415–21

36. Lippman M. Growth regulation of breast cancer. In Hammond CB, Haseltine FP, Schiff I, eds. *Menopause: Evaluation, Treatment and Health Concerns. Progress in Clinical and Biological Research.* New York: Alan R Liss, 1989:111–19

37. Franzén S, Zajicek J. Aspiration biopsy in diagnosis of palpable lesions of the breast. Critical review of 3479 consecutive biopsies. *Acta Radiol* 1968;7:241–62

38. Skoog L, Rutqvist LE, Wilking N. Analysis of hormone receptors and proliferation fraction in fine-needle aspirates from primary breast carcinomas during chemotherapy or tamoxifen treatment. *Acta Oncol* 1992;31:139–41

39. Isaksson E, von Schoultz E, Odlind V, *et al.* Effects of oral contraceptives on breast epithelial proliferation. *Breast Cancer Res Treat* 2001;65:163–9

40. Conner P, Skoog L, Söderqvist G. Breast epithelial proliferation in postmenopausal women, evaluated through fine-needle aspiration cytology. *Climacteric* 2001;4:7–12

41. Conner P, Cristow A, Kersemaekers W, *et al.* A comparative study on breast cell proliferation during HRT: effects of tibolone and continuous combined estrogen/progestogen treatment. *Breast Cancer Res Treat* 2003; in press

42. Raafat AM, Hofseth LJ, Haslam SZ. Proliferative effects of combination estrogen and progesterone replacement therapy on the normal postmenopausal mammary gland in a murine model. *Am J Obstet Gynecol* 2001;184:340–9

43. Raafat AM, Songjiang L, Bennet JM, *et al.* Estrogen and estrogen plus progestin act directly on the mammary gland to increase proliferation in a postmenopausal mouse model. *J Cell Physiol* 2001;187:81–9

44. Cline JM, Söderqvist G, Register TC, *et al.* Assessment of hormonally active agents in the reproductive tract of female primates. *Toxicol Pathol* 2001;29:84–9

45. Tsubura A, Hatano T, Hayama S, *et al.* Immunophenotypic difference on keratin expression in normal mammary glandular cells from five different species. *Acta Anat* 1991;140:287–93

46. Cline JM, Söderqvist G, von Schoultz E, *et al.* Effects of conjugated estrogens, medroxyprogesterone acetate, and tamoxifen on the mammary glands of macaques. *Breast Cancer Res Treat* 1998;48:221–9

47. Nyström L, Rutqvist LE, Wall S, *et al.* Breast cancer screening with mammography: overview of Swedish randomized trials. *Lancet* 1993;341: 973–8

48. Boyd NF, Lockwood GA, Byng JW, *et al.* Mammographic densities and breast cancer risk. *Cancer Epidemiol Biomark Prev* 1998;7: 1133–44

49. Wolfe JN. Breast patterns as an index of risk for developing breast cancer. *AJR Am J Roentgenol* 1976;126:1130–9

50. Wolfe JN. Risk for breast cancer development determined by mammographic parenchymal pattern. *Cancer* 1976;37:2486–92

51. Rutter C, Mandelson M, Laya M, *et al.* Changes in breast density associated with initiation, discontinuation and continuing use of hormone replacement therapy. *J Am Med Assoc* 2001; 285:171–6

52. Lundström E, Wilczek B, von Palffy Z, *et al.* Mammographic breast density during hormone replacement therapy: differences according to treatment. *Am J Obstet Gynecol* 1999; 181:348–52

53. Lundström E, Wilczek B, von Palffy Z, *et al.* Mammographic breast density during hormone replacement therapy: effects of continuous combination, unopposed transdermal and low potency estrogen regimens. *Climacteric* 2001;4: 1–7

54. Greendale GA, Reboussin BA, Sie A, *et al.* Postmenopausal Estrogen/Progestin Interventions (PEPI) investigators. Effects of estrogen and estrogen–progestin on mammographic density. *Ann Intern Med* 1999;130:262–9

55. Lundström E, Christow A, Kersemaekers W, *et al.* Effects of tibolone and continuous combined hormone replacement therapy on mammographic breast density. *Am J Obstet Gynecol* 2002;186:717–22

8

Mammographic density and breast cancer

G. Svane

INTRODUCTION

Breast cancer is the most common malignancy in women in numerous industrialized countries, and its incidence is increasing in many countries around the world. Breast cancer is more common in elderly women with incidence increasing after the age of 40 years and especially after the menopause, but breast cancer sometimes develops in very young women, even, albeit rarely, before the age of 20. A woman's menstrual and reproductive history may have a substantial impact on her risk of developing breast cancer. Early age at menopause, also due to oophorectomy, has been reported to be a protective factor in breast cancer. Parity, age at first childbirth, length of menstrual cycle and regularity, late menopause, breast-feeding, etc. also seem to be related to breast cancer incidence, but no factors have yet been found that can be used to prevent breast cancer or reduce breast cancer incidence. During the past decade, interest in hereditary reasons for breast cancer development has increased, especially since women with the *BRCA1* and/or *BRCA2* gene have been shown to have a high risk of developing breast cancer during their lifetime, especially at an early age.

BREAST CANCER PROGNOSIS AND EARLY DETECTION

Since there is no way as yet to prevent women from developing breast cancer, most interest has stemmed from reducing the effects of breast cancer, which, especially in young women, is an important cause of death. Numerous studies have shown the prognosis of breast cancer to vary according to the size of the tumor and the presence or absence of metastases to axillary lymph nodes at the time of diagnosis. In many patients who die from breast cancer, distal metastases are already present at the time of diagnosis. The best way to reduce mortality from breast cancer is to detect and treat tumors at an early stage before any metastases have occurred. Self-breast examination is important, but it is very difficult for a woman to find a tumor that is less than 1 cm in size. Such a small tumor can only be detected if it is superficially sited close to the skin, or in a small breast which is soft and easy to examine. Even clinical examination performed by experienced physicians rarely detects cancers less than 1 cm in diameter. In large breasts and in breasts with only little fatty tissue and rich in glandular tissue, even tumors with a diameter exceeding 2 cm are readily concealed by surrounding tissue.

Mammography has been used for almost 40 years to diagnose breast cancer in patients with various breast-related symptoms. This method has proved to be excellent for detecting breast tumors less than 1 cm in size, and many tumors, especially in fatty breasts, of less than 5 mm size have been detected. During the past three decades, mammography has been the method of choice to detect breast cancer at a non-palpable stage. Screening programs have shown that mammography is an excellent tool for early detection of breast cancer as well as a mass survey examination method. A 20–40% reduced breast cancer mortality rate has been noted in randomized screening programs[1,2] when the study group has been compared with a control group. In the above randomized screening studies, comparison of mortality was made between women who received an invitation to undergo mammography examination, the study group, and those who were not invited, the control group. Comparison was not performed between those who accepted the invitation and underwent a mammography examination and those who were not examined. Other studies have compared mortality rates for women who accepted the invitation and actually underwent a mammography examination and for those who did not. These studies have found the reduction in breast cancer mortality to be over 40%[3,4]. In another study, Tabár and colleagues[5] compared breast cancer-specific mortality for three different time periods in women 20–69 years old. The first period was when no mammography screening was taking place, the second when a randomized screening trial in women 40–74 years was ongoing and the last period when service screening had started for women aged 40–69 years of age. The invitation to mammography screening seemed to have reduced mortality from breast cancer by 50%. However, breast cancer mortality decreased by 63% among women who were actually screened. Mammography is now widely used as a population-based screening tool in many countries to detect breast cancer at an early stage, before any clinical symptoms have occurred. However, the age group invited to or included in the screening program differs not only between countries but also sometimes within the same country. Nevertheless, women older than 50 years of age are invited to participate in most screening programs.

MAMMOGRAPHIC BREAST DENSITY

Most breasts have both radiologically translucent and dense areas. The dense parts consist of fibrous connective tissue and glandular tissue, while the translucent parts consist of mainly fat. In general, the proportion of dense tissue will decrease with age owing to fatty involution of the breast. In a study from Finland, Salminen and co-workers[6,7] found the incidence of fatty breasts to be two times higher among women aged 45 or more, compared with women under 45 years.

Mammography screening programs today mostly include the whole female population within a specific age group. Most of these women will never develop breast cancer, and it would be more efficient, if possible, to invite just a high-risk group of women to mammography examination instead of inviting everyone as in current screening programs. Just who is at high risk, and whether the mammographic appearance of the breast parenchyma can be used to predict the risk of developing breast cancer in the future are questions that have been asked many times. In the 1970s, Wolfe[8] suggested the answer to the latter question to be yes. He classified the breast parenchymal pattern into four categories depending upon the proportions of fat tissue and fibroglandular tissue, and also the pattern of the fibroglandular tissue. The four classes were: N1, the breast is composed of primarily fat; P1, ducts and glandular tissue occupy up to 25% of the breast volume; P2, ducts and glandular tissue occupy more than 25% of the breast volume; and DY, extremely dense breast with hyperplasia or dysplasia (Figures 1–4). Breast density can also be classified in percentages, usually in steps of 20%. Wolfe[9] suggested that the radiologic appearance of the breast parenchyma could be useful in the appraisal of a predisposition to cancer of the breast. He reported a 30-fold increase in breast cancer incidence for patients with the DY pattern, compared with patients with the N1 pattern, over a 3-year period. The P1 and P2 patterns were associated with an intermediate risk. Other studies have also found an increased risk for women with the P2/DY pattern. Salminen and colleagues[10] reported the age-adjusted relative risk of breast cancer to be 2.5 among women with the P2/DY pattern, compared with women with N1 and P1 patterns. Salminen's group[7] also found that the odds ratio of the P2/DY pattern for women with body mass index (BMI) 25 kg/m^2 or more was

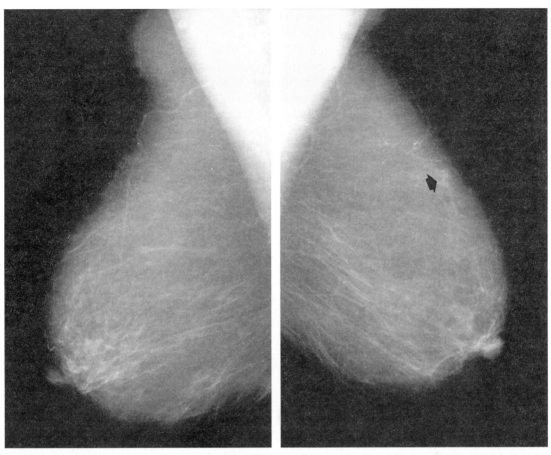

Figure 1 Mediolateral oblique views showing breasts with mostly fatty tissue, an N1 pattern. In the upper-outer quadrant of the left breast is a 6-mm irregular density representing invasive ductal cancer

0.2 (95% confidence interval (CI) 0.1–0.6), compared with women with BMI less than 20. In a randomized mammography screening study from Malmö, women between 45 and 69 years of age were invited to screening. Andersson[11] reported the overall attendance rate in this study to be 74%. He classified mammograms as N1 in 11%, P1 in 38%, P2 in 16.2% and DY in 34.8%. P2 and DY patterns were found to correlate with an increased risk for cancer. The percentage of women with P2 and DY patterns decreased with advancing age, and also correlated with the age of the woman's first childbirth.

EVALUATION OF BREAST DENSITY

The density of the parenchyma can be evaluated visually using more or less subjective methods. The most frequent method of evaluating density is visually, by the naked eye, from the mammograms. The proportions of dense and fatty parts are evaluated from one or two views. Today there are also computerized methods, which might turn out to be more precise and more reproducible. A quantitative assessment of mammographic density can be carried out using digitized mammograms[12]. However, there are difficulties with all methods, and the precision of the evaluation might be influenced by choice of mammographic view, craniocaudal or mediolateral oblique or both. High variation between individual women, concerning not only the amount of dense tissue but also the distribution, makes assessment even more difficult. The dense tissue might be situated in all quadrants of the breast, only centrally or in the upper-outer quadrant, or be more

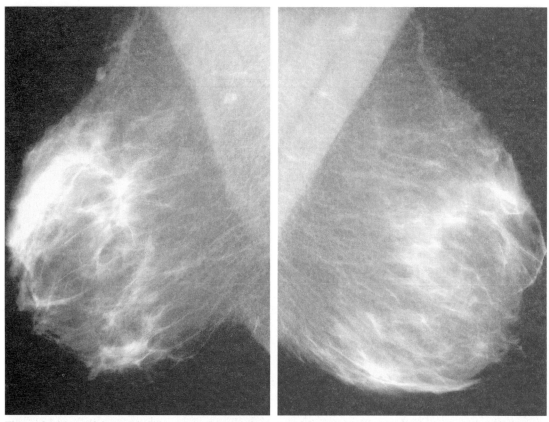

Figure 2 Normal breasts with mostly fatty tissue but also moderately dense tissue spread in both the upper and lower parts of the breasts. Some lymph nodes of ordinary appearance can be seen in both axillae. This is most probably a P1 pattern but is not easy to assess from only mediolateral oblique views. A more precise assessment could be made if the craniocaudal view was also evaluated

irregularly spread in the breast and split by small or large fatty lobules. In some women the mammograhic pattern appears very irregular, and in such cases breast density is more difficult to evaluate both with the naked eye and using a computerized system. However, the difference in assessment of density when two experienced radiologists visually evaluate the mammograms has been shown to be minor. In a prospective, randomized, double-blind placebo-controlled study[13] of 166 patients, one-third were given tibolone 2.5 mg, one-third estradiol 2 mg plus norethisterone acetate 1 mg and one-third placebo. Patients were examined by mammography before inclusion in the study and 6 months later. All mammograms were evaluated visually using both a percentage scale and Wolfe's system. Only five mammography

examinations were evaluated differently by the two radiologists. The difference occurred when a percentage scale in five steps was used, and not when Wolfe's classification was used. Nevertheless, the differences were minor, for example one radiologist suggested slightly less than 20% and P1 and the other suggested also P1 but slightly over 20%.

INFLUENCE OF ENDOGENOUS AND EXOGENOUS HORMONES ON BREAST DENSITY

It is well established that breast density decreases with age, but individual variations are enormous. Endogenous and exogenous hormones may influence mammographic density. Riza and co-workers[14] studied urinary

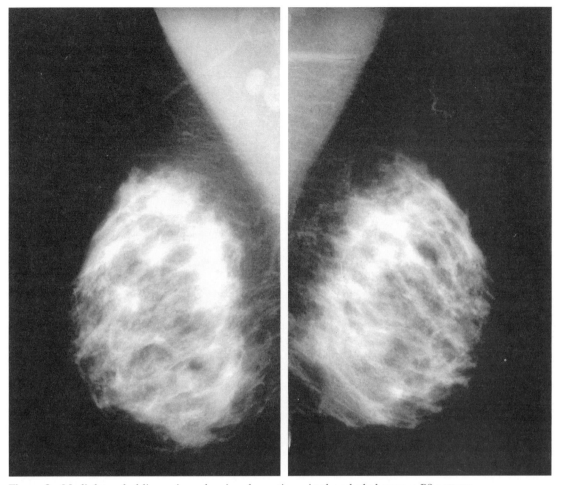

Figure 3   Mediolateral oblique views showing dense tissue in the whole breast, a P2 pattern

estrogen metabolites and mammographic patterns in postmenopausal women participating in a population-based breast screening program in Northern Greece. Seventy women with a P2/DY pattern were individually matched with 70 women with an N1 pattern. Urinary levels of 2-hydroxyestrone (2-OHE_1) and 16α-hydroxyestrone ($16\alpha\text{-OHE}_1$) were measured. These authors found that women with a P2/DY pattern had 58% higher levels of 2-OHE_1 and 15% higher levels of $16\alpha\text{-OHE}_1$ than women with an N1 pattern. They suggested that a high ratio of $2\text{-OHE}_1/16\alpha\text{-OHE}_1$ might be associated with an increase in breast cancer risk in postmenopausal women, since this ratio was 35% higher in the studied women with P2/DY patterns.

Women in the highest one-third of this ratio were six times more likely to have P2/DY patterns than those in the lowest one-third. The odds ratio was 6.2. In another study, Boyd and colleagues[15] examined the association of circulating levels of hormones and growth factors with mammographic density. Mammograms were digitized, and the density was measured by a computer-assisted method. These authors found that in postmenopausal women, serum levels of prolactin and in premenopausal women, serum insulin-like growth factor-I levels were significantly and positively associated with percentage density. In postmenopausal women, sex hormone-binding globulin was positively and free estradiol was

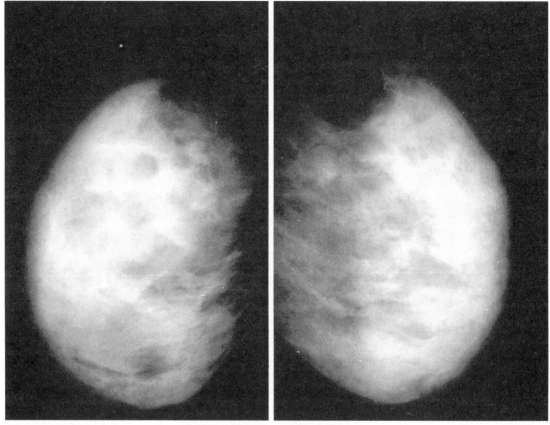

Figure 4 Very dense breasts with a DY pattern according to Wolfe's classification

negatively associated with percentage density. These results suggest a biologic basis for mammographic density which is associated with increased risk of breast cancer. In another study, Boyd and associates[16] studied 353 pairs of monozygotic and 246 pairs of zygotic twins from the Australian Twin Registry, and 218 pairs of monozygotic twins and 134 pairs of dizygotic twins in Canada and the USA. The mammograms were digitized. They were then randomly ordered and read by a blinded investigator. The authors found the correlation coefficient for percentage of dense tissue to be 0.67 for monozygotic pairs in North America and 0.61 for monozygotic pairs in Australia, and 0.27 for dizygotic pairs in North America and 0.25 for dizygotic pairs in Australia, after adjustment for age and measured covariates. They suggested

that the percentage of dense tissue on mammograms at a given age has high heritability, and that 'finding the genes responsible for this phenotype could be important for understanding the causes of the disease'.

Saftlas and Szklo[17] reported an increased proportion of N1 and P1, the low-risk patterns, in women who ever used contraceptive pills (OCs). However, in another study, Gram and colleagues[18] found that ever-users of OCs were 20% more likely to have high-risk mammographic patterns compared with those who had never used OCs. They did not find any dose–response differences. Nulliparous women who had used OCs had a four times increased risk of having high-risk patterns. De Stavola and associates[19] also found an association between mammographic breast density and the use of contraceptive pills. However, they reported different effects for premenopausal and post-menopausal women.

Hormone replacement therapy (HRT) may increase mammographic density. It may also increase the size and the number of cysts and fibroadenomas. HRT might inhibit involutional processes within the breast, and therefore women with ongoing HRT have higher-risk mammographic patterns compared with women without HRT and, hence, a higher risk of developing breast cancer. Some authors have suggested that mammographically dense breasts may be a contraindication to HRT. However, the risk of an increase in mammographic density differs between different hormonal therapies and also between individuals. The highest risk of increased density seems to be associated with estrogen in continous combination with progesterone, where up to 50% of postmenopausal women showed increased density. The mammographic pattern can change from N1 to P2 in some women. Women receiving estrogen in cyclic combination with progesterone and those receiving estrogen-only treatment showed a less frequent increase in breast density of around 6–20%. Only very few (2%) women using transdermal treatment showed an increase in density[13,20–22]. Some studies found an increased risk of breast cancer after many years of HRT. Persson and colleagues[23] carried out multivariate analyses which showed an increased risk among users of HRT of any type for more than 10 years. The odds ratio was 2.1. The risk was higher for women using estradiol–progestin combined treatment, compared with women using estradiol or conjugated estrogens alone. The odds ratio was 2.4 and 1.3, respectively. In a population-based case–control study of women aged 50–74 years of age, Magnusson and co-workers[24] found breast cancer risk to increase with duration of HRT use. The odds ratio for women treated for at least 10 years with estrogen with and without progestins was 2.23, compared with women who had never used HRT. An excess risk was shown for both women who were current users and those who had used HRT in the past. The increase was less pronounced with

cyclic compared with continuous combinations. The use of oral estriol and topical treatment was not associated with increased breast cancer risk.

In a study from Florence, Ciatto and associates[25] showed that both radiologic density and exposure to HRT were found to correlate with age, radiologic density decreasing with increasing age. They also found the duration of HRT to be associated with radiologic density, a higher density occurring in women using HRT for many years. Boyd and co-workers[26] suggested that mammographic density may be a short-term marker of the effect on the breast of potential preventive interventions for breast cancer, and that a variety of interventions such as tamoxifen, gonadotropin-releasing hormone inhibitor, stopping HRT and adopting a low-fat, high-carbohydrate diet might influence and reduce the density of the breast.

MAMMOGRAPHIC SENSITIVITY AND SPECIFICITY

Salminen and co-workers[7] found the sensitivity of mammography to increase statistically significantly with increasing age of the woman. An increase in sensitivity of mammography was also found to occur with a decrease in density of the breast. However, the effect of age was larger than the effect of density on sensitivity when considered simultaneously. It is well known that it is easier to read mammograms when the breast is mostly composed of fatty tissue than when the breast is very dense with much glandular and fibrous tissue. Technical progress in recent decades has resulted in improved image quality, and dense breasts can be examined more efficiently today than 20 years ago. However, dense breasts are in general still more difficult to examine than fatty breasts, and the examination might be slightly painful. It is sometimes more difficult to position and compress the breast properly in the case of a dense breast and more views are sometimes needed. The standard views usually used are the mediolateral oblique, the lateromedial and the craniocaudal views. Special views such as coned-down views, rolled views or magnification views can sometimes allow correct prediction of palpable masses not seen on standard views. The experience of the radiologist reading the mammograms is more important in dense breasts, compared with fatty breasts. Some types of cancer, such as lobular cancer, can be more difficult to detect in a dense breast compared with a more fatty breast. However, ductal cancer *in situ*, which mostly presents as micro-calcifications only (Figure 5), and invasive cancers with microcalcifications in combination with distortion or increased density, can be found quite easily even in a dense breast. In an overview study, Banks[27] found an increased risk of interval cancer and also false positive recall for more mammographic views and further investigations in current users of HRT, compared with women without HRT. In a study from Uppsala, Thurfjell and colleagues[28] estimated differences in sensitivity and specificity of screening in women who had previously

used and in women who had never used HRT. They found a marginal decrease in specificity varying with the HRT regimen and duration of treatment, but there was no decrease in sensitivity of screening in women using HRT. However, the sensitivity of mammography might be different for women with the *BRCA1/2* gene. These carriers develop breast cancer before age 50 years in up to 50% of cases. In a study from Rotterdam, Tilanus-Linthorst and co-workers[29] compared 34 sporadic cases of breast cancer in patients matched for age and year of diagnosis with 34 cases of breast cancer in patients with *BRCA1/2*. Mammography resulted in more false negatives in carriers than in controls, despite comparable mammo-graphic density, but false-negative mammo-graphy correlated with high density. These authors also found that breast cancer in women with *BRCA1/2* showed more prominent push-ing margins of the tumor than in tumors of non-carriers. This mammographic appearance caused the tumor to resemble a benign lesion rather than cancer.

FUTURE RESEARCH

There is a reported association between P2 and DY mammographic density patterns and an increased risk of developing cancer in the future. The risk of breast cancer in general increases with age, while a fatty involution of the breast takes place after the menopause and the percentage of P2 and DY patterns decreases with advancing age. HRT increases breast density in some women. However, there seems to be no increased breast cancer risk for women who have used HRT in the short term but a moderately increased risk after long-term use. Whether this increased risk is associated only with women in whom an increase in breast density has occurred is still not known. Salminen and colleagues[30] found that women taking HRT and with DY patterns had a relative risk of 11.6 (95% CI 2.5–53.6) of developing breast cancer, compared with women not using HRT and with an N1 pattern. Some studies have reported that an increase in density, especially at older ages, due to HRT will further increase

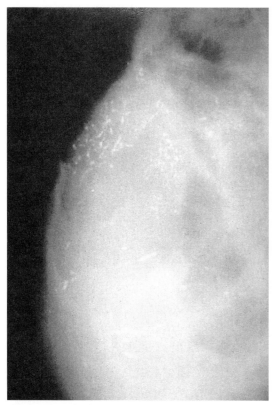

Figure 5 Part of a very dense breast with irregular microcalcifications representing intraductal cancer *in situ*

the breast cancer incidence. Further studies are needed to evaluate this. Nevertheless, an increase in breast density seems to be an unwanted side effect of HRT. There is a need to clarify the significance of a change in mammographic density and its relation to breast cancer risk, and to improve knowledge about the effects of both endogenous and exogenous hormones on breast density, breast parenchymal pattern and breast cancer risk.

References

1. Tabár L, Fagerberg CJG, Gad A, *et al.* Reduction in mortality from breast cancer after mass screening with mammography. Randomised trial from the Breast Cancer Screening Working Group of the Swedish National Board of Health and Welfare. *Lancet* 1985;1:829–32

2. Bjurstam N, Björneld L, Duffy SW, *et al.* The Gothenburg breast screening trial: first results on mortality, incidence, and mode of detection for women aged 39–49 years at randomisation. *Cancer* 1997;80:2091–9

3. Palli D, Roselli del Turco M, Buiatti E, *et al.* A case–control study of the efficacy of a non-randomised breast cancer screening program in Florence (Italy). *Int J Cancer* 1986;38:501–4

4. Collette HJA, Day NE, Rombach JJ, *et al.* Evaluation of screening for breast cancer in a non-randomised study (the DOM project) by means of a case–control study. *Lancet* 1984;I: 1224–6

5. Tabár L, Vitak B, Chen HH, *et al.* Beyond randomised controlled trials: organised mammographic screening substantially reduces breast carcinoma mortality. *Cancer* 2001;91:1724–31

6. Salminen T, Hakama M, Heikkilä M, *et al.* Favourable change in mammographic parenchymal patterns and breast cancer risk factors. *Int J Cancer* 1998;78:410–14

7. Saarenmaa I, Salminen T, Geiger U, *et al.* The effect of age and density of the breast on the sensitivity of breast cancer diagnostic by mammography and ultrasonography. *Breast Cancer Res Treat* 2001;67:117–23

8. Wolfe JN. Risk for breast cancer development determined by mammographic parenchymal pattern. *Cancer* 1976;37:2486–92

9. Wolfe JN. Breast pattern as an index of risk for developing breast cancer. *Am J Roentgenol* 1976; 126:1130–9

10. Salminen TM, Saarenmaa IE, Heikkilä MM, *et al.* Risk of breast cancer and changes in mammographic parenchymal patterns over time. *Acta Oncol* 1998;37:547–51

11. Andersson I. Radiographic patterns of the mammary parenchyma; variations with age at examination and age at first birth. *Radiology* 1981;138:59–62

12. Byng JW, Yaffe MJ, Jong RA, *et al.* Analysis of mammographic density and breast cancer risk from digitised mammograms. *Radiographics* 1998;18:1587–98

13. Lundström E, Christow A, Kersemaekers W, *et al.* Effects of tibolone and continuous combined hormone replacement therapy on mammographic breast density. *Am J Obstet Gynecol* 2002;186:717–22

14. Riza E, dos Santos Silva I, De Stavola B, *et al.* Urinary estrogen metabolites and mammographic parenchymal patterns in postmenopausal women. *Cancer Epidemiol Biomarkers Prev* 2001;10:627–34

15. Boyd NF, Stone J, Martin LJ, *et al.* The association of breast mitogens with mammographic densities. *Br J Cancer* 2002;87:876–82

16. Boyd N, Dite G, Stone J, *et al.* Heritability of mammographic density, a risk factor for breast cancer. *N Engl J Med* 2002;347:886–93

17. Saftlas AF, Szklo M. Mammographic parenchymal pattern and breast cancer risk. *Epidemiol Rev* 1987;9:146–74

18. Gram IT, Funkhouser E, Nordgard L, *et al.* Oral contraceptive use and mammographic patterns. *Eur J Cancer Prev* 2002;11:265–70

19. De Stavola BL, Gravelle IH, Wang DY, *et al.* Relationship of mammographic parenchymal patterns with breast cancer risk factors and risk of breast cancer in a prospective study. *Int J Epidemiol* 1990;19:247–54

20. Schairer C, Lubin J, Troisi R, *et al.* Menopausal estrogen and estrogen–progestin replacement therapy and breast cancer risk. *J Am Med Assoc* 2000;283:485–91

21. Lundström E, Wilczek B, von Palffy Z, *et al.* Mammographic breast density during hormone replacement therapy: differences according to treatment. *Am J Obstet Gynecol* 1999;181:348–52

22. Lundström E, Wilczek B, von Palffy Z, *et al.* Mammographic breast density during hormone replacement therapy: effects of continuous combination, unopposed transdermal and low-

potency estrogen regimens. *Climacteric* 2001;4: 42–8

23. Persson I, Thurfjell E, Bergström R, *et al.* Hormone replacement therapy and the risk of breast cancer. Nested case–control study in a cohort of Swedish women attending mammography screening. *Int J Cancer* 1997;72:758–61

24. Magnusson C, Persson I, Baron J, *et al.* Breast cancer risk following long-term estrogen and estrogen–progestin replacement therapy. *Int J Cancer* 1999;81:339–44

25. Ciatto S, Bonardi R, Zappa M. Impact of replacement hormone therapy in menopause on breast radiologic density and possible complications of mammography in the assessment of breast masses. *Radiol Med (Torino)* 2001; 101:39–43

26. Boyd NF, Martin LJ, Stone J, *et al.* Mammographic densities as a marker of human breast cancer risk and their use in chemoprevention. *Curr Oncol Rep* 2001;3:314–21

27. Banks E. Hormone replacement therapy and the sensitivity and specificity of breast cancer screening: a review. *J Med Screen* 2001;8:29–34

28. Thurfjell EL, Holmberg LH, Persson IR. Screening mammography: sensitivity and specificity in relation to hormone replacement therapy. *Radiology* 1997;203:339–41

29. Tilanus-Linthorst M, Verhoog L, Obdeijn IM, *et al.* A *BRCA1/2* mutation, high breast density and prominent pushing margins of a tumour independently contribute to a frequent false-negative mammography. *Int J Cancer* 2002;102: 91–5

30. Salminen T, Saarenmaa IE, Heikkilä M, *et al.* Is dense mammographic parenchymal pattern a contraindication to hormonal replacement therapy? *Acta Oncol* 2000;39:969–72

9

Estrogen replacement therapy in the endometrial- and breast-cancer patient

W. T. Creasman and M. F. Kohler

ENDOMETRIAL CANCER

It has been recognized for many years that an aberration of endogenous estrogen may have an impact upon the endometrium. The association of feminizing ovarian tumors and endometrial cancer is well documented in the literature. Over a quarter of a century ago, studies appeared which suggested an increased incidence of endometrial cancer in patients who used unopposed exogenous estrogen. Although publications noted risk ratios (RRs) into the teens, most were much less than that, and a recent meta-analysis of 29 observational studies noted an RR of 2.3 (95% confidence interval (CI) 2.1–2.5)[1]. In cases in which unopposed estrogen, either endogenous or exogenous, has been associated with endometrial cancer, the malignancy is usually well differentiated and superficially invasive without extrauterine disease. These individuals have an excellent survival prognosis. Studies have indicated that adenocarcinoma in patients with a history of estrogen replacement therapy (ERT) is associated with just as good survival, if not better, than that of cohorts on ERT but without cancer and much better than that of patients not on ERT and without cancer. It is also well recognized that the combination of estrogen and progestogen decreases the risk of endometrial cancer back to, if not below, the normal incidence of the disease. This is particularly true if the progestin is given for 12–14 days cyclically or as continuous therapy along with the estrogen.

HORMONE REPLACEMENT THERAPY AFTER ENDOMETRIAL CANCER

Historically, hormone replacement therapy (HRT) has been contraindicated in patients who have been treated for adenocarcinoma of the uterus. However, when one evaluates the literature, there are no data that substantiate the detrimental effect of estrogen in these patients. It is our observation that many postmenopausal women who had been successfully treated for adenocarcinoma of the endometrium experienced significant vasomotor symptoms after removal of their ovaries. Subsequent evaluation concluded that even in the quiescent ovary, the stroma produces androgen which is peripherally converted to estrone. The removal of this source of estrogen apparently resulted in the vasomotor symptoms. Other end-organ effects of estrogen deprivation were also noted such as vaginal dryness, post-coital bleeding and dyspareunia. Since it had been noted for many years that a progestin could alleviate vasomotor symptoms, these patients were treated post-therapy with a progestin, which alleviated their vasomotor symptoms. Several months after therapy had begun, the side-effects of the progestin, mainly atrophy in the vagina with subsequent local symptoms, became apparent. At that point, topical estrogen was used to manage the vaginal symptoms as it was felt that appreciable estrogen was not absorbed. Subsequently, it was learned that local estrogen is absorbed from the vagina and can have a systemic effect. As a result, almost 30 years ago, we began treating individual patients with estrogen as necessary. The indication for HRT was essentially vasomotor symptoms. Between 1975 and 1980, 221 women with clinical stage I adenocarcinoma of the endometrium were treated, and many of our patients were given estrogen[2]. After a minimum of 5 years' follow up, 47 patients who had been given post-treatment estrogen were compared with 174 who had not received estrogen. Multiple prognostic factors were evaluated, and the only significant variant was a larger number of estrogen-treated women with positive progesterone receptors compared with non-estrogen-treated patients, although there was no difference in estrogen receptors between the two groups. Only one (2%) of the estrogen-treated patients had developed recurrence compared with 26 (15%) of the non-estrogen-treated women ($p < 0.05$). Patients who had historically the highest risk of recurrence (grade 3 and deep myometrial invasion) showed considerably less recurrence if estrogen was given, compared with the non-estrogen-receiving patients. In those not receiving estrogen, 26 died, compared with only one among those taking estrogen ($p = 0.014$). Of the non-estrogen-treated patients, 16 died from cancer and ten from intercurrent disease. One estrogen-treated patient whose cancer recurred and who died received only 3 months of estrogen therapy, a year and a half before recurrence was noted. In a multivariate analysis, it was noted that those patients who had metastasis to the pelvic nodes, poorly differentiated cancers and malignant cells present on peritoneal cytology were at risk for recurrence. Those patients who had received estrogen appeared to be protected from recurrence ($p = 0.0336$). Based upon this retrospective study, a history of adenocarcinoma of the endometrium did not appear to be an absolute contraindication to ERT.

In 1989, Lee and his associates reported a similar study describing 114 patients with clinical stage I endometrial cancer treated over an 11-year period[3]. After surgical staging, 44 selected patients were placed on oral estrogen for a medium duration of 64 months. In the estrogen group, there were no recurrences or intercurrent deaths. Of the 99 non-estrogen users there were eight recurrences and eight intercurrent deaths. Patients on ERT had low-recurrence risk factors such as a well-differentiated tumor and superficial invasion. None of the patients were found to have extrauterine disease. These authors felt that postoperative ERT was safe in selected low-risk patients.

A third retrospective study evaluated 132 patients with stage I or II adenocarcinoma of the endometrium, of whom 65 (49%) received HRT after diagnosis and therapy[4]. The same physicians treated control patients during the same time period, who were not interested in HRT. The HRT patients were given medroxyprogesterone 2.5 mg daily. The mean duration of follow-up for the HRT group was 58 months, and 31 months for the controls. There were two (3%) recurrences in the HRT group versus six (9%) in the control group.

A recent preliminary analysis of patients with surgical stages I, II and III adenocarcinoma has been performed at the authors' institutions. Approximately 130 patients received replacement therapy and others did not. The reason for the difference was mainly the philosophy of the treating physicians. Similar numbers of patients in both groups were noted with regard to stage, grade and depth of invasion. There were fewer recurrences in the patients who had been on ERT. A recent match-control study evaluated 259 women with surgical stages I, II and III endometrial cancer of whom 130 received ERT after primary cancer treatment[5]. Among these, 75 matched treatment controls were identified. There were two recurrences (1%) among the estrogen users compared with 11 (14%) recurrences in the 75 non-hormone users. Hormone users showed a statistically significant longer disease-free interval than non-users ($p = 0.005$) (Figure 1).

Many of the present authors' patients have now been on replacement therapy after successful treatment for their adenocarcinoma of the endometrium for over 20 years. The benefits of this treatment with regard to chronic diseases

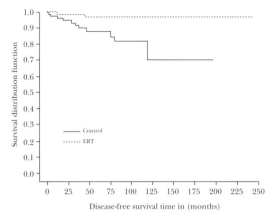

Figure 1 Survival in endometrial cancer, estrogen replacement therapy (ERT) users vs. non-users ($p = 0.0052$). Reproduced with permission from Suriano KA, *et al.* Estrogen replacement therapy in endometrial cancer patients: a matched control study. *Obstet Gynecol* 2001;97:555–60[5]

such as colon cancer and osteoporosis with subsequent fractures are well documented, and these are without detrimental effects concerning replacement therapy and recurrent disease. A large prospective, randomized, double-blind study sponsored by the Gynecologic Oncology Group and the National Cancer Institute in the USA is currently ongoing, which should allow a definitive statement to be made about the safety and efficacy of HRT in patients who have had adenocarcinoma of the endometrium. To date, HRT in this patient population appears to be beneficial.

The American College of Obstetricians and Gynecologists (ACOG), in a Committee Opinion, noted that in women with a history of endometrial cancer, estrogen could be used for the same indications as in any other women, except selection of appropriate candidates should be based on prognostic indicators and the risk that the patient is willing to assume[6]. The statement again emphasizes the importance of informed consent, and giving our patients information concerning the benefits and risks so that they can make an educated decision concerning their health-care. In women who have experienced the disease, many (> 90%) will show long-term survival. It certainly appears that the benefits of HRT are

considerable and at least should be considered by all.

ESTROGEN AND BREAST CANCER

The role of ERT and its possible relationship to several chronic diseases, for example of the breast, heart and bone, have been topics of discussion for many years. Some studies have shown benefit, others risk and the vast majority no relationship, particularly to breast cancer. Recently, the discussion has intensified with the publication of the Heart and Estrogen/ progestin Replacement Study II (HERS II)[7], the first report from the Women's Health Initiative (WHI) study[8] and the 'scientific review' of postmenopausal HRT[1]. The lay public, as well as the medical community, have been bombarded with reports of 25–35% or even higher increased risk of developing breast cancer if one takes ERT for any prolonged period of time (> 5 years), while on the other hand there is no beneficial effect with regard to the prevention of adverse heart events, as either primary or secondary prevention.

The interaction of estrogen and breast cancer has been known for over 100 years. In 1896, Beatson reported remission in premenopausal women with breast cancer who underwent bilateral oophorectomy[9]. Since that time, hundreds if not thousands of articles, at both the basic science level and the clinical level, have implicated estrogens, both endogenous and exogenous, in the pathogenesis of breast cancer. Other authors, however, have suggested that the early observations concerning the relationship of estrogen and breast cancer may not be entirely valid. Some studies have shown more favorable situations in breast-cancer patients who have been exposed to estrogen. The role of progestogens has been implicated by some but not supported by others.

During the last quarter of the 20th century, Bush, Whiteman and Flaws[10] were able to identify 65 articles that had been published concerning the possible relationship between ERT or HRT (estrogen plus progestogen) and breast cancer. Forty-five of these articles addressed ERT, and over 80% noted neither increased nor decreased risk. Of the remaining, some showed an increased risk while others showed a decreased risk. Of the 20 articles concerning HRT and breast cancer, again 80% showed no benefit or risk, while four of these reported statistical significance, two showing increased risk and two others showing decreased risk. There have been at least six meta-analyses performed on this subject in an attempt to reconcile the differences[11–16]. All six of these note no increased risk of developing breast cancer with replacement therapy (Table 1).

The Collaborative Group on Hormonal Factors in Breast Cancer reanalyzed 51 studies (49 published and two unpublished), which included over 52 000 women with invasive breast cancer (cases) and over 108 000 women without breast cancer (controls)[17]. Among the current users of ERT/HRT, the relative risk (RR) of having breast cancer diagnosed was 1.023 for each year of use. The RR was 1.35 for women who had used ERT/HRT for 5 years or longer (average duration of use was 11 years). This 35% increased risk has been reported widely in the lay press, which has generated considerable concern among physicians and women alike. Unfortunately, relative risks do not translate into meaningful clinical data, and absolute risk portrays a more accurate picture. In women between the ages of 50 and 70 years, the cumulative incidence of breast cancer in never users is about 45/1000 women. The data from the collaborative study would suggest an excess number of breast cancers

in ERT/HRT users to be two (0.2%), six (0.6%) and 12 (1.2%) if used for 5, 10 and 15 years, respectively.

The WHI is a prospective, randomized, double-blind study of HRT versus placebo in over 16 000 postmenopausal women. After a median of 5.2 years' follow-up, the study was stopped. The hazard ratio for invasive breast cancer was 1.26 (CI 1.00–1.59 nominal, 0.83–1.92 adjusted), indicating a 26% increase observed in the HRT group. As the authors noted, this 'almost reached' nominal statistical significance. It is of interest that the incidence of breast cancer according to the duration of years in the study showed no increase in years 1–3, an increase in year 4 and 5 but not an increase in year 6 or later. Since it is known that breast cancer is present for 6, 8 or 10 years before diagnosis, the role of HRT may be that of enhancing diagnosis at an earlier stage than would be observed otherwise.

ESTROGEN REPLACEMENT THERAPY POST-BREAST CANCER

One of the dichotomies of the possible association between ERT/HRT and breast cancer is that several studies have noted a reduced mortality in breast-cancer patients who had used HRT prior to the diagnosis of breast cancer. These include large cohort studies from the Nurses' Health Study as well as the Iowa Women's Health Study[18,19]. The latter study evaluated the association between HRT and mortality in women with and without a family history of breast cancer, and the adjusted RR for total mortality in women with family history of breast cancer who were currently using HRT for greater than 5 years was 0.55 (CI 0.28–1.07), not different from the established RR for women without a family history of breast cancer. Many patients who took ERT before diagnosis had smaller, better-differentiated tumors and less cellular proliferation than women who developed breast cancer and had not taken ERT.

Is there any rationale for giving women ERT after the diagnosis of breast cancer, considering the possible relationship between ERT and breast cancer? Conventional wisdom would

Table 1 Meta-analysis of estrogen replacement therapy and relative risk (RR) for breast cancer

	RR	(95% CI)
Armstrong[14]	1.01	(0.95–1.08)
Steinberg et al.[16]	1.0	(0.96–1.20)
Dupont and Page[11]	1.08	(0.96–1.20)
Sillero-Arenas et al.[13]	1.06	(1.00–1.12)
Colditz et al.[15]	1.02	(0.93–1.02)
Grady et al.[12]	1.01	(0.97–1.03)

CI, confidence interval

suggest that to do so would be detrimental. In fact, the Physicians' Desk Reference (PDR) notes that breast cancer is a contraindication to replacement therapy. The data to substantiate that contraindication, however, are lacking. None of the references in the PDR include data from the last quarter of the 20th century, and none of those present discuss the post-breast-cancer patient. If there are no data to support the non-use of ERT/HRT in the breast-cancer patient, are there data to support its use? There are some data, although limited, but the amount is increasing with time. It is interesting to note that there are at least six prospective randomized studies comparing tamoxifen with estrogen in the postmenopausal patient with advanced breast cancer. All six studies report that the response rate with tamoxifen and estrogen is similar, as is the response duration. The median survival days in three of the studies reporting this information implied that those who had taken estrogen had a considerably longer survival time than those women who were on tamoxifen, with one study noting over 13.5 months' longer survival. There are about a dozen studies which have evaluated a progestin and the treatment of metastatic breast cancer, and their results are equivalent to the overall response rate with tamoxifen.

Several retrospective studies have been published (Table 2)[20–25]. They have demonstrated that ERT/HRT in the post-breast-cancer patient can be given without a negative impact upon survival. The retrospective studies show very low recurrence and death rates. The potential bias of retrospective studies is appreciated. In many instances, women are seeking information and advice concerning replacement therapy because of significant vasomotor symptoms, or are interested in the prevention of chronic disease such as osteoporosis or colon cancer. To a large degree, these retrospective studies show a selection bias, but the selection bias is due to the patients themselves. There have been at least three case-controlled studies in which recurrences and deaths in breast-cancer in patients taking replacement therapy after diagnosis were not different from those in non-estrogen users. A recent cohort study was published by DiSaia and associates[26]. There were 125 breast-cancer patients identified who received HRT after the diagnosis of breast cancer. These were matched with 362 controls from the same geographical region. Almost three-quarters of the patients were on estrogen plus a progestogen. The risk of death was considerably lower in estrogen users compared with non-estrogen users, with an odds ratio of 0.28 (CI 0.11–0.71), $p = 0.01$ (Figure 2).

The largest study to date evaluated 2755 women with breast cancer enrolled in a large health maintenance organization[27]. Medical and pharmacy records were reviewed concerning hormone use after breast cancer diagnosis. Of the women, 174 eligible ERT/HRT users were identified for analysis. Four matched controls were identified for each of the breast-cancer patients. Both estrogen alone and

Table 2 Hormone replacement therapy in women with breast cancer

	Recurrences	Deaths
Stoll and Parbhoo[22]	0/65 (0%)	0
Powles et al.[21]	2/35 (6%)	0
Vassilopoulou-Sellin et al.[23]	1/49 (2%)	0
Bluming et al.[20]	12/189 (6%)	1 (1%)
Brewster et al.[25]	13/145 (9%)	3 (2%)
Natrajan et al.[24]	2/50 (4%)	3 (6%)
Total	30/533 (6%)	7 (1%)

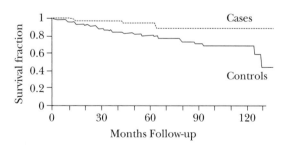

Figure 2 Survival in breast cancer, estrogen replacement therapy users vs. non-users ($p = 0.01$). Reproduced with permission from DiSaia PJ, et al. Breast cancer survival and hormone replacement therapy: a cohort analysis. *Am J Clin Oncol* 2000;23:541–5[26]

estrogen plus a progestogen were used. Breast cancer recurrence was diagnosed in 16 hormone users (9%) compared with 101 (15%) non-users. The rate of recurrence was 17/1000 person-years in users and 30/1000 women-years in non-users. Comparison of rates adjusted for multiple factors noted an RR of 0.50 (CI 0.30–0.85). Five users (3%) and 59 non-users (8%) died of their disease (5/1000 person-years versus 15/1000 person-years, respectively). The adjusted RR was 0.34 (CI 0.13–0.91). Total mortality was associated with an adjusted RR of 0.48 (CI 0.29–0.78) (Table 3).

This year in the USA, almost 50 000 women 50 years of age or younger will develop breast cancer. Most will undergo chemotherapy. The vast majority will develop chemotherapeutically induced amenorrhea. Very few will have resumption of their menstrual periods after their chemotherapy has been completed. This results in a premature chemotherapeutically induced menopause. It is well known that a premature surgical menopause usually results in more significant vasomotor symptoms than a natural menopause and they last for a longer period of time. There is no reason to believe that this would not occur also in chemotherapeutically induced menopause. To state that HRT is absolutely contraindicated in this group of women who want replacement therapy because of significant symptoms may not be in their best interest. Without any data to indicate deleterious effects of replacement therapy in the post-breast-cancer patient, to deny such

therapy for life-disturbing symptoms does not appear to be in their best self-determined interest. Today, mortality from breast cancer occurs in only 20% of those who develop the disease, and, in women with early-stage disease, over 90% long-term survival is expected.

The data to date would suggest that ERT/HRT in patients who have had breast cancer does not appear to be detrimental. In fact, some of the larger studies found significantly fewer recurrences of breast-cancer deaths and total mortality in hormone users compared with matched controls. The 'gold standard' clinical trials (double-blind, prospective, randomized studies) have not been completed. There are two such ongoing studies in Europe at present; HABITS in Sweden and a similar trial in the UK. Several smaller studies are also ongoing in the USA. The fact that trials are ongoing suggests that previous admonition of detrimental effects in the breast-cancer patient, if she uses HRT, is not substantiated. In the mean time, should HRT be denied to patients based upon the concept of opinion only? The ACOG states in its Committee Opinion that, 'There is no conclusive data to indicate an increased risk of recurrent breast cancer in postmenopausal women taking HRT. No woman can be guaranteed protection from recurrence. Late manifestations of recurrent disease and apparent predisposition to recur as shown by selective subgroups of women cannot be ignored; however, the benefits of HRT are well recognized in contributing to the quality and length of life in postmenopausal women[28]'. Many women who have had breast cancer may be interested in HRT. Not even to discuss this and to reject it out of hand for a patient who may be having significant vasomotor symptoms, or who is several years beyond breast-cancer therapy and may be interested in preventive measures for bone and cancer that HRT can provide, is unrealistic and not in the patient's best interest. Women want information so that they can make appropriate choices for themselves. As health-care providers, we must be sensitive to their desires and supportive of their decisions.

Table 3 Hormone replacement therapy in women after breast cancer

	OR or RR (95% CI)	
	Recurrence	Death
DiSaia et al.[26]		0.28* (0.11–0.71)
O'Meara et al.[27]	0.50** (0.30–0.85)	0.34** (0.13–0.91)

*OR, odds ratio; **RR, relative risk; CI, confidence interval

References

1. Nelson HD, Humphrey LL, Nygen P, *et al.* Postmenopausal hormone replacement therapy. *J Am Med Assoc* 2002;288:872–81
2. Creasman WT, Henderson D, Hinshaw W, *et al.* Estrogen replacement therapy in the patient treated for endometrial cancer. *Obstet Gynecol* 1986;67:326–30
3. Lee RB, Burke TW, Park RC. Estrogen replacement therapy following treatment for stage I endometrial carcinoma. *Gynecol Oncol* 1990;36: 189–91
4. Chapman JA, DiSaia PJ, Osann K, *et al.* Estrogen replacement in surgical stage I and II endometrial cancer survivors. *Am J Obstet Gynecol* 1996; 175:1195–2000
5. Suriano KA, McHale M, McClaren C, *et al.* Estrogen replacement therapy in endometrial cancer patients: a matched control study. *Obstet Gynecol* 2001;97:555–60
6. American College of Obstetricians and Gynecologists. Committee Opinion, Number 126, 1993, reaffirmed 1996; Washington, DC
7. Hulley S, Furberg C, Barrett-Conner E, *et al.* Noncardiovascular disease outcomes during 6.8 years of hormone therapy. *J Am Med Assoc* 2002;288:58–66
8. Writing Group for the Women's Health Initiative Investigators. Risks and benefits of estrogen plus progestin in healthy postmenopausal women. *J Am Med Assoc* 2002;288:321–33
9. Beatson GT. On the treatment of inoperable cases of carcinoma of the mamma: suggestions for a new method of treatment with illustrative cases. *Lancet* 1896;2:104–7
10. Bush TL, Whiteman M, Flaws JA. Hormone replacement therapy and breast cancer: a qualitative review. *Obstet Gynecol* 2001;98:498–508
11. Dupont WD, Page DL. Menopausal estrogen replacement therapy and breast cancer. *Arch Intern Med* 1991;151:67–72
12. Grady D, Rubin SM, Petitti DB, *et al.* Hormone therapy to prevent disease and prolong life in postmenopausal women. *Ann Intern Med* 1992; 117:1038–41
13. Sillero-Arenas M, Delgado-Rodriguez M, Rodigues-Conteras R, *et al.* Menopausal hormone replacement therapy and breast cancer: a meta-analysis. *Obstet Gynecol* 1992;79: 286–94
14. Armstrong BK. Oestrogen therapy after the menopause – boon or bane? *Med J Aust* 1988;148: 213–14
15. Colditz GA, Egan KM, Stampfer MJ. Hormone replacement therapy and risk of breast cancer. Results from epidemiologic studies. *Am J Obstet Gynecol* 1993;168:1473–80
16. Steinberg KK, Thacker SB, Smith SJ, *et al.* A meta analysis of the effect of estrogen replacement therapy on the risk of breast cancer. *J Am Med Assoc* 1991;265:1985–90
17. Collaborative Group on Hormonal Factors in Breast Cancer. Breast cancer and hormone replacement therapy: collaborative reanalysis of data from 51 epidemiological studies of 52 705 women with breast cancer and 108 411 women without breast cancer. *Lancet* 1997; 350:1047–59
18. Holli K, Isola J, Cuzick J. Low biologic aggressiveness in breast cancer in women using hormone replacement therapy. *J Clin Oncol* 1998;16: 3115–20
19. Sellers TA, Mink PJ, Cerhan JR, *et al.* The role of hormone replacement therapy in the risk for breast cancer and total mortality in women with a history of breast cancer. *Ann Intern Med* 1997;127:973–80
20. Bluming VAZ, Waishman JR, Doski GM, *et al.* Hormone replacement therapy in women with previously treated primary breast cancer. Update. Presented at the *18th Meeting of the American Society of Clinical Oncology* 1999:471.
21. Powles TJ, Hickish T, Casey S, *et al.* Hormone replacement after breast cancer. *Lancet* 1993; 342:60–1
22. Stoll BA, Parbhoo S. Treatment of menopausal symptoms in breast cancer patients. *Lancet* 1988;1:1278–9
23. Vassilopoulou-Sellin R, Asmur L, Hortobagyi GN, *et al.* Estrogen replacement therapy after localized breast cancer: clinical outcome of 319 women followed prospectively. *J Clin Oncol* 1999; 17:1482–7
24. Natrajan PK, Soumakis K, Gambrell RD, *et al.* Estrogen replacement therapy in women with previous breast cancer. *Am J Obstet Gynecol* 1999;181:288–95
25. Brewster WR, DiSaia PJ, Grosen EA, *et al.* An experience with estrogen replacement therapy in breast cancer survivors. *Int J Fertil* 1999; 44:186–92
26. DiSaia PJ, Brewster WR, Ziogas A, *et al.* Breast cancer survival and hormone replacement therapy: a cohort analysis. *Am J Clin Oncol* 2000; 23:541–5
27. O'Meara ES, Rossing MA, Daling JR, *et al.* Hormone replacement therapy after a diagnosis of breast cancer in relation to recurrence and mortality. *J Natl Cancer Inst* 2001;93:754–61
28. American College of Obstetricians and Gynecologists. Committee Opinion, Number 226, November 1999; Washington, DC

10

Oral contraceptives and ovarian cancer: a review

C. La Vecchia

INTRODUCTION

Over recent years in several developed countries, younger women have demonstrated substantial declines in ovarian cancer incidence and mortality[1-4].

Cohort analyses based on data from Switzerland[5], Britain[6], Sweden[7], England and Wales[8] and The Netherlands[9], as well as systematic analyses of mortality trends in 16 major European countries[2,3,10] and in the USA[11], showed that women born from 1920 onwards, i.e. the generations who had used oral contraceptives (OCs), demonstrated consistently reduced ovarian cancer rates. The downward trends were larger in countries where OCs had been more widely utilized[3].

There are still open issues regarding the relationship between OCs and ovarian cancer, including a clearer understanding of biological mechanism(s), the potentially different roles of various types of OC formulations and the very long-term implications of OC use, as well as possible interactions with menopausal hormone replacement therapy (HRT) and other exogenous hormones in the assessment of a woman's global exposure to such compounds[4,12,13].

COHORT STUDIES

Four cohort studies on OCs conducted in the USA and Britain provided data on OC use and risk of epithelial ovarian cancer (Table 1). These included the US Walnut Creek Study[14], recruitment into which was carried out in 1968–72, including 10 638 women aged 18–54 years. Up to 1977, a total of 16 cases of ovarian cancer were reported, corresponding to an age-adjusted relative risk (RR) for ever-use of OCs of 0.4.

The Royal College of General Practitioners' study was based on 47 000 women recruited in 1968 in 1400 British general practices[15,16]. Thirty cases of ovarian cancer were observed up to 1987, corresponding to multivariate RRs of 0.6 (95% confidence interval (CI) 0.3–1.4) for

Table 1 Selected cohort studies on combined oral contraceptives and ovarian cancer, 1980–2000

| Reference | Number of cases (age in years) | Relative risk | |
		Ever-use	Longest use
Ramcharan *et al.*, 1981, USA[14]	16 (18–54)	0.4	—
Beral *et al.*, 1988, 1999, UK[15,16]	55 (25–55)	0.6	0.2
Vessey and Painter, 1995, UK[17]	42 (all ages)	0.4	0.3
Hankinson *et al.*, 1995, USA[18]	260 (30–65)	1.1	0.6

ever-users of OCs and of 0.3 for ≥ 10 years of use. Allowance in the analysis was made for age, parity, smoking and social class. At the 25-year follow-up for mortality[16], 55 deaths from ovarian cancer were observed, corresponding to a RR of 0.6 for ever-use and of 0.2 for long-term use of OCs. The protection persisted for ≥ 20 years after stopping OC use (RR 0.6).

The Oxford Family Planning Association study was based on 17 032 women enrolled between 1968 and 1976 from various family planning clinics in the UK[17]. Up to October 1993, 42 cases of ovarian cancer were registered, corresponding to RRs of 0.4 (95% CI 0.2–0.8) for ever-use of OCs and of 0.3 (95% CI 0.1–0.7) for > 8 years of use. Adjustment was made for age and parity.

Furthermore, in the Nurses' Health Study, based on 121 700 registered nurses aged 30–55 in 1976, 260 cases of ovarian cancer were prospectively observed between 1976 and 1988[18]. The multivariate RR for ever-use, which essentially reflected former use, was 1.1 (95% CI 0.83–1.43), but declined to 0.6 (95% CI 0.32–1.07) for use ≥ 5 years. Adjustment was made for age, tubal ligation, age at menarche, age at menopause, smoking and body mass index.

Thus, the overall RR from cohort studies is around 0.7 for ever-use and 0.4 for long-term use, on the basis of approximately 400 cases of ovarian cancer.

CASE–CONTROL STUDIES

At least 25 of 26 studies published between 1980 and 2001 found relative risks of ovarian cancer in OC users to be below unity, the sole apparent outlier being a study conducted in China[19]. Table 2 gives their main results.

Willett and colleagues[20], in a case–control study of 47 cases of ovarian cancer and 470 controls nested in the Nurses' Health Study cohort (based on 121 694 registered nurses aged 30–55 in 1986 and residing in 11 larger American states), found an age-adjusted RR of 0.8 (95% CI 0.4–1.5) for ever-use of OCs, and of 0.2 (95% CI 0.1–1.0) for women aged 35 or

younger, who were more likely to be current or recent users.

Hildreth and associates[21] considered 62 cases of epithelial ovarian cancer and 1068 hospital controls aged 45–74 from Connecticut, diagnosed between 1977 and 1978. The response rate was 71% for both cases and controls. The multivariate RR for ever-use of OCs, after allowance for age and parity, was 0.5 (95% CI 0.2–1.5).

Weiss and colleagues[22], in a population-based case–control study of 112 cases diagnosed between 1975 and 1979 from Washington State and Utah, found a RR (adjusted for demographic factors and parity) of 0.6 for ever-use and of 0.4 (95% CI 0.15–1.28) for longest use, of borderline statistical significance ($p = 0.04$). Response rate was 66% for cases and 92% for controls.

Franceschi and co-workers[23] considered data on 161 cases of epithelial ovarian cancer and 561 hospital controls interviewed in Milan, Italy in 1979–80. The age-adjusted RR for ever-use of OCs was 0.7 (95% CI 0.4–1.1).

Cramer and colleagues[24], in a population-based case–control study of 144 cases and 139 population controls conducted during the period 1978–81 in the Greater Boston area, found a RR, adjusted for age and parity, of 0.4 (95% CI 0.2–1.0) for ever-use of OCs, in the absence of a consistent duration–risk relationship (RR 0.6 for > 5 years). This could, however, be due to the small number of cases, and hence to the influence of chance. Response rate was around 50% for both cases and controls.

Rosenberg and associates[25], in a hospital-based case–control study of 136 cases and 539 controls collected between 1976 and 1980 from various areas of the USA and Canada, found an age-adjusted RR of 0.6 (95% CI 0.4–0.9) for ever-use and of 0.3 for OC use of ≥ 5 years. Response rate was 94% for both cases and controls, and the results were not materially modified by multivariate analysis.

Risch and co-workers[26] provided data from a case–control study of 284 cases and 705 controls from Washington and Utah diagnosed between 1975 and 1979. The multivariate RR was 0.5 for

Table 2 Selected case–control studies on combined oral contraceptives and ovarian cancer, 1980–2001

Reference	Type of study	Number of cases (age in years)	Relative risk Ever-use	Relative risk Longest use
Willett et al., 1981, USA[20]	nested in a cohort	47 (< 55)	0.8	0.8
Hildreth et al., 1981, USA[21]	hospital-based	62 (45–74)	0.5	0.3
Weiss et al., 1981, USA[22]	population-based	112 (36–55)	0.6	0.4
Franceschi et al., 1982, Italy[23]	hospital-based	161 (19–69)	0.7	—
Cramer et al., 1982, USA[24]	population-based	144 (< 60)	0.4	0.6
Rosenberg et al., 1982, USA[25]	hospital-based	136 (< 60)	0.6	0.3
Risch et al., 1983, USA[26]	population-based	284 (20–75)	0.5	—
Tzonou et al., 1984, Greece[27]	hospital-based	150 (34–64)	0.4	—
CASH, 1987, USA[28]	population-based	546 (20–54)	0.6	0.2
Harlow et al., 1988, USA[29]	population-based	92 (20–59)	0.4	0.4
Wu et al., 1988, USA[30]	hospital-based	299 (18–85)	0.7	0.4
Shu et al., 1989, China[19]	population-based	172 (18–79)	1.8	1.9
WHO, 1989, seven countries[31]	hospital-based	368 (< 63)	0.8	0.5
Hartge et al., 1989, USA[32]	hospital-based	296 (20–79)	1.0	0.8
Booth et al., 1989, UK[33]	hospital-based	213 (< 65)	0.5	0.1
Parazzini et al., 1991, Italy[34]	hospital-based	505 (22–59)	0.7	0.5
Parazzini et al., 1991, Italy[35]	hospital-based	91 (23–64)	0.3	0.2
Polychronopoulos et al., 1993, Greece[36]	hospital-based	189 (< 75)	0.8	—
Rosenberg et al., 1994, USA[37]	hospital-based	441 (< 65 years)	0.8	0.5
Risch et al., 1994, 1996, Canada[38,39]	population-based	450 (35–79)	0.9 (for each year of use)	—
Purdie et al., 1995, Australia[40]	population-based	824 (18–79)	0.6	0.3
Narod et al., 1998, USA[41]	hereditary cancers	207 (< 75)	0.5	0.4
Beard et al., 2000, USA[42]	population-based	103	0.8	—
Ness et al., 2000, USA[43]	population-based	767 (< 70)	0.6	0.3
Greggi et al., 2000, Italy[44]	hospital-based	440 (≤ 80)	0.4	0.3
Chiaffarino et al., 2001, Italy[45]	hospital-based	1031 (< 80)	0.9	0.5
Overviews				
Franceschi et al., 1991, Bosetti et al., 2002, Greece, Italy, UK[46,47]	three hospital-based case–control studies	2768 (< 65) 2197 (all ages)	0.7 0.7	0.5 0.3
Whittemore et al., 1992, USA[48]	12 US population- and hospital-based case–control studies			
Harris et al., 1992, USA[49]	as above	327	0.8	0.6
John et al., 1993, USA[50]	as above	110	0.7	0.6

CASH, Cancer and Steroid Hormone Study; WHO, World Health Organization

ever-use. Response rate was 68% for cases and 95% for controls.

In a case–control study conducted in 1980–89 on 150 cases and 250 hospital controls from Athens, Greece, Tzonou and colleagues[27] found a multivariate RR (adjusted for age, age at menopause and use of HRT) of 0.4 (95% CI 0.1–1.1). The lack of significance is explainable through the low frequency of OC use in that population.

The Cancer and Steroid Hormone (CASH) study[28] was a population-based investigation conducted between December 1980 and December 1982 in eight areas of the USA on 546 women, 20–54 years of age, with ovarian cancer and 4227 controls. The response rate was 71% for cases and 83% for controls. The multivariate RR, adjusted for age and parity, was 0.6 (95% CI 0.5–0.2) for ever-use of OCs, and 0.2 (95% CI 0.1–0.4) for use ≥ 10 years. The results were consistent when different formulations of OCs were considered separately. However, no meaningful protection was evident for short-term use, i.e. 3–6 years[51].

Harlow and associates[29] provided information on OC use for 92 cases of borderline malignancy epithelial ovarian cancer and 124 controls diagnosed between 1980 and 1985. The RR for ever-use, adjusted for age and parity, was 0.4, in the absence however of a consistent duration–risk relationship.

Wu and colleagues[30], in a hospital-based case–control study of 299 cases and 752 controls diagnosed in 1983–85 from the San Francisco Bay area, found a RR, adjusted for parity, of 0.7 (95% CI 0.5–1.1) for ever-use and of 0.4 (95% CI 0.3–0.7) for > 3 years of OC use. The overall RR per year of use was 0.88 (95% CI 0.83–0.94). The response rate was about 70% for both cases and controls.

Shu and colleagues[19], in a case–control study conducted in 1984–86 in Shanghai, China, on 229 ovarian cancer cases (172 epithelial) and an equal number of controls, found a RR (adjusted for education, parity, ovarian cysts and age at menarche) of 1.8 (95% CI 0.8–4.1) for ever-use of OCs. However, only 21 cases and 12 controls had ever used OCs. The response rate was 89% for cases and 100% for controls.

The World Health Organization (WHO) Collaborative Study of Neoplasia and Steroid Contraceptives[31] included data on 368 cases of histologically confirmed epithelial ovarian cancer and 2397 hospital controls interviewed between 1979 and 1986 in seven (mainly developing) countries of the world. The response rate was 73% for cases and 94% for controls. The multivariate RR (adjusted for age, center, year of interview and parity) for ever-use of OCs was 0.75 (95% CI 0.56–1.01), and decreased to 0.54 (95% CI 0.33–0.58) for 10 years of use or longer. The protection was of similar magnitude in developed and developing countries[52].

In a case–control study conducted in 1978–81 in the Washington, DC area, on 296 patients with epithelial ovarian cancer and 343 hospital controls, Hartge and colleagues[32] found RRs (adjusted for age and race) of 1.0 (95% CI 0.7–1.7) for ever-use, and 0.8 (95% CI

0.4–1.5) for ≥ 5 years of OC use. Response rate was 74% for cases and 78% for controls.

Booth and co-workers[33], in a hospital-based case–control study of 213 cases < 65 years and 451 controls interviewed between 1978 and 1983 in London and Oxford, England, found multivariate RRs of approximately 0.5 for ever-use, and of 0.1 (95% CI 0.01–1.0) for > 10 years of OC use, with a significant inverse trend in risk with duration of use. Allowance was made for age, social class, gravidity and duration of unprotected intercourse.

Parazzini and associates[34] provided data on 505 cases of epithelial ovarian cancer under 60 years of age and 1375 hospital controls interviewed between 1983 and 1989 in northern Italy. The multivariate RR (adjusted for socio-demographic factors, parity, age at menarche, lifelong menstrual pattern, menopausal status and age at menopause) for ever-use of OCs was 0.7 (95% CI 0.5–1.0), and decreased to 0.5 (95% CI 0.3–0.9) for ≥ 2 years of use, with a significant inverse trend in risk with duration.

Parazzini and associates[35] also considered 91 cases of borderline malignancy epithelial ovarian cancer and 237 hospital controls interviewed between 1983 and 1990 in northern Italy. The multivariate RR (adjusted for age, education, parity and age at menopause) for ever-use of OCs was 0.3 (95% CI 0.2–0.6), and that for ≥ 2 years of use was 0.2 (95% CI 0.08–0.6). Response rate was 98% for both cases and controls.

In a case–control study of 189 cases and 200 controls conducted in 1989–91 in Greater Athens, Greece[36], only three cases and seven controls reported ever-use of OCs, corresponding to a multivariate RR of 0.80 (95% CI 0.11–3.67). Response rate for cases was about 90%.

Rosenberg and colleagues[37] updated their 1982 report, providing data collected between 1977 and 1998 on 441 cases of epithelial ovarian cancer and 2065 hospital controls from various US areas. The response rate was 94% for both cases and controls. The multivariate RR for ever-use was 0.8 (95% CI 0.6–1.0). No appreciable protection was observed up to 3 years of use, but the RR declined to 0.5

(95% CI 0.2–0.9) for ≥ 10 years of use. The risk estimates were similar for various types of OC formulations.

Risch and co-workers[38,39] provided data on 450 cases of epithelial ovarian cancer aged 35–79 and 564 controls diagnosed between 1989 and 1992 in Ontario, Canada. The response rate was 71% for cases and 65% for controls. The overall multivariate RR per year of pill use, adjusted for age, parity, lactation, HRT use, tubal ligation, hysterectomy and family history of breast cancer, was 0.90 (95% CI 0.86–0.94), and protection was stronger for serous and endometrioid than for mucinous neoplasms.

Purdie and colleagues[40], in a population-based study of 824 cases and 860 controls diagnosed between 1990 and 1993 in three Australian states found a RR around 0.6 for ever-use, which declined to 0.26 (95% CI 0.18–0.38) for ≥ 10 years of OC use. Response rate was 90% for cases and 73% for controls. Allowance was made for sociodemographic factors, family history of cancer, talc use, smoking, and reproductive and hormonal factors.

A study conducted in North America and Europe on 207 women with hereditary ovarian cancer (179 with BRCA1 and 28 with BRCA2 mutations) and 161 sister controls found a RR of 0.5 for ever-use of OCs, and the risk decreased with increasing duration of use[41].

A study of 103 cases from Olmsted County, Minnesota, found a RR for ever-use of OCs of 0.8[42].

A study conducted in Delaware Valley and contiguous counties between 1994 and 1998 on 767 cases and 7347 controls below age 70 found a RR of 0.6 for ever-use and 0.3 for ≥ 10 years of use. The protection was similar for use of low-estrogen/low-progestin pills and high-estrogen/ high-progestin pills (RR 0.5)[43].

A subsequent report from the same dataset[53] showed an appreciably stronger protection of long-term use (> 48 months) for women with positive family history of ovarian cancer (RR 0.12) than for those with negative family history (RR 0.51), although absolute numbers of women with positive family history were small (three cases, nine controls among long-term

users), and the estimates were therefore not significantly heterogeneous.

In contrast, in a population-based case–control study including 240 ovarian cancer cases with BRCA1 or BRCA2 mutations and 592 without mutations from Israel[54], duration of OC use was inversely related to ovarian cancer risk in women without, but not in those with, BRCA1 or BRCA2 mutations.

No appreciable difference in the relationship between OC use and ovarian cancer risk between women without and those with family history of ovarian and breast cancer was observed in a large case–control study from Italy[55].

Two hospital-based case–control studies of ovarian cancer were conducted in Italy in the 1990s. One of these[44] was conducted in the Rome area and included 440 cases and 868 controls, with a response rate of 97%. The multivariate RR for ever-use of OCs was 0.4, and for long-term use was 0.3. The second was a multicentric study, conducted in four areas of northern, central and southern Italy, and included 1031 cases and 2441 controls below age 80. The response rate was over 95%. The multivariate RR was 0.9 for ever-use and 0.5 for ≥ 5 years of use[45].

The findings of two collaborative reanalyses of case–control studies on the issue are also included in Table 2. These were conducted on 2768 cases and 6274 controls from three European countries[46,47] and on 2197 cases and 8893 controls in white women from 12 US studies[48] (i.e. a total of almost 5000 cases, and over 15 000 controls).

In the European meta-analysis[46,47], the multivariate RR was 0.7 (95% CI 0.6–0.8) for ever-use and 0.5 (95% CI 0.2–0.8) for longest OC use. Allowance was made for age and other sociodemographic factors, menopausal status and parity. The protection appeared to persist for at least 20 years from last OC use[47].

In the American meta-analysis[48], corresponding values were 0.7 (95% CI 0.5–0.6) for ever-use and 0.3 (95% CI 0.2–0.4) for OC use > 6 years. Adjustment was made for age, study and parity. The results were similar when hospital-based or population-based studies were considered separately. The RRs were 0.7 for both types of studies for ever-use of OCs, 0.6 for hospital-based and 0.3 for population-based for longest use (> 6 years), and 0.95 and 0.90 (significant) per added year of use. An inverse association was also observed in a further analysis of 110 black cases and 251 black controls (RR 0.7 for ever-use and 0.6 for ≥ 6 years of use)[50].

The US meta-analysis also included data on 327 borderline malignancy epithelial ovarian neoplasms in white women. The RRs were 0.8 (95% CI 0.6–1.1) for ever-use, and 0.6 (95% CI 0.4–0.9) for > 5 years of OC use[49].

DISCUSSION

The overall estimate of protection with ever-use of OCs in terms of ovarian cancer risk is approximately 40%, and a steady inverse relationship is observed with duration of use. Protection of around 60% for long-term use (i.e. over 5 years) was observed for various types of combined OCs[56].

The inverse relationship between OCs and ovarian cancer was observed also after allowance for parity in most studies, and was consistently reproduced in several studies across separate strata of parity, as well as age and other potential covariates, including marital status, education, menopausal status, other types of contraceptive use, and other selected menstrual and reproductive factors. In particular, protection was also observed in women with hereditary ovarian cancer[41], although the issue remains open to discussion[54]. Potential selection or indication biases, including selective exclusion of OC use by smokers and by women at risk of liver and thromboembolic diseases[57], were also unlikely to modify materially the inverse association observed between OC use and ovarian cancer risk.

At least two studies[29,35], and the meta-analysis of 12 US studies[49], also considered borderline epithelial ovarian tumors. An inverse relationship was also evident for these neoplasms, suggesting that OCs exert a protective effect on the whole spectrum of epithelial ovarian carcinogenesis. Likewise, the limited information available on different histological types of epithelial invasive ovarian cancer does not indicate any histotype-specific effect[12].

With reference to non-epithelial ovarian cancers, 38 germ-cell neoplasms and 45 sex cord-stromal neoplasms were considered from the collaborative re-analysis of 12 US case–control studies[58]. The multivariate RRs among ever-users of OCs were 2.0 (95% CI 0.8–5.1) for germ-cell cancers and 0.4 (95% CI 0.2–0.8) for sex cord-stromal neoplasms. The data were inadequate for evaluating duration – or any other time–risk relationship.

The few available data indicate a consistent protection of OCs against benign epithelial tumors, i.e. ovarian cysts[59,60], but not against benign ovarian teratomas[61,62].

The favorable effect of OCs on epithelial ovarian cancer seems to persist for at least 20 years after OC use has ceased[12,28,37,46,48], and is not confined to any particular type of OC formulation[37,63].

Very limited information is available on progestin-only oral contraceptives. In a hospital-based case–control study of 441 cases and 2065 controls recruited between 1977 and 1991 from various US areas[37], 1% of cases versus 3% of controls had ever used progestin-only oral contraceptives. The unadjusted RR was 0.3. Another two studies[64,65] gave RRs of 0.8 and 1.1. The overall evidence on progestogen-only contraception is therefore broadly compatible with the well-known inverse relationship between combined OCs and ovarian cancer[66].

From a biological viewpoint, the beneficial effect of OCs on ovarian cancer risk has been interpreted chiefly within the framework of the incessant ovulation theory, i.e. the multistage theory of ovarian carcinogenesis[67]. Ovariostasis, induced by oral contraceptives as well as by pregnancy and menopause, avoids the exposure of ovarian epithelium to recurrent trauma and contact with follicular fluid[1].

OCs may also protect against ovarian cancer by reducing exposure to pituitary gonadotropins, which stimulate the growth of cell lines derived from human ovarian carcinoma[68]. The lack of apparent protection by menopausal HRT[1,48,69], however, does not support the existence of a favorable role of gonadotropin stimulation on ovarian carcinogenesis. Indeed, several recent studies have demonstrated a direct association between menopausal HRT and ovarian cancer risk, including the American Cancer Society (ACS) prospective study[70], a collaborative re-analysis of European case–control studies based on over 2900 cases[71], an additional case–control study from Sweden[72] and a cohort study based on the Breast Cancer Demonstration Project[73]. The best estimate for the RR of ovarian cancer among long-term users of HRT is between 1.3 and 1.6[74,75], but there are still uncertainties on the role of duration, type of preparation (estrogen versus combined therapy progestogens) and schedule used.

Since the incidence of ovarian cancer is already appreciable in middle age, and survival from the disease is unsatisfactory, the protection of OC use corresponds to a far from negligible number of deaths, and is therefore one of the major issues in any risk–benefit and public-health evaluation of the OC[76,77]. The long-term persistence (at least 20 years) of the protection from OCs against ovarian carcinogenesis has important implications for individual risk assessment and on a public-health scale[47].

ACKNOWLEDGEMENTS

This work was conducted with contributions from the Italian Association for Cancer Research and the Italian League against Cancer. The authors thank Mrs M. P. Bonifacino for editorial assistance.

References

1. Parazzini F, Franceschi S, La Vecchia C, Fasoli M. The epidemiology of ovarian cancer. *Gynecol Oncol* 1991;43:9–23

2. La Vecchia C, Lucchini F, Negri E, *et al.* Trends of cancer mortality in Europe, 1955–1989: III. Breast and genital sites. *Eur J Cancer* 1992; 28A:927–98

3. La Vecchia C, Negri E, Levi F, Decarli A, Boyle P. Cancer mortality in Europe: effects of age, cohort of birth and period of death. *Eur J Cancer* 1998;34:118–41

4. La Vecchia C, Franceschi S. Oral contraceptives and ovarian cancer. *Eur J Cancer Prev* 1999;8: 297–304

5. Levi F, Gutzwiller F, Decarli A, La Vecchia C. Oral contraceptive use and breast and ovarian cancer mortality in Switzerland. *J Epidemiol Community Health* 1987;41:267–8

6. Villard-Mackintosh L, Vessey MP, Jones L. The effects of oral contraceptives and parity on ovarian cancer trends in women under 55 years of age. *Br J Obstet Gynaecol* 1989;96:783–8

7. Adami H-O, Bergström R, Persson I, Sparén P. The incidence of ovarian cancer in Sweden, 1960–1984. *Am J Epidemiol* 1990;132:446–52

8. dos Santos Silva I, Swerdlow AJ. Recent trends in incidence of and mortality from breast, ovarian and endometrial cancers in England and Wales and their relation to changing fertility and oral contraceptive use. *Br J Cancer* 1995;72:485–92

9. Koper NP, Kiemeney LALM, Massuger LFAG, *et al.* Ovarian cancer incidence (1989–1991) and mortality (1954–1993) in The Netherlands. *Obstet Gynecol* 1996;88:387–93

10. Levi F, Lucchini F, Negri E, Boyle P, La Vecchia C. Cancer mortality in Europe, 1990–94, and an overview of trends from 1955 to 1994. *Eur J Cancer* 1999;35:1477–516

11. Tarone RE, Chu KC. Age-period-cohort analyses of breast-, ovarian-, endometrial- and cervical-cancer mortality rates for Caucasian women in the USA. *J Epidemiol Biostat* 2000;5:221–31

12. World Health Organization. *Hormonal Contraception and Post-menopausal Hormonal Therapy.* IARC Monographs on the Evaluation of Carcinogenic Risks to Humans, Vol 72. Lyons: IARC, 1999

13. La Vecchia C. Oral contraceptives and ovarian cancer. In Neves-e-Castro M, Wren BG, eds. *Menopause. Hormones and Cancer.* Lancaster, UK Parthenon Publishing, 2002:77–85

14. Ramcharan S, Pellegrin FA, Ray R, Hsu JP. *The Walnut Creek Contraceptive Study. A Prospective Study of the Side Effects of Oral Contraceptives.* NIH publication no 81–564, Vol iii. Bethesda, MD: National Institutes of Health, 1981

15. Beral V, Hannaford P, Kay C. Oral contraceptive use and malignancies of the genital tract. Results of the Royal College of General Practitioners' Oral Contraception Study. *Lancet* 1988;1:1331–5

16. Beral V, Hermon C, Kay C, *et al.* Mortality associated with oral contraceptive use: 25 year follow up of cohort of 46 000 women from Royal College of General Practitioners' Oral Contraception Study. *Br Med J* 1999;318:96–100

17. Vessey MP, Painter R. Endometrial and ovarian cancer and oral contraceptives – findings in a large cohort study. *Br J Cancer* 1995;71:1340–2

18. Hankinson SE, Colditz GA, Hunter DJ, *et al.* A prospective study of reproductive factors and risk of epithelial ovarian cancer. *Cancer* 1995;76:284–90

19. Shu XO, Brinton LA, Gao YT, Yuan JM. Population-based case–control study of ovarian cancer in Shangai. *Cancer Res* 1989;49:3670–4

20. Willett WC, Bain C, Hennekens CH, Rosner B, Speizer FE. Oral contraceptives and risk of ovarian cancer. *Cancer* 1981;48:1684–7

21. Hildreth NG, Kelsey JL, LiVolsi VA, *et al.* An epidemiologic study of epithelial carcinoma of the ovary. *Am J Epidemiol* 1981;114:398–405

22. Weiss NS, Lyon JL, Liff JM, Vollmer WM, Daling JR. Incidence of ovarian cancer in relation to the use of oral contraceptives. *Int J Cancer* 1981;28:669–71

23. Franceschi S, La Vecchia C, Helmrich SP, Mangioni C, Tognoni G. Risk factors for epithelial ovarian cancer in Italy. *Am J Epidemiol* 1982;115:714–19

24. Cramer DW, Hutchison GB, Welch WR, Scully RE, Knapp RC. Factors affecting the association of oral contraceptives and ovarian cancer. *N Engl J Med* 1982;307:1047–51

25. Rosenberg L, Shapiro S, Slone D, *et al.* Epithelial ovarian cancer and combination oral contraceptives. *J Am Med Assoc* 1982;247:3210–12

26. Risch HA, Weiss NS, Lyon JL, Daling JR, Liff JM. Events of reproductive life and the incidence of epithelial ovarian cancer. *Am J Epidemiol* 1983;117:128–39

27. Tzonou A, Day NE, Trichopoulos D, *et al.* The epidemiology of ovarian cancer in Greece: a case–control study. *Eur J Cancer Clin Oncol* 1984;20:1045–52

28. CASH (Cancer and Steroid Hormone Study of the Centers for Disease Control and the National Institute of Child Health and Human Development). The reduction in risk of ovarian cancer associated with oral contraceptive use. *N Engl J Med* 1987;316:650–5

29. Harlow BL, Weiss NS, Roth GJ, Chu J, Daling JR. Case–control study of borderline ovarian tumors: reproductive history and exposure to exogenous female hormones. *Cancer Res* 1988;48:5849–52

30. Wu ML, Whittemore AS, Paffenbarger RS Jr, *et al.* Personal and environmental characteristics related to epithelial ovarian cancer. I. Reproductive and menstrual events and oral contraceptive use. *Am J Epidemiol* 1988;128:1216–27

31. World Health Organization Collaborative Study of Neoplasia and Steroid Contraceptives. Epithelial ovarian cancer and combined oral contraceptives. *Int J Epidemiol* 1989;18:538–45

32. Hartge P, Schiffman MH, Hoover R, *et al.* A case–control study of epithelial ovarian cancer. *Am J Obstet Gynecol* 1989;161:10–16

33. Booth M, Beral V, Smith P. Risk factors for ovarian cancer: a case–control study. *Br J Cancer* 1989;60:592–8

34. Parazzini F, La Vecchia C, Negri E, *et al.* Oral contraceptives use and the risk of ovarian cancer: an Italian case–control study. *Eur J Cancer* 1991;27:594–8

35. Parazzini F, Restelli C, La Vecchia C, *et al.* Risk factors for epithelial ovarian tumours of borderline malignancy. *Int J Epidemiol* 1991;20:871–7

36. Polychronopoulou A, Tzonou A, Hsieh C, *et al.* Reproductive variables, tobacco, ethanol, coffee and somatometry as risk factors for ovarian cancer. *Int J Cancer* 1993;55:402–7

37. Rosenberg L, Palmer JR, Zauber AG, *et al.* A case–control study of oral contraceptive use and invasive epithelial ovarian cancer. *Am J Epidemiol* 1994;139:654–61

38. Risch HA, Marrett LD, Howe GR. Parity, contraception, infertility, and the risk of epithelial ovarian cancer. *Am J Epidemiol* 1994;140:585–97

39. Risch HA, Marrett LD, Jain M, Howe GR. Differences in risk factors for epithelial ovarian cancer by histologic type. Results of a case–control study. *Am J Epidemiol* 1996;144:363–72

40. Purdie D, Green A, Bain C, *et al.* for the Survey of Women's Health Group. Reproductive and other factors and risk of epithelial ovarian cancer: an Australian case–control study. *Int J Cancer* 1995;62:678–84

41. Narod SA, Risch H, Moslehi R, *et al.*, for the Hereditary Ovarian Cancer Clinical Study Group. Oral contraceptives and the risk of hereditary ovarian cancer. *N Engl J Med* 1998;339:424–8

42. Beard CM, Hartmann LC, Atkinson EJ, *et al.* The epidemiology of ovarian cancer: a population-based study in Olmsted County, Minnesota, 1935–1991. *Ann Epidemiol* 2000;10:14–23

43. Ness RB, Grisso JA, Klapper J, *et al.*, and the Steroid Hormones and Reproduction (SHARE) Study Group. Risk of ovarian cancer in relation to estrogen and progestin dose and use characteristics of oral contraceptives. *Am J Epidemiol* 2000;152:233–41

44. Greggi S, Parazzini F, Paratore MP, *et al.* Risk factors for ovarian cancer in central Italy. *Gynecol Oncol* 2000;9:50–4

45. Chiaffarino F, Pelucchi C, Parazzini F, *et al.* Reproductive and hormonal factors and ovarian cancer. *Ann Oncol* 2001;12:337–41

46. Franceschi S, Parazzini F, Negri E, *et al.* Pooled analysis of three European case–control studies of epithelial ovarian cancer. III. Oral contraceptive use. *Int J Cancer* 1991;49:61–5

47. Bosetti C, Negri E, Trichopoulos D, *et al.* Long-term effects of oral contraceptives on ovarian cancer risk. *Int J Cancer* 2002;102:262–5

48. Whittemore AS, Harris R, Itnyre J, and the Collaborative Ovarian Cancer Group. Characteristics relating to ovarian cancer risk: collaborative analysis of 12 US case–control studies. II. Invasive epithelial ovarian cancers in white women. *Am J Epidemiol* 1992;136:1184–203

49. Harris R, Whittemore AS, Itnyre J, the Collaborative Ovarian Cancer Group. Characteristics relating to ovarian cancer risk: collaborative analysis of 12 US case–control studies. III. Epithelial tumors of low malignant potential in white women. *Am J Epidemiol* 1992;136:1204–11

50. John EM, Whittemore AS, Harris R, Itnyre J, the Collaborative Ovarian Cancer Group. Characteristics relating to ovarian cancer risk: collaborative analysis of seven US case–control studies. Epithelial ovarian cancer in black women. *J Natl Cancer Inst* 1993;85:142–7

51. Gross TP, Schlesselman JJ, Stadel BV, Yu W, Lee NC. The risk of epithelial ovarian cancer in short-term users of oral contraceptives. *Am J Epidemiol* 1992;136:46–53

52. Thomas DB, World Health Organization Collaborative Study of Neoplasia and Steroid Contraceptives. The influence of combined oral contraceptives on risk of neoplasms in developing and developed countries. *Contraception* 1991; 43:695–710

53. Walker GR, Schlesselman JJ, Ness RB. Family history of cancer, oral contraceptive use, and ovarian cancer risk. *Am J Obstet Gynecol* 2002; 186:8–14

54. Modan B, Hartge P, Hirsh-Yechezkel G, *et al.*, for the National Israel Ovarian Cancer Study Group. Parity, oral contraceptives, and the risk of ovarian cancer among carriers and noncarriers of a *BRCA1* or *BRCA2* mutation. *N Engl J Med* 2001;345:235–40

55. Tavani A, Ricci E, La Vecchia C, *et al.* Influence of menstrual and reproductive factors on ovarian cancer risk in women with and without family history of breast or ovarian cancer. *Int J Epidemiol* 2000;29:799–802

56. La Vecchia C, Altieri A, Franceschi S, Tavani A. Oral contraceptives and cancer. An update. *Drug Safety* 2001;24:741–54

57. Fioretti F, La Vecchia C, Tavani A, Parazzini F. Package inserts of oral contraceptives in Italy. *Pharmacoepidemiol Drug Safety* 1996;5:315–19

58. Horn-Ross PL, Whittemore AS, Harris R, Itnyre J, the Collaborative Ovarian Cancer Group. Characteristics relating to ovarian cancer risk: collaborative analysis of 12 US case–control studies. VI. Nonepithelial cancers among adults. *Epidemiology* 1992;3:490–5

59. Parazzini F, La Vecchia C, Franceschi S, Negri E, Cecchetti G. Risk factors for endometrioid, mucinous and serous benign ovarian cysts. *Int J Cancer* 1989;18:108–12

60. Booth M, Beral V, Maconochie N, Carpenter L, Scott C. A case–control study of benign ovarian tumours. *J Epidemiol Community Health* 1992;46: 528–31

61. Westhoff C, Pike M, Vessey M. Benign ovarian teratomas: a population-based case–control study. *Br J Cancer* 1988;58:93–8

62. Parazzini F, La Vecchia C, Negri E, Moroni S, Villa A. Risk factors for benign ovarian teratomas. *Br J Cancer* 1995;71:644–6

63. Rosenblatt KA, Thomas DB, Noonan EA, the WHO Collaborative Study of Neoplasia and Steroid Contraceptives. High-dose and low-dose combined oral contraceptives: protection against epithelial ovarian cancer and the length of the protective effect. *Eur J Cancer* 1992; 28A:1872–6

64. Liang AP, Levenson AG, Layde PM, *et al.* Risk of breast, uterine corpus, and ovarian cancer in women receiving medroxyprogesterone injection. *J Am Med Assoc* 1983;249:2909–12

65. World Health Organization Collaborative Study of Neoplasia and Steroid Contraceptives. Depot medroxyprogesterone acetate (DMPA) and risk of epithelial ovarian cancer. *Int J Cancer* 1991; 49:191–5

66. La Vecchia C, Franceschi S. Progestogen-only contraceptives and cancer risk. *Eur J Cancer Prev* 2002;11:113–15

67. Casagrande JT, Louie EW, Pike MC, *et al.* Incessant ovulation and ovarian cancer. *Lancet* 1979;2:170–3

68. Simon WE, Albrecht M, Hänsel M, Dietel M, Hölzer F. Cell lines derived from human ovarian carcinomas: growth stimulation by gonadotropic and steroid hormones. *J Natl Cancer Inst* 1983; 70:839–45

69. Negri E, Tzonou A, Beral V, *et al.* Hormonal therapy for menopause and ovarian cancer in a collaborative re-analysis of European studies. *Int J Cancer* 1999;80:848–51

70. Rodriguez C, Patel AV, Calle EE, Jacob EJ, Thun MJ. Estrogen replacement therapy and ovarian cancer mortality in a large prospective study of US women. *J Am Med Assoc* 2001; 285:1460–5

71. Bosetti C, Franceschi S, Trichopoulos D, Beral V, La Vecchia C. Relationship between postmenopausal hormone replacement therapy and ovarian cancer. *J Am Med Assoc* 2001; 285:3089

72. Riman T, Dickman PW, Nilsson S, *et al.* Hormone replacement therapy and the risk of invasive epithelial ovarian cancer in Swedish women. *J Natl Cancer Inst* 2002;94:497–504

73. Lacey JV, Mink PJ, Lubin JH, *et al.* Menopausal hormone replacement therapy and risk of ovarian cancer. *J Am Med Assoc* 2002;288:334–41

74. Vecchia C, Brinton LA, McTiernan A. Menopause, hormone replacement therapy and cancer. *Maturitas* 2001;39:97–115

75. Noller KL. Estrogen replacement therapy and risk of ovarian cancer. *J Am Med Assoc* 2002; 288:368–9

76. Gross TP, Schlesselman JJ. The estimated effect of oral contraceptive use on the cumulative risk of epithelial ovarian cancer. *Obstet Gynecol* 1994;83:419–24

77. La Vecchia C, Tavani A, Franceschi S, Parazzini F. Oral contraceptives and cancer. *Drug Safety* 1996;14:260–72

11

Mood and the menopause

P. Klein

INTRODUCTION

The relationship of mood changes and the menopause/perimenopause continues to be a controversial topic that has been the subject of a number of recent reviews and commentaries[1–4]. While in the past, clinical experience had led physicians to recognize that the time of perimenopause/menopause was a period of increased susceptibility to depression and other affective disorders[5], over the last two to three decades a number of epidemiological, correlational and therapeutic studies have cast doubt on this association. Since 'involutional melancholia' was dropped from the Diagnostic and Statistical Manual of Mental Disorders (DSM) classification of psychiatric diseases in 1980, the view has prevailed that the climacteric and depression are not associated; that emotive symptoms associated with the climacteric are more likely to be due to psychosocial than biological causes; and that hormonal treatment of affective disturbances experienced by women during the climacteric is, with the possible exception of postsurgical menopause, ineffective[1,2]. To quote two recent reviews, 'involutional melancholia seems to be of vanishing interest to psychiatry'[6] because 'there is no substantial evidence that a natural menopause causes depression'[7]. Instead, depressed mood during the climacteric has been attributed to middle age-related life events and associated psychosocial changes such as the departure of children from home, illness and death of parents, and marital separation/divorce.

Yet, the experience of many clinicians continues to be that some women are susceptible to clinically significant symptoms of affective and anxiety disorders and that some of these women improve with the appropriate hormone replacement therapy (HRT)[3,8,9]. Furthermore, gonadal steroids have profound effects on the central nervous system (CNS) and it would be surprising if major changes in their secretion associated with the climacteric did not affect at least some women. The issue is of considerable clinical importance, because treatment is readily available in the form of HRT. If hormone secretion changes associated with the climacteric do not influence affective and anxiety symptoms, then HRT should not be used to treat mood changes. If, however, they do, then denying HRT as is currently common practice would be wrong; and determining which hormones or combination of hormones should be included in HRT used for affective symptom treatment would be important.

This chapter will first review briefly the effects of gonadal steroidal hormones on the CNS as pertaining to depression and anxiety and then discuss the evidence relating to the climacteric, mood and hormonal changes. The term climacteric will be used to refer to both perimenopause and menopause and the terms perimenopause and menopause will be used when discussing each state separately. Finally three cases which illustrate different ways of managing some patients with menopausal affective and anxiety disorders in the clinic will be presented.

GONADAL HORMONES AND THE BRAIN

Estrogens, progesterone and androgens all have neuroactive and psychoactive properties. They affect neurons both via receptor-mediated genomic mechanisms, which alter neuronal protein synthesis, and by non-genomic mechanisms, which have a direct effect on the neuronal membrane and excitability[10]. Essentially, estrogens and progesterone have opposite effects on most neuronal functions and on behavior. The effect of androgens is complex[11] and more varied because neuronal function is affected both by androgens and by their neuroactive metabolites, dehydroandrogens, 3α,5α-17-androstanediol or estrogens, which have opposite effects on neuronal functions and behavior. In the following paragraphs, the effects of estrogens and progesterone will be discussed.

Estrogen cytoplasmic receptors are found in neurons in a number of different areas of the brain, including those that are involved in the expression and modulation of emotions and pain perception, such as the cortical and medial amygdala, cingulate cortex and central gray area of the brain stem[12]. In estrogen receptor (ER) containing neurons, estradiol co-localizes with other neurotransmitters, including γ-amino-butyric acid (GABA)[13] and opioids[14]. By regulating the expression of genes affecting the synthesis, release, post-synaptic action and breakdown of different neurotransmitters and neuromodulators, estrogens act to increase the excitability of neurons which concentrate estradiol. For instance, estradiol reduces GABA synthesis in the amygdala by decreasing the activity of glutamic acid decarboxylase[15]. It increases the synthesis of 5-hydroxytryptamine (serotonin) by up-regulating the genomic expression of the rate-limiting enzyme tryptophan hydroxylase[16], and reduces breakdown of 5-hydroxytryptamine and noradrenaline by inhibiting or competing for the activity of the mono-aminergic catabolic enzymes, monoamine

oxidase (MAO) and catechol-O-methyl transferase (COMT)[17–19]. As a result, it increases the availability at the synapse of these monoamines linked to the maintenance of normal emotional tone. Estrogens may further enhance the effect of 5-hydroxytryptamine and noradrenaline by increasing the affinity of certain types of noradrenergic and serotonergic receptors for these neurotransmitters[20] and also potentiate the activity of opiate-containing neurons[21].

Estrogens also modulate neuronal plasticity and synaptogenesis in the adult as well as the developing brain[22]: estradiol increases the number of excitatory synapses in a number of different brain areas, including the hippocampus; surgical menopause results in reduced formation of such synapses in animal models[22].

Finally, estrogens also affect neuronal firing by acting directly on the neuronal membrane. They exert an excitatory neuronal effect by augmenting both the N-methyl-D-asparate (NMDA) and non-NMDA glutamate receptor activity[23,24].

Behaviorally, estrogens have arousing and antidepressant effects in animal models of depression. In surgically menopausal (i.e. castrated) rats, this effect is similar in magnitude to the effect of tricyclic antidepressants[25]. This may be due to potentiation of the serotonergic, noradrenergic and opioidergic activity described above.

Progesterone receptors are found in most ER-containing brain regions, and in some areas such as cerebral cortex that lack ERs[26]. Progesterone has a slightly negative effect on the serotonergic and noradrenergic systems[16,17,20,27], by downregulating the genomic expression of tryptophan hydroxylase and by increasing the activity of MAO. It may thus reduce the amount of 5-hydroxytryptamine and noradrenaline available at the synapse. It decreases the number of dendritic spines and synapses on hippocampal CA1 pyramidal neurons, counteracting the stimulatory effects of estradiol[22].

Progesterone's most profound neuronal effect, however, results from its direct effect on the neuronal membrane. Progesterone has an inhibitory effect on neuronal excitation, depressing neuronal firing[10,28,29]. Most of the membrane effect of progesterone is due to the action of its metabolites, the 3α,5β-hydroxylated metabolite pregnanolone and, in particular, the 3α,5α-hydroxylated metabolite, 3α-hydroxy-5α-pregnane-20-one or allopregnanolone[28,29]. Allopregnanolone hyperpolarizes neurons by potentiating GABA-mediated synaptic inhibition[28–30]. It acts at a neurosteroid-specific site on the GABA$_A$ receptor to facilitate chloride channel opening and prolong the inhibitory action of GABA on neurons[28–30]. Allopregnanolone is one of the strongest ligands of GABA$_A$ receptors in the CNS, with a potency similar to that of the most potent benzodiazepines and approximately a thousand times higher than pentobarbital[28,30]. The parent steroid, progesterone, enhances GABA-induced chloride currents only weakly and only in high concentrations[28]. Allopregnanolone is devoid of hormonal effects and may, together with other related neuroactive steroids, be thought of as an endogenous regulator of brain excitability with anxiolytic, anticonvulsant and sedative-hypnotic properties[28,29]. Both plasma and brain levels of allopregnanolone rise rapidly in animals exposed to acute stress[28]. In rats, acute withdrawal of progesterone mimicking the premenstrual fall of serum progesterone in humans causes anxiety-like behavior and seizures. This may result from an increased expression of one of the subunits of the GABA$_A$ receptor (the α-4 subunit), which desensitizes the GABA$_A$ receptor to GABA as well as to benzodiazepines[31]. Plasma and brain levels of allopregnanolone parallel those of progesterone in rats throughout the estrous cycle, pregnancy and senescence. In normal women, plasma levels of allopregnanolone correlate with progesterone levels during the menstrual cycle and pregnancy[28]. However, brain activity of progesterone and allopregnanolone is not dependent solely on ovarian and adrenal production, as they are both synthesized *de novo* in the brain[32].

Behaviorally, allopregnanolone has a potent anxiolytic effect in animal models of anxiety which resembles the effect of diazepam[33,34]. In higher doses, progesterone and allopregnanolone have sedating, depressant and potentially anesthetic effects similar to those of the benzodiazepines and barbiturates[28,35]. As already mentioned, acute withdrawal of progesterone can cause anxiety and seizures[31].

In summary, estrogens have arousing, antidepressant and, in excess, potentially anxiogenic effects, while progesterone has, via its metabolite allopregnanolone, potent anxiolytic properties. In addition, it is possible that the rate of change (e.g. withdrawal) of these hormones and the ratio of the hormones may be as important as their absolute levels in determining their overall effect on emotional behavior, as has been shown to occur in epilepsy[36].

There are a number of other steroids with potent and often diverse neuroactive properties. Some of the sulfated neuroactive steroids, for instance, have excitatory neuronal effects. These include pregnenolone sulfate and dehydroepiandrosterone sulfate (DHEAS), the naturally occurring sulfated esters of pregnenolone and of the pregnenolone metabolite DHEA[28]. DHEAS increases neuronal firing when directly applied to neurons by antagonizing the action of GABA at the GABA$_A$ receptor and by facilitating glutamate-induced excitation at the NMDA receptor[28]. By contrast, another metabolite of DHEA and of androstenedione, 3α,5α-17-androstanediol, has GABA$_A$ receptor potentiating properties similar to those of allopregnanolone.

EPIDEMIOLOGICAL STUDIES

A number of epidemiological studies in normal populations have failed to show an increase in the incidence of depression during and after the menopause[37–45]. In large studies in the 1970s, Winokur[37] and Hallstrom[38] showed that women were not at greater risk for depression at the time of their menopause compared to other times during the lifespan. These findings have been confirmed by more recent, even larger studies of general population surveys of women in the 45–55 age bracket[39,40,45]. A number of longitudinal follow-up studies have reached similar conclusions[41–43]. In a 5-year longitudinal follow-up of a cohort of 2565 women aged 45–55 at baseline, Avis and associates[44] showed that the onset of menopause was not associated with increased risk of depression. In some other studies, the data were not as clearly negative. Hunter[43] followed 36 premenopausal women drawn from a cross-sectional survey of women aged 45–55 for 3 years into peri-menopause and menopause. Although the incidence of clinical depression during perimenopause and menopause was 16% versus 2.9% during premenopause, this was not statistically significant because of the small population sample. Kaufert and colleagues[41] followed 477 women aged 45–59, drawn from a survey of 2500 women from the general population, for a period of 3 years with 6 monthly interviews. Although 26% of all women were depressed at least once in the course of the five interviews and 25% of women who were depressed at one interview were also depressed at two or more other inter-views, they concluded that natural menopause did not increase the risk that a woman may become depressed.

Based on all these studies, the American College of Obstetricians and Gynecologists has concluded that 'the climacteric is not associated with an increased risk of depressive disorder in general female population'[46]. However, several studies, including some of those above, have shown that there may be an increased risk for depression in women during the perimeno-pause as opposed to the menopause[44,47–51]. For instance, Avis and associates[44] found that a perimenopausal period of > 27 months duration was associated with increased risk of depression. They termed such perimenopause 'prolonged' and felt that it affected a minority of women[44]. However, perimenopause lasting for more than 2 years is not uncommon. Jaszman[48] showed that the highest incidence of depression and the most severe depression occurred 2–3 years before the cessation of periods[48]. An increase in more minor psycho-logical morbidity as distinct from clinical depression has also been reported in associa-tion with the perimenopause rather than with menopause[42,48,50].

In addition, a number of studies have demonstrated that women with pre-existing depression are more likely to suffer from depression at the time of the climacteric[44,51,52]. This may hold particularly true for women in whom premenopausal depression was associ-ated with reproductive life events. Finally, women with surgical, as distinct from natural, menopause may have an increased risk for depression[53].

The largely negative findings from the general population surveys are in marked con-trast with clinical experience which shows that between 33 and 45% of women who seek medical attention in the menopausal clinic suffer from major depression[47,52,54,55]. In a recent study, Hay and co-workers[51] showed that 37% of women attending menopause clinics were depressed, with a life-long peak of first episode of depression in the 4 years before and after the last menstrual period.

The variance between the negative epidemi-ological and the positive clinical studies may be due to a number of reasons. Methodological problems with the epidemiological studies include definitions of menopause and peri-menopause, and subject inclusion/exclusion criteria. Definition of menopause and of peri-menopause differs between studies. Some studies use cessation of menses as the beginning of menopause and ignore the perimeno-pause[2,7]. Yet the perimenopausal state may begin with somatic symptoms years before amenorrhea and affective/anxiety disorders associated with the climacteric may be most severe or only present during the perimeno-pause[38,44,48,51,54]. Thus, studies that include only amenorrheic women may be excluding a large proportion of the population at risk for depres-sion[40]. Furthermore, most of the epidemio-logical studies that do include pre-, peri- and menopausal groups define premenopause simply by the presence of regular menses, some-times for as short a period as 3 months[39,44], and perimenopause by irregular menses[41–43]. However, women with regular menses may be perimenopausal as determined by the pres-ence of somatic symptoms and altered bio-chemical parameters such as elevation of follicle stimulating hormone (FSH) or decrease in inhibin levels[56]. Inadequate classification of patient groups may lead to erroneous grouping of patients and to erroneous conclusions.

Subject selection may also affect results. Population-based epidemiological studies typically select women in the 45–55 age group[39,40,42–44], often exclude women receiving HRT[40,42,43] and women with a history of hysterectomy and oophorectomy[40,42–44], or fail to provide information about HRT[41,44]. Yet, Harlow and associates[57] have shown that women with natural premature menopause (i.e. menopause at < 46 years) are twice as likely to suffer from treated depression than women with normal menopausal age, 6.6 times so if the menopause occurs before the age of 40[57]. Similarly, women between the age of 50 and 59 who use estrogen have an approximately three times higher rate of depression compared with untreated women[58]. Thus, by excluding these groups, the studies selectively exclude women with affective disorders and are biased towards normalcy.

The nature of the information collected in large epidemiological studies may also not be optimal to evaluate complex clinical conditions such as depression. The surveys are typically done by postal questionnaires with or without subsequent telephone interviews. There is generally a 15–30% response failure[39,40–44]. By contrast, the data from clinic-based studies are derived from detailed clinical encounters with physicians and are likely to contain more detailed, and therefore more accurate clinical information. For all these reasons, the data available from general population surveys may not provide an ideal basis for drawing conclusions about the relationship between mood changes and the climacteric.

Even so, it can be concluded from the epidemiological studies that the majority of women go through the climacteric without clinically significant mood changes. This contrasts with the experience in the clinic where such changes are commonly encountered. One way of reconciling this discrepancy is to consider the possibility that only certain women are at risk for significant affective changes at the time of the climacteric, and that while these women make up a substantial proportion of the clinically evaluated population, their numbers are very small compared to the larger pool of asymptomatic women in the general population surveys. A search for possible subpopulations at risk might be useful in this respect. It has already been established that women with previous depression are at increased risk for suffering from depression at the time of the climacteric[43,51]. Emotional disturbance related to reproductive endocrine changes could result from abnormality in either the brain sites on which hormones act or in the quantity or nature of hormones to which the brain is exposed. Other groups at increased risk might therefore include women with previous history of affective/anxiety disorders in the setting of endocrine fluctuation such as menarche, premenstrual phase and puerperium[59]; women with chronic reproductive endocrine disorders such as polycystic ovarian syndrome, hypothalamic hypogonadism, endometriosis, etc.; and women with altered brain substrate, for instance women with temporal or frontal lobe epilepsy, structural temporal or frontal lobe brain lesions or developmental central nervous system abnormalities[60].

CORRELATIONAL STUDIES

A small number of studies have attempted to correlate serum levels of gonadal hormones with mood during the climacteric. Coope[61] found no correlation between depression, symptoms of well-being and serum estrone and estradiol levels in women treated with estrogen. Furuhjelm and colleagues[62] showed no difference in estradiol levels between postmenopausal women with and without depression. Ballinger and co-workers[63] found no difference in serum levels of estradiol, progesterone, testosterone, androstenedione, prolactin, cortisol, FSH and luteinizing hormone (LH) between depressed and non-depressed perimenopausal and menopausal women. More recent surveys of menopausal and perimenopausal women have confirmed a lack of association between serum estradiol levels and depression[65–67]. By contrast, Sherwin[53,64] and

Gelfand[53] found that in healthy non-depressed women treated with estrogen, mood covaried with circulating estradiol levels and a recent study of women with Alzheimer's disease demonstrated a negative correlation between depression scores and estradiol levels in this group of women[68].

These studies have been interpreted as showing that 'There is no link between estrogen concentrations and depression'[2]. This view has been extrapolated to a belief that there is no relationship between hormone changes and mood changes at the time of the climacteric[1,2].

For a number of reasons, such a conclusion may not be warranted. First, gonadal hormone profiles differ in different stages of the climacteric[69–71]. The perimenopause may last for years and gonadal hormonal secretion may change during it. Estrogen secretion remains normal through most of the perimenopause and may even *increase* episodically during it when, as a result of erratic follicular development, multiple follicles develop during some menstrual cycles[69–71]. Periods of hypo- and hyperestrogenism may alternate[70]. Estrogen levels only drop consistently late in the perimenopause, chiefly during the last few months before cessation of menses as the follicle pool becomes exhausted[69–71]. Random sampling of estrogen levels of a population of perimenopausal women may result in some women with normal, some with increased and some with low estrogen levels, producing a normal average for the group. Reflecting individual fluctuation in estrogen profiles during the perimenopause, somatic symptoms of both estrogen excess and deficiency have been reported in the same individual[69,70]. Psychological symptoms could conceivably also vary in the same individual during the climacteric, *pari passu* with fluctuation of hormone levels. None of the correlational studies specify the time during the course of the climacteric when the levels were drawn. The relationship of fluctuations of estrogen levels longitudinally through the climacteric to psychological symptoms has not been examined.

Second, the menopause is often thought of as an 'estrogen deficiency disease'. The consequences of altered secretion of progesterone and other ovarian hormones have often been neglected[61,66]. In fact, during the perimenopause, the decline in progesterone levels precedes that of estrogens[69,70] as menstrual cycles change from ovulatory to anovulatory[70]. Thus, for a period of time that may last several years, there may be relative excess of serum estrogen levels compared to serum progesterone levels, even though the absolute levels of both may decline[69,70]. Correlation studies which examine only serum estrogen levels in relation to depression[39,63] examine only one of the endocrine variables.

Androgens need also to be considered. Most studies have shown no clear patterns of testosterone and androstenedione changes in menopausal women, and no relationship of androgen levels to well-being or depression[63,67]. But these studies are also subject to methodological limitations. In most studies, androgen levels are drawn randomly at all times of day. Yet there is a diurnal pattern to testosterone secretion (highest levels early in the morning, with a smaller peak in mid-afternoon), with more than two-fold difference between the peak and trough levels. Some studies measure only total testosterone and not the free or bioavailable testosterone[63]. However, clinical status, for instance hyposexuality, correlates not with total testosterone levels but with levels of free or bioavailable testosterone – in certain cases of hyposexuality, total testosterone levels may even be elevated even as free testosterone levels are low[71].

By contrast, a number of studies have shown that DHEA, as well as its metabolite, $3\alpha,5\alpha$, 17-androstanediol, may be altered during the perimenopause/menopause and may contribute to mood changes seen at this time[66,67]. Berr and associates[65] found low DHEAS concentrations correlated with depressive symptomatology in a cross-section of women over 65 years of age. This finding was confirmed in a recent study which showed an association of low levels of DHEAS and depression but no association of depression with estradiol, total and bioavailable testosterone, androstenedione and cortisol in a survey of community-dwelling postmenopausal women (90% of whom were older than 65 years)[66,72]. Cawood and Bancroft[67] also showed DHEA to be positively related to well-being in 141 women aged 40–60 recruited from the community. Estradiol, estrone, progesterone, total testosterone, free androgen index, androstenedione, DHEAS, FSH and LH did not correlate with well-being[67]. The α-reduced metabolite of androstenedione (and, indirectly, of DHEA), 3α,5α,17-androstanediol, a positive modulator of the $GABA_A$ receptor, is lower in menopausal women with anxiety compared with asymptomatic menopausal women. Its serum levels correlate inversely with anxiety scores[73]. Thus, these androgens may affect mood during the climacteric.

Third, most correlational studies have based their conclusions on a small number of serum or urine samples, usually one to four, drawn over a short period of time[61,63,66,67]. No studies have attempted to correlate the rate of change of hormone profiles to evolution of affective symptoms. Yet, it may be that the rate of change (i.e. fall) of hormone secretion and levels may be as important or more important than the absolute (low) hormone levels in the manifestation of affective symptoms[74,75]. Gangar and associates[76] showed that hot flushes occur in perimenopausal women receiving estrogen implants when estrogen levels are in the high-normal range but decreasing. Brincat and co-workers[55,77] described similar findings with depressive symptoms in postmenopausal women. These symptoms improved with treatment with estradiol and testosterone implants, returned after 4–6 months of treatment when estradiol and testosterone levels fell from moderately high to the normal premenopausal range, and were relieved again with further implant treatment. Longitudinal studies to determine the correlation of hormone levels and psychological symptoms are needed.

THERAPEUTIC STUDIES

A large number of therapeutic studies have investigated the effect of hormone replacement on mood, depression and well-being in both clinically depressed and in healthy women, in both natural menopause and in women with post-surgical menopause. These have been reviewed recently[1,8,52].

In healthy menopausal women, estrogen replacement improves mood and increases a sense of well-being[62,64,66,78–81]. The positive mood is associated with higher levels of circulating estrogens[64]. It is enhanced by the addition of testosterone[64] and possibly also by DHEA[81].

There is a consensus that estrogen is effective in treating depressive symptoms and depression in surgically menopausal women[53,82,83]. This effect, too, is increased by the addition of androgens[53,84].

The effect of HRT on clinical depression in naturally perimenopausal/menopausal women is less clear. A number of studies have shown a beneficial effect of estrogen, with or without added androgens[9,52,55,62,75,84,85]. In the most striking of these studies, Klaiber[85] administered very large doses of oral conjugated estrogen to women, including menopausal women with severe depression refractory to standard antidepressant drugs of the 1970s, and found improvement in depression scores compared to placebo. The improvement in depression scores correlated with lowering of levels of the enzyme MAO, the catabolic enzyme of noradrenaline and serotonin. Furuhjelm and co-workers[62] also showed significant improvement in depression in postmenopausal women treated with estradiol. Montgomery and colleagues[55] showed that treatment with high dose of percutaneous estrogens, which produced plasma estradiol levels of higher than 600 pmol/l, was beneficial in climacteric depression, but only in perimenopausal, not menopausal women. Testosterone increased the effect. Schneider and associates[86] showed that postmenopausal women differed in their response to estrogen therapy depending on the degree of their depression. Nine out of ten women with initial scores of less than 18 on the Beck Depression Inventory improved with Premarin® 1.25 mg daily, while six of the ten women whose scores were above 20 at baseline actually became more depressed. A number of recent studies have added to this experience. Thirty-five women using estrogen replacement therapy had lower anxiety symptoms than untreated women in an uncontrolled study[87]. Sixty postmenopausal women treated prospectively with conjugated equine estrogen combined with different doses of medroxyprogesterone improved in their Beck Depression Inventory[88]. A recent double-blind, placebo-controlled study showed a decrease in anxiety during estradiol treatment of postmenopausal women compared with placebo[89]. Another recent double-blind, placebo-controlled study of 34 women with perimenopausal depression showed a decrease in depression scores in 80% of estradiol-treated versus 22% of placebo-treated subjects. Depression scores were lower in the estradiol-treated women compared both to their baseline and to the placebo-treated group[90]. This effect was independent of hot flushes.

By contrast, other studies have shown no difference between estrogens and placebo[61,91,92]. Sherwin[78] found that while estrogen had mood-enhancing effects in non-depressed menopausal women, conventional estrogen doses were ineffective in women with more severe depressive symptoms.

The argument has sometimes been made that response of depressive symptoms to estrogen therapy may be secondary to concomitant improvement in vasomotor and other somatic symptoms (the 'domino theory'). However, Chakravarti and associates[93] showed no association between response of the vasomotor symptoms and depressive symptoms to treatment with Premarin and concluded that vasomotor symptoms were not the cause of depressive symptoms seen during the climacteric. This was confirmed in two recent studies, including one study of 499 women with natural or surgical menopause whose depressive feelings and symptoms of well-being improved independently of symptomatic treatment of vasomotor symptoms with estradiol[80,90].

Estrogen may be effective as an adjunct to the treatment of depression in menopausal women resistant to treatment with tricyclic antidepressants[86], although another study failed to confirm these findings[94]. Recently, estrogen therapy was found to potentiate significantly the antidepressant effect of the selective serotonin re-uptake inhibitors (SSRIs) fluoxetine and sertraline in elderly depressed women[95,96]. A synergistic effect of estrogen with both these classes of antidepressant drugs may relate to the fact that serotonergic activity is reduced in the menopause and is increased with estrogen replacement therapy[27].

Sherwin[83] has stated that 'discrepancies in the results of different studies may be related both to the psychiatric status of the populations that were investigated in individual studies and to the dosages of estradiol administered'. Failure to distinguish between different affective/anxiety disorders may be particularly important. Many studies lump all emotional symptoms into one group. In fact, the emotional changes attending the climacteric are quite diverse. They may include different forms of depression including an agitated form of depression, atypical depression with vegetative symptomatology or a combination of the two, as well as anxiety disorders including general anxiety disorder, panic attacks, phobias and obsessive compulsive disorders. This distinction is important, for different emotional changes could be associated with different gonadal hormonal alterations. During natural perimenopause, when failure of progesterone secretion precedes the decline in estrogen levels and there may be a relative excess ratio of estrogen to progesterone, depression with agitated components or anxiety disorders may be expected to predominate. In contrast, in menopause or late perimenopause, when there is a loss of production of both hormones, vegetative depressive symptoms may be expected to be more common. If estrogen increases the level of arousal, it is possible that it could have a beneficial effect on depressive symptoms associated with lack of energy ('vegetative' depression, according to older psychiatric nomenclature), but exacerbate depressive symptoms associated with increased arousal and anxiety ('agitated' depression). This might explain the finding that depression worsened in some women even in some of the positive studies[85,86]. In Klaiber's study, a small number of women became significantly worse on Premarin®. Furuhjelm, also, found that while the majority of depressed women improved with estradiol treatment 10/28 became worse, in conjunction with very high serum estradiol levels[62]. De Ligniere and Vincens[9] found that in postmenopausal women, a moderate increase of estradiol levels (to physiological luteal levels of 50–150 pg/ml) was associated with improvement in depressive symptoms and a sense of well-being, but an 'excessive' increase in plasma estradiol levels (to > 150 pg/ml) was associated with increase in anxiety, aggressiveness and irritability[9]. There are also reports of patients with refractory depression in whom estrogen treatment precipitated rapid mood cycling and mania[97].

Almost all the hormone replacement trials aimed at treatment of affective symptoms have targeted estrogen replacement, sometimes combined with androgen replacement[1,52]. Progesterone therapy has been neglected. A small number of estrogen trials have included adjunct synthetic progestational therapy, usually with negative mood effects[1,27,88,89]. Grant and Pryse-Davies[98] showed that progestational oral contraceptives exacerbated depression. This was associated with enhanced MOA activity. Magos and co-workers[99] showed that norethisterone added to treatment with subcutaneous estradiol and testosterone implants in menopausal women had adverse behavioral effects compared to placebo. In another study, medroxyprogesterone acetate added to conjugated equine estrogen treatment in 48 healthy, naturally menopausal women dampened mood in a dose-dependent manner[78], a finding that was recently confirmed[100]. However, synthetic progestins may affect the brain and behavior differently from natural progesterone. The metabolic pathways of synthetic progestins and of natural progesterone differ. Natural progesterone is converted to allopregnanolone[28,32], while the synthetic progestins are not. Allopregnanolone is much more potent than progesterone in eliciting the benzodiazepine-like GABA-ergic neuronal[28,30] and behavioral anxiolytic

effects[33,35]. Replacement therapy with synthetic progestins may therefore not have the same psychoactive effects as replacement therapy with natural progesterone. Thus, appropriate progestational HRT has not yet been tried.

To summarize, the findings to date show that estrogen replacement therapy alone is insufficient to treat the majority of women with depression occurring at the time of the climacteric, although it may be useful treatment in women with surgical menopause and may improve the sense of well-being in clinically non-depressed menopausal women; that androgen therapy may be beneficial in addition to estrogen; and that synthetic progestins have a negative effect on the mood of women in the climacteric. It is also apparent, however, that there are certain women with depression at the time of perimenopause/menopause who do improve with estrogen treatment; that estrogen may be useful adjunct antidepressant therapy with standard antidepressant treatment such as SSRIs and tricyclics; and, finally, that some women with depression at the time of the climacteric may actually get worse with estrogen replacement therapy. The questions that remain unanswered are:

(1) Whether there are certain subgroups of women with affective and anxiety symptoms who are likely to improve and others who may get worse with estrogen therapy;

(2) What role natural progesterone may have in treatment of women with depression and anxiety, both alone and in conjunction with estrogen;

(3) Whether there may be a role for a more physiological HRT with combined treatment of estrogen, cyclical natural progesterone and androgens.

An intriguing thought is the possibility that affective/anxiety symptoms might change in a given woman in the course of the climacteric as her hormonal profile changes and that she might benefit from different combination of HRT at different points of the climacteric.

OTHER CONSIDERATIONS

The role of the brain

The role of the brain often gets overlooked. The effects of gonadal hormones on the brain depend not only on the hormones themselves but also on the specific brain sites with which the hormones interact. Abnormality in either the brain sites on which the hormones act or in the quantity or nature of hormones to which the brain is exposed may result in abnormal emotional manifestation in the context of reproductive endocrine change. The majority of women have normal hormones acting on normal brains, and adjust to the altered perimenopausal hormonal milieu without difficulties. In contrast, in women suffering from abnormal hormonal environment (for instance in polycystic ovarian syndrome) or abnormal brain substrate, fluctuation of gonadal hormones during the climacteric may produce emotional imbalance. Brain abnormalities may include not only such clinically distinct entities as seizures or structural lesions affecting temporal or frontal lobes, but also clinically asymptomatic women with subtle neurological findings disclosed only on examination or with electroencephalography (EEG) or neuroimaging[60]. In fact, markers of anomalous brain substrates such as left-handedness, subtle neurological findings of hemispheric dysfunction, significant lateralized skeletal asymmetry and paroxysmal EEG abnormalities are significantly more common among women with perimenopausal depression than among unaffected controls[60]. Hormonal effects, therefore, may tend to be exaggerated in women with an abnormal or anomalous temporolimbic brain substrate and psychiatric disorders at the time of the climacteric[60,63].

Different subtypes of affective disorders

Distinction needs to be made in correlational and therapeutic studies between different subsets of affective symptoms. Estrogen has antidepressant, arousing and potentially anxiogenic properties, while progesterone has anxiolytic and potentially sedating and depressive properties. Fluctuation of the two sets of hormones may therefore be expected to correlate with different sets of symptoms. Relative progesterone deficiency, perimenopausal increase in estrogen secretion and increase in the estrogen to progesterone ratio might be expected to be associated with symptoms of anxiety and agitated depression and exacerbation of hypomania. Decline in estrogen secretion, on the other hand, might be expected to be associated more with vegetative depressive symptoms.

EXAMPLE CASE REPORTS

A few example case reports may help to illustrate the kinds of problems encountered in the clinic and how they may be dealt with.

Patient 1

A 44-year-old woman presented with an 8-month history of 'constant PMS (premenstrual syndrome)', and a 4-month history of anxiety, agitation, irritability, of feeling depressed and of rare panic attacks. She had had irregular menses for 1 year, with hot flushes and sweating for 2 months. Past history was positive for premenstrual syndrome (anxiety, irritability, crying) and postpartum depression with panic attacks. Family history was positive for left-handedness and autoimmune disorders. Treatment had included nortriptyline, clonazepam and, for 3 weeks, premarin which had increased her irritability and anxiety. Serum estradiol was 69 ng/l, (estrone level not determined) and mid-luteal progesterone was normal at 13.3 μg/l. FSH was 15 IU. She was felt to have agitated depression in the setting premature perimenopause. Treatment with micronized oral progesterone 200 mg three times a day led to resolution of psychiatric symptoms (while vasomotor symptoms persisted). Hamilton Depression Rating Scale scores improved from 11 to 2, and profile of mood scale tension subscore improved from 20/36 to 9/36. Post-treatment estradiol level was 76 ng/l, progesterone 35.7 μg/l, with estradiol/progesterone ratio dropping from

0.0051 pretreatment to 0.0021 after treatment. The patient was drowsy on this dose. Drowsiness abated with progesterone dose reduction to 100 mg four times a day. The patient stopped nortriptyline and clonazepam and has remained well during a 3-year follow-up.

Patient 2

A 55-year-old woman was referred for a second neurological evaluation of possible dementia. She had undergone hysterectomy and bilateral oophorectomy for ovarian carcinoma 5 years previously, with no relapse. She had suffered from depression for 15 years. The depression became worse after the oophorectomy. She had passive suicidal thoughts, impaired motivation and concentration, leading to the loss of a highly demanding job. Medroxyprogesterone caused fatigue. Unsuccessful psychiatric treatments had included doxepin, imipramine and trifluoperazine. Past medical history was positive for prematurity and well-substituted hypothyroidism, PMS with irritability and insomnia, and postpartum depression in two out of two pregnancies, with crying and lack of energy. Examination showed the patient to be depressed and neurologically normal. Serum estradiol level was 10 ng/l, progesterone 0.4 µg/l. Within 1 week of starting treatment with Estraderm® patch 0.05 mg twice weekly her symptoms resolved. She started a new job and discontinued imipramine and Stelazine®. Her Hamilton Depression Rating Scale score improved from 21 pretreatment to 2. Serum estradiol increased to 92 ng/l with unchanged progesterone level. Estradiol/progesterone ratio increased from 0.025 pretreatment to 0.23 on treatment. She has remained symptom-free for 2½ years.

Patient 3

A 59-year-old woman was seen because of a 14-month history of compulsive behavior (incessant apologizing for what she considered to be intrusive behavior), leading to job loss and virtual house-incarceration. She also had mild anxiety and depression. The symptoms started at the same time as sweating, hot flushes and loss of libido. Past history included 6 months of compulsive cleaning, aged 50, after the death of her brother, anorexia–bulimia at the age of 15, secondary amenorrhea, ovarian cysts and fibroids, agitation and anxiety with oral contraceptive treatment. She had not had postpartum depression or PMS. Her mother had suffered from depression at the time of menopause. Past unsuccessful treatment had included sertraline, loxapine and nortriptyline. Fluoxetine had exacerbated the symptoms. Clomipramine and fluvoxamine were partially effective but were associated with drowsiness. Current HRT included estropipate. Serum estradiol was 281 ng/l and progesterone was 0.20 µg/l. The patient was diagnosed as having obsessive compulsive disorder, anxiety and mild agitated depression coincidental with perimenopause. The symptoms improved with treatment with progesterone 100 mg p.o. t.i.d. on calendar days 1–15 and resolved completely with 200 mg three times a day. Hamilton Depression Rating Scale score improved from 18 to 11, and the Yale–Brown obsessive-compulsive questionnaire score improved from 20/40 to 5/40. Progesterone level rose to 29 µg/l (serum estradiol of 275 ng/l) and serum estradiol/progesterone ratio dropped from 1.402 pretreatment to 0.009. The patient has remained well for 3 years.

CONCLUSION

Despite the considerable research efforts that have been directed at the relationship of mood changes to the climacteric over the recent decades, the basic question as to whether hormonal changes are associated with mood changes during the climacteric remains unanswered. Future research needs to incorporate recent advances in our knowledge of the CNS action of gonadal steroid hormones and related neurosteroids, and to study susceptible populations of women to supplement the studies of general population. In particular, greater attention needs to be paid to the possible role of progesterone and allopreg-nanolone, in addition to that of estrogen and androgens. In the meantime, the clinician should keep an open mind to the fact that both biological and psychosocial factors might contribute, individually or in combination, to the patient's emotional lability at the time of the climacteric and manage her accordingly.

References

1. Pearce J, Hawton K, Blake F. Psychological and sexual symptoms associated with the menopause and the effects of hormone replacement therapy. *Br J Psychiatry* 1995;167:163–73
2. Hunter MS. Depression and the menopause. *Br Med J* 1996;313:1043–4
3. Barlow DH. Who understands the menopause? *Br J Obstet Gynaecol* 1997;107:879–80
4. Klein P, Versi E, Herzog AG. Mood and the menopause. *Br J Obstet Gynaecol* 1999;106:1–4
5. Jackson SW. *Melancholia and Depression: from Hippocratic Times to Modern Times.* New Haven, CT: Yale University Press, 1986
6. Gitlin MJ, Pasnau RO. Psychiatric syndromes linked to reproductive function in women: a review of current knowledge. *Am J Psychiatry* 1989;146:1413–22
7. Nicol Smith L. Causality, menopause and depression: a critical review of the literature. *Br Med J* 1996;313:1129–32
8. Panay N, Studd JWW. The psychotherapeutic effects of estrogens. *Gynecol Endocrinol* 1998; 12:353–65
9. de Lignieres B, Vincens M. Differential effects of exogenous oestradiol and progesterone on mood in different post-menopausal women: individual dose/effect relationship. *Maturitas* 1982;4:67–72
10. McEwen BS. Nongenomic and genomic effects of steroids on neural activity. *Trends Pharmacol Sci* 1991;12:141–7
11. Frye CA, Reed TAW. Androgenic neurosteroids: anti-seizure effects in animal model of epilepsy. *Psychoneuroendocrinology* 1998;23:385–99
12. Simerly RB, Chang C, Muramatsu M, *et al.* Distribution of androgen and estrogen receptor mRNA-containing cells in the rat brain: an *in situ* hybridization study. *J Comp Neurol* 1990; 294:76–95
13. Flugge G, Oertel WH, Wuttke W. Evidence for oestrogen-receptive GABAergic neurons in the preoptic/anterior hypothalamic area of the rat brain. *Neuroendocrinology* 1986;43:1–5
14. Morrell JI, McGinty JF, Pfaff DW. A subset of 5β-endorphin- or dynorphin-containing neurons in the medial basal hypothalamus accumulates estradiol. *Neuroendocrinology* 1986; 41:417–26
15. Wallis GJ, Luttge WG. Influence of estrogen and progesterone on glutamic acid decarboxylase activity in discrete regions of rat brain. *J Neurochem* 1980;34:609–13
16. Pecins-Thompson M, Brown NA, Kohama SG, *et al.* Ovarian steroid regulation of tryptophan hydroxylase mRNA expression in rhesus macaques. *J Neurosci* 1996;16:7021–9
17. Luine VN, Khylchevskaya R, McEwen BS. Effect of gonadal steroids on activities of monoamine oxidase and choline acetyl transferase in rat brain. *Brain Res* 1975;86:293–306
18. Briggs M, Briggs M. The relationship between monoamine oxidase activity and sex hormone concentrations in human blood plasma. *J Reprod Fertil* 1972;29:447–50
19. Fishman J. Biological action of catechol estrogens. *J Endocrinol* 1981;89:59–65
20. Biegnon A, Reches A, Snyder L, McEwen BS. Serotonergic and noradrenergic receptors in the rat brain: modulation by chronic exposure to ovarian hormones. *Life Sci* 1983;32:2015–21
21. Barden N, Merand Y, Ruleau D, *et al.* Changes in the β-endorphin content of discrete hypothalamic nuclei during the estrous cycle of the rat. *Brain Res* 1981;204:441–5
22. Woolley CS, McEwen BS. Roles of estradiol and progesterone in regulation of hippocampal dendritic spine density during the estrous cycle in the rat. *J Comp Neurol* 1993;336:293–306
23. Smith SS. Estrogen administration increases neuronal responses to excitatory amino acids as a long term effect. *Brain Res* 1989;503:354–7
24. Wong M, Moss RL. Long-term and short-term electrophysiological effects of estrogen on

the synaptic properties of hippocampal CA1 neurons. *J Neurosci* 1992;12:3217–25

25. Bernardi M, Vergoni AV, Sandrini M, *et al.* Influence of ovariectomy, estradiol and progesterone on the behavior of mice in an experimental model of depression. *Physiol Behav* 1989; 45:1067–8

26. McEwen BS, Davis P, Gerlach J, *et al.* Progestin receptors in the brain and pituitary gland. In: Bardin CW, Mauvais-Jarvis J, Milgrom R, eds. *Progesterone and Progestins.* New York: Raven Press, 1983:59–76

27. Halbreich U. Role of estrogen in post-menopausal depression. *Neurology* 1997;48 (Suppl 7):S16–20

28. Paul SM, Purdy RH. Neuroactive steroids. *FASEB J* 1992;6:2311–22

29. Gee KW, McCauley LD, Lan NC. A putative receptor for neurosteroids on the GABA receptor complex: the pharmacological properties and therapeutic potential of epalons. *Crit Rev Neurobiol* 1995;8:207–27

30. Majewska MD, Harrison NL, Schwartz RD, *et al.* Steroid hormone metabolites and barbiturate-like modulators of the GABA receptor. *Science* 1986;232:1004–7

31. Smith SS, Gong QH, Hsu FC, *et al.* GABA-A receptor α-4 subunit suppression prevents withdrawal properties of an endogenous steroid. *Nature* 1998;392:926–9

32. Cheney DL, Uzunov D, Costa E, Guidotti A. Gas chromatographic-mass fragmentographic quantitation of 3α-hydroxy-5α-pregnan-20-one (allopregnanolone) and its precursors in blood and brain in adrenalectomised and castrated rats. *J Neurosci* 1995;15:4641–50

33. Bitran D, Purdy RH, Kellogg CK. Anxiolytic effect of progesterone is associated with increases in cortical allopregnanolone and GABA-A receptor function. *Pharmacol Biochem Behav* 1993;45:423–8

34. Carboni E, Wieland S, Lan NC, Gee KW. Anxiolytic properties of endogenously occurring pregnanediols in two rodent models of anxiety. *Psychopharmacol* 1996;126:173–8

35. Selye H. The anesthetic effect of steroid hormones. *Proc Soc Exp Biol Med* 1941;46:116–21

36. Backstrom T. Epileptic seizures in women related to plasma estrogen and progesterone during the menstrual cycle. *Acta Neurol Scand* 1976;54:321–47

37. Winokur G. Depression and the menopause. *Am J Psychiatry* 1973;130:92–3

38. Hallstrom T. Sexuality in the climacteric. *Clin Obstet Gynecol* 1977;4:227–39

39. McKinlay JB, McKinlay SM, Brambilla DJ. The relative contributions of endocrine changes and social circumstances to depression in mid-aged women. *J Health Soc Behav* 1987;28:345–63

40. Holte A. Influences of natural menopause on health complaints; a prospective study of healthy Norwegian women. *Maturitas* 1992;14:127–41

41. Kaufert PA, Gilbert P, Tate R. The Manitoba project: a re-examination of the link between menopause and depression. *Maturitas* 1992;14:143–56

42. Hunter MS. Somatic experience of the menopause: a prospective study. *Psychosom Med* 1990;52:357–67

43. Hunter M. The South-East England longitudinal study of the climacteric and postmenopause. *Maturitas* 1992;14:117–26

44. Avis NE, Brambilla D, McKinlay SM, Vass KA. A longitudinal analysis of the association between menopause and depression. *Ann Epidemiol* 1994;4:214–20

45. Kessler RC, McGonagle KA, Swartz M, *et al.* Sex and depression in the National Comorbidity Survey. I. Lifetime prevalence, chronicity and recurrence. *J Affect Disord* 1993;29:85–96

46. American College of Physicians. Guidelines for counseling postmenopausal women about preventive hormone therapy. *Ann Int Med* 1992;117:1038–41

47. Stewart DE, Boydell KM. Psychologic distress during menopause: associations across the reproductive life cycle. *Int J Psychiatry Med* 1993;23:157–62

48. Jaszman L. Epidemiology of the climacteric complaints. *Horm Res* 1973;2:220–34

49. Ballinger CB. Psychiatric morbidity and the menopause; screening of general population sample. *Br Med J* 1975;3:344–6

50. Hallstrom T, Samuelsson S. Mental health in the climacteric. The longitudinal study of women in Gothenburg. *Acta Obstet Gynecol Scand Suppl* 1985;130:13–18

51. Hay AG, Bancroft J, Johnstone EC. Affective symptoms in women attending a menopause clinic. *Br J Psychiatry* 1994;164:513–16

52. Pearlstein TB. Hormones and depression: what are the facts about premenstrual syndrome, menopause, and hormone replacement therapy? *Am J Obstet Gynecol* 1995;173:646–53

53. Sherwin BB, Gelfand MM. Differential symptom response to parental estrogen and/or androgen administration in the surgical menopause. *Am J Obstet Gynecol* 1985;151:153–60

54. Ballinger CB. Psychiatric morbidity and the menopause: survey of a gynaecological outpatient clinic. *Br J Psychistry* 1977;131:83–9

55. Montgomery JC, Brincat M, Tapp A, *et al.* Effect of estrogen and testosterone implants on psychological disorders in the climacteric. *Lancet* 1987;1:297–9

56. Santoro N, Adel T, Skumick JH. Decreased inhibin tone and increased activin A secretion characterize reproductive ageing in women. *Fertil Steril* 1999;71:658–62

57. Harlow BL, Cramer DW, Annis KM. Association of medically treated depression and age at natural menopause. *Am J Epidemiol* 1995;141: 1170–6

58. Palinkas LA, Barrett-Connor E. Estrogen use and depressive symptoms in postmenopausal women. *Obstet Gynecol* 1992;80:30–6

59. Sherwin BB. Estrogenic effects on the central nervous system: clinical aspects. In: Lindsay R, Dempster DW, Jordan CV, eds. *Estrogens and Antiestrogens.* Philadelphia: Lippincott-Raven Publishers, 1997

60. Herzog AG. Perimenopausal depression: possible role of anomalous brain substrates. *Brain Dysfunct* 1989;2:146–54

61. Coope J. Is oestrogen therapy effective in the treatment of menopausal depression? *J Royal Coll Pract* 1981;31:134–40

62. Furuhjelm M, Karlgren E, Carlstrom K. The effect of estrogen therapy on somatic and psychical symptoms in postmenopausal women. *Acta Obstet Gynecol Scand* 1984;63: 655–61

63. Ballinger CB, Browning MCK, Smith AHW. Hormone profiles and psychological symptoms in perimenopausal women. *Maturitas* 1987;9: 235–51

64. Sherwin BB. Affective changes with estrogen and androgen replacement therapy in surgically menopausal women. *J Affect Disord* 1988; 14:177–87

65. Berr C, Lafont S, Debuire B, *et al.* Relationship of dehydroepiandrosterone sulfate in the elderly with functional, psychological, and mental status, and short-term mortality: a French community-based study. *Proc Natl Acad Sci USA* 1996;93:13410–15

66. Barrett-Connor E, Kritz-Silverstein D. Estrogen replacement and cognitive function in older women. *J Am Med Assoc* 1993;269:2637–41

67. Cawood EHH, Bancroft J. Steroid hormone, the menopause, sexuality and well-being of women. *Psychol Med* 1996;26:925–36

68. Carlson LE, Sherwin BB, Chertkow HM. Relationships between mood and estradiol (E2) levels in Alzheimer's disease (AD) patients. *J Gerontol B Psychol Sci Soc Sci* 2000; 55:P47–53

69. Burger HC, Dudley EC, Hopper JL, *et al.* The endocrinology of the menopausal transition: a cross-sectional study of a population-based sample. *J Clin Endocrinol Metab* 1995;80:3537–45

70. Santoro N, Brown JR, Adel T, *et al.* Characterization of reproductive hormonal dynamics in the perimenopause. *J Clin Endocrinol Metab* 1996; 81:1495–1501

71. Herzog AG. Hormonal changes in epilepsy. *Epilepsia* 1995;36:323–6

72. Barrett-Connor E, von Muhlen D, Laughlin GA, Kripke A. Endogenous levels of dehydroepiandrosterone sulfate, but not other sex hormones, are associated with depressed mood in older women: the Rancho Bernardo Study. *J Am Geriatr Soc* 1999;47:685–91

73. Barbaccia ML, Lello S, Sidiropoulou T, *et al.* Plasma 5alpha-androstane-3 alpha, 17betadiol, an endogenous steroid that positively modulates GABA (A) receptor function, and anxiety: a study in menopausal women. *Psychoneuroendocrinology* 2000;25:659–75

74. Schmidt PJ, Rubinow DR. Menopausal mood disorders. In Demers LM, Phillips A, McGuire JL, Rubinow DR, eds. *Premenstrual, Postpartum, and Menopausal Mood Disorders.* Baltimore, MD: Urban & Schwarzenberg, 1997

75. Khasttgir G, Studd JWW. Is there a hormonal basis to hysterectomy-related depression? *Br J Obstet Gynaecol* 1999;106:620–2

76. Gangar KF, Cust MP, Whitehead MI. Symptoms of oestrogen deficiency associated with supraphysiological plasma oestradiol concentrations in women with oestradiol implants. *Br Med J* 1989;299:601–2

77. Brincat M, Studd JWW, O Dowd T, *et al.* Subcutaneous hormone implants for the control of climacteric symptoms. *Lancet* 1984;i:16–17

78. Sherwin B. The impact of different doses of estrogen and progestin on mood and sexual behavior in postmenopausal women. *J Endocrinol Metab* 1991;72:336–43

79. Ditkoff EC, Cary WG, Cristo M, Lobo R. Estrogen improves psychological function in asymptomatic postmenopausal subjects. *Obstet Gynecol* 1991;78:991–5

80. Limouzin-Lamothe MA, Mairon N, Joyce CRB, Le Gal M. Quality of life after the menopause: influence of hormonal replacement therapy. *Am J Obstet Gynecol* 1994;170:618–24

81. Morales AJ, Nolan JJ, Nelson JA, Yen SS. Effect of replacement dose of dehydroepiandrosterone in men and women of advancing age. *J Clin Endocrinol Metab* 1994;78:1360–7

82. Dennerstein L, Burrows GD, Hyman GJ, Sharpe K. Hormone therapy and affect. *Maturitas* 1979; 1:247–59

83. Sherwin B. Hormones, mood and cognitive functioning in post-menopausal women. *Obstet Gynecol* 1996;87(Suppl):20S–6S

84. Sarrel PM. Psychosexual effects of menopause: role of androgens. *Am J Obstet Gynecol* 1999;180: S319–24

85. Klaiber EL, Broverman DM, Vogel W, *et al.* Estrogen therapy for severe persistent

depression in women. *Arch Gen Psychiatry* 1979;36:550–4

86. Schneider MA, Brotherton PL, Hailes J. The effect of oestrogens on depression in menopausal women. *Med J Aust* 1977;2:162–3

87. Boyle GJ, Murrihy R. A preliminary study of hormone replacement therapy and psychological mood states in perimenopausal women. *Psychol Rep* 2001;88:160–70

88. Bukhulmez O, Al A, Gurdal H, *et al.* Short-term effects of three continuous hormone replacement therapy regimens on a platelet tritiated imipramine binding and mood scores: a prospective randomized trial. *Fertil Steril* 2001; 75:737–43

89. Linzmayer L, Semluitsch HV, Saletu B, *et al.* Double-blind, placebo-controlled psychometric studies on the effects of a combined estrogen-progestin regimen versus estrogen alone on performance, mood and personality of menopausal syndrome patients. *Arzneimittelforschung* 2001;51:238–45

90. Schmidt PJ, Nieman L, Danaceau MA, *et al.* Estrogen replacement in perimenopause-related depression: a preliminary report. *Am J Obstet Gynecol* 2000;183:414–20

91. Strickler RC, Borth R, Cecutti A, *et al.* The role of oestrogen replacement in the climacteric syndrome. *Psychol Med* 1977;7:631–9

92. Coope J, Thomson JM, Poller L. Effects of 'natural oestrogen' replacement therapy on menopausal symptoms and blood clotting. *Br Med J* 1975;4:139–43

93. Chakravarti S, Collins WP, Thom MH, Studd JWW. Relation between plasma hormone profiles, symptoms, and response to oestrogen treatment in women approaching the menopause. *Br Med J* 1979;1:983–5

94. Shapira B, Oppenheim G, Zohar J, *et al.* Lack of efficacy of estrogen supplementation to imipramine in resistant female depressives. *Biol Psychiatry* 1985;20:576–9

95. Schneider LS, Small GW, Hamilton SH, *et al.* Estrogen replacement and response to fluoxetine in multicenter geriatric depression trial. Fluoxetine collaborative study group. *Am J Geriatr Psych* 1977;5:97–106

96. Schneider LS, Small GW, Clary CM. Estrogen replacement therapy and antidepressant response to sertaline in older depressed women. *Am J Geriatr Psychiatr* 2001;9:393–9

97. Oppenheim G. A case of rapid mood cycling with estrogen: implication for therapy. *J Clin Psychiatr* 1984;45:34–5

98. Grant ECG, Pryse-Davies J. Effect of oral contraceptives on depressive mood changes and on endometrial monoamine oxidase and phosphatases. *Br Med J* 1968;3:777–80

99. Magos AL, Brewster E, Singh R, *et al.* The effects of norethisterone in postmenopausal women on oestrogen replacement therapy: a model for the premenstrual syndrome. *Br J Obstet Gynaecol* 1986;93:1290–6

100. Natale V, Albertazzi P, Zini M, Di Micco R. Exploration of cyclical changes in memory and mood in postmenopausal women taking sequential combined oestrogen and progestogen preparations. *Br J Obstet Gynaecol* 2001;108:286–90

12

Premenstrual syndrome and the menopause

S. O'Brien, K. M. K. Ismail and K. Jain

INTRODUCTION

Many women develop premenstrual syndrome (PMS) in the years before the menopause, and treatment of their symptoms may be difficult. Many other women on reaching the menopause require treatment with conventional, cyclical estrogen–progestogen hormone replacement therapy (HRT) preparations. A good understanding of premenstrual disorders is essential to those who manage patients at the menopause. It is also true that those who manage PMS must understand the mechanism and management of the menopause. There are several reasons for this:

(1) For many women premenstrual syndrome and the natural pre- menopause appear to dovetail.

(2) Several treatment methods for PMS involve producing a surgical or medical menopause, the symptoms and consequences of which may require treating.

(3) The introduction of sequential HRT frequently reintroduces premenstrual symptoms in susceptible women

The aim of this chapter is to provide a PMS update and to introduce the concept that this syndrome could be reintroduced by HRT. The first part of the chapter outlines what is considered to be the current status of knowledge concerning terminology, diagnosis, etiology and management of PMS. The management section includes treatment methods, which involve the induction of a menopausal state, be

it permanent or temporary. The second part introduces the concept of HRT-induced PMS and its possible etiology, and highlights some strategies that could be adopted in the clinical setting to avoid it. This is an important section, because HRT-induced PMS seems to be a frequent reason for discontinuation of HRT.

PREMENSTRUAL DISORDERS

The terminology is confusing; general practitioners, gynecologists and psychiatrists have different views.

Premenstrual symptoms occur in 95% of all women of reproductive age, and are thus physiological. The term 'premenstrual symptoms' covers everything, but is not a diagnosis. So many women have symptoms to some degree that they can probably be considered as physiological changes of the ovulatory menstrual cycle.

Premenstrual tension (PMT) was first described in the USA (Frank, 1931), but is now considered an old-fashioned term used predominantly in the lay press.

Premenstrual syndrome (PMS) is a severe form of premenstrual symptoms having a major impact on the patient's normal functioning[1]. Psychiatrists often use this term for the milder symptoms but it is the term used by gynecologists in the case of severely affected patients.

Late luteal phase dysphoric disorder (LLPDD) is a term no longer used, and is replaced by the term *premenstrual dysphoric disorder (PMDD)*.

Table 1 Research criteria for premenstrual dysphoric disorder. Reproduced with permission from the Diagnostic and Statistical Manual of Mental Disorders, 4th edn. Washington: American Psychiatric Association, 1994[2]

A   In most menstrual cycles during the past year, five (or more) of the following symptoms were present for most of the time during the last week of the luteal phase, began to remit within a few days after the onset of the follicular phase, and were absent in the week post-menses, with at least one of the symptoms being either (1), (2), (3) or (4):

(1)   Markedly depressed mood, feelings of hopelessness, or self-deprecating thoughts;

(2)   Marked anxiety, tension, feelings of being 'keyed up,' or 'on edge';

(3)   Marked affective lability (e.g. feeling suddenly sad or tearful or increased sensitivity to rejection);

(4)   Persistent and marked anger or irritability or increased interpersonal conflicts;

(5)   Decreased interest in usual activities (e.g. work, school, friends, hobbies);

(6)   Subjective sense of difficulty in concentrating;

(7)   Lethargy, easy fatigability or marked lack of energy;

(8)   Marked change in appetite, overeating or specific food cravings;

(9)   Hypersomnia or insomnia;

(10)   A subjective sense of being overwhelmed or out of control;

(11)   Other physical symptoms, such as breast tenderness or swelling, headaches, joint or muscle pain, a sensation of bloating, weight gain.

Note In menstruating females, the luteal phase corresponds to the period between ovulation and the onset of menses, and the follicular phase begins with menses. In non-menstruating females (e.g. those who have had a hysterectomy), the timing of luteal and follicular phases may require measurement of circulating reproductive hormones.

B   The disturbance markedly interferes with work or school or with usual social activities and relationships with others (e.g. avoidance of social activities, decreased productivity and efficiency at work or school).

C   The disturbance is not merely an exacerbation of the symptoms of another disorder, such as major depressive disorder, panic disorder, dysthymic disorder or a personality disorder (although it may be superimposed on any of these disorders).

D   Criteria A, B and C must be confirmed by prospective daily ratings during at least two consecutive symptomatic cycles. (The diagnosis may be made provisionally prior to this confirmation.)

PMDD is an important term devised by the American Psychiatric Association Advisory Committee to the Workshop group for the 4th edition of the *Diagnostic and Statistical Manual of Mental Disorders* (DSM-IV)[2]. PMDD has very strict criteria and represents the extreme end of the PMS spectrum; it relates almost exclusively to psychological symptoms (Table 1). Although this definition only reluctantly acknowledges the existence of physical symptoms, it would be reasonably safe to consider severe PMS and PMDD as being synonymous.

SYMPTOMS AND DIAGNOSIS

Over 200 PMS symptoms have been documented. Irritability, aggression, tearfulness, loss of control, fatigue and depression are typical psychological symptoms. Breast swelling, abdominal bloatedness and headache are typical physical symptoms. The precise character is less important than the timing of their occurrence. Symptoms must have occurred in the luteal phase of most cycles over the last year.

They must resolve by the end of menstruation. There must be a symptom-free week, i.e. no symptoms in the follicular phase.

An underlying psychological diagnosis must not coexist, and the symptoms must not merely be an accentuation of an underlying disorder such as depression.

The symptoms must be so severe that the patient's normal functioning, her work and her family relationships are disturbed. It is this that distinguishes PMS/PMDD from milder premenstrual symptoms. The patient history is insufficient to make a diagnosis and prospective charts should be given. Figure 1 represents a chart completed prospectively by a patient suffering from PMS.

ETIOLOGY OF PREMENSTRUAL SYNDROME

There have been many theories of PMS etiology. Progesterone deficiency[3] and water retention were popular, but have been largely discredited. Factors other than differences in the levels of individual hormones must be important. Interactions with other endocrine, neuro-endocrine or biochemical systems may operate, or differences in receptor status may be relevant.

Ovulation, suppression of ovulation and PMS

PMS does not exist before puberty, during pregnancy or in the untreated postmenopause. It disappears during gonadotropin-releasing hormone (GnRH) therapy and after bilateral oophorectomy. Therefore, ovulation seems to be the trigger for PMS.

For many gynecological problems, ovulation is suppressed by GnRH analogs, danazol, estradiol, progestogen or removal of the ovaries. In the following paragraphs, the effects of these interventions on the course of PMS are discussed.

GnRH analogs

Suppression of ovulation using injected depot GnRH analogs is highly effective[4]. Unfortunately, discontinuation of therapy results in the return of symptoms, and the long-term effect of such combinations is untested. Therefore, GnRH analogs are mainly used as a diagnostic test for PMS, to exclude an underlying physical or psychological problem. While this test has been shown scientifically to eliminate PMS

Day of cycle	1	2	3	4	5	6	7	8	9	1	1	1	1	1	1	1	1	1	1	2	2	2	2	2	2	2	2	2	2	3	3	3	3	3
										0	1	2	3	4	5	6	7	8	9	0	1	2	3	4	5	6	7	8	9	0	1	2	3	4
Day of month	■	■	■	■	■	■																								■	■	■	■	■
Irritability	3	3	3	1	1	1	0	0	0	0	0	0	0	0	0	0	0	0	0	1	1	3	3	3	2	3	3	2	3	2	3	2	1	1
Mood swings	3	3	3	1	1	1	0	0	0	0	0	0	0	0	0	0	0	0	0	1	1	3	3	3	2	3	3	2	3	2	3	2	1	1
Depression	0	0	0	1	1	0	0	0	0	0	0	0	0	0	0	0	0	0	0	0	0	0	0	0	0	0	0	0	0	0	0	0	0	0
Hostility	3	3	3	1	1	1	0	0	0	0	0	0	0	0	0	0	0	0	0	1	1	3	3	3	2	3	3	2	3	2	3	2	1	1
Sadness	3	3	3	1	1	1	0	0	0	0	0	0	0	0	0	0	0	0	0	1	1	3	3	3	2	3	3	2	3	2	3	2	1	1
Negative thoughts	3	3	3	1	1	1	0	0	0	0	0	0	0	0	0	0	0	0	0	1	1	3	3	3	2	3	3	2	3	2	3	2	1	1
Bloating	3	3	3	1	1	1	0	0	0	0	0	0	0	0	0	0	0	0	0	1	1	3	3	3	2	3	3	2	3	2	3	2	1	1
Breast pain	3	3	3	1	1	1	0	0	0	0	0	0	0	0	0	0	0	0	0	1	1	3	3	3	2	3	3	2	3	2	3	2	1	1
Appetite changes	3	3	3	1	1	1	0	0	0	0	0	0	0	0	0	0	0	0	0	1	1	3	3	3	2	3	3	2	3	2	3	2	1	1
Carbohydrate cravings	3	3	3	1	1	1	0	0	0	0	0	0	0	0	0	0	0	0	0	1	1	3	3	3	2	3	3	2	3	2	3	2	1	1
Hot flushes	0	0	0	1	1	0	0	0	0	0	0	0	0	0	0	1	0	0	0	1	0	0	0	0	1	0	0	0	0	0	0	0	0	1
Insomnia	3	3	3	1	1	1	0	0	0	0	0	0	0	0	0	0	0	0	0	1	1	3	3	3	2	3	3	2	3	2	3	2	1	1
Headache	0	0	0	1	1	0	0	0	0	0	0	0	0	0	0	0	0	0	0	0	0	0	0	0	0	0	0	0	0	0	0	0	0	0
Fatigue	3	3	3	1	1	1	0	0	0	0	0	0	0	1	1	1	1	1	1	0	1	3	3	3	2	3	3	2	3	2	3	2	1	1
Confusion	0	0	0	1	1	0	0	0	0	0	0	0	0	0	0	0	0	0	0	0	0	0	0	0	0	0	0	0	0	0	0	0	0	0
Poor concentration	0	0	0	1	1	0	0	0	0	0	0	0	0	0	0	0	0	0	0	1	0	0	0	2	0	3	0	0	0	0	0	2	1	1
Social withdrawal	0	0	0	1	1	0	0	0	0	0	0	0	0	0	0	0	0	0	0	0	0	0	0	0	0	0	0	0	0	0	0	0	0	0
Hyperphagia	0	0	0	1	1	0	0	0	0	0	0	0	0	0	0	0	0	0	0	0	0	0	0	0	0	0	0	0	0	0	0	0	0	0
Arguing	3	3	3	1	1	1	0	0	0	0	0	0	0	0	0	0	0	0	0	1	1	3	3	3	2	3	3	2	3	2	3	2	1	1
Decreased interest	0	0	0	1	1	0	0	0	0	0	0	0	0	0	0	0	0	0	0	0	0	0	0	0	0	0	0	0	0	0	0	0	0	0

Day 1 is the first day of cycle (ie first day of menses)
Use one chart for each menstrual cycle
luteal phase and, thus, ovulation occurs 14 days before menses

Severity code: 0 none, 1 = mild, 2 = moderate, 3 = severe

Figure 1 Calendar of premenstrual experiences (COPE): a chart completed prospectively by a patient suffering from premenstrual syndrome (PMS). Note the cyclicity of symptoms, occurring mainly premenstrually. The patient also has at least a week free of symptoms

symptoms, it has not been used in the preoperative test scenario in any scientific way.

Danazol

There is good evidence to show that danazol in doses that suppress ovulation is effective for many PMS symptoms, particularly for cyclical mastalgia[5–7]. Unfortunately, this drug has limited use in the long term because of its androgenic side-effects, particularly those on the lipid profile. Studies have attempted to reduce these adverse effects by using a lower dose (200 mg/day) during the luteal phase of the cycle; a positive effect is seen for breast symptoms only and no others[7]. Probably the persistence of ovulation in the latter method of administration is the reason for the inadequate therapeutic effect.

Estrogen

There is good evidence showing that ovulation suppression with estradiol implants or patches (100 and 200 mg) effectively treats PMS[8].

However, estrogen alone incurs the risk of endometrial hyperplasia, and, as discussed below, administration of progestogens can restimulate PMS symptoms. This can be avoided by administering the progestogen via the intra-uterine route (levonorgestrel intrauterine system (IUS)) when systemic levels are low, and thus central nervous system (CNS) stimulation is very unlikely. Data relating to this approach have yet to be published.

Bilateral oophorectomy

Randomized trials of oophorectomy are probably not ethical, and although the procedure is the only curative treatment, it can only rarely be justified. However, it is worth considering if there is an indication for hysterectomy when the patient with extremely severe PMS has to make the decision to conserve or lose her ovaries. The patient must make this well-documented choice after appropriate counseling and informed consent. Undertaking a 'GnRH test' may help this decision.

Progesterone, progestogens and PMS

Because of the previous popularity of the progesterone deficiency theory, progesterone pessaries and progestogens are the most commonly prescribed preparations for PMS in the UK and USA. This is surprising, as there is no evidence to support their continued use; meta-analysis of randomized clinical trials shows them to be no more effective than placebo[9].

Smith and colleagues[10] studied the symptomatology of progesterone intolerance. The commonest symptoms of progesterone intolerance were bloating, mastalgia, mood swings, fatigue, depression, irritability, skin disorders, weight gain and anxiety. The similarity of these symptoms to those of PMS lends support to the theory that progesterone is most probably the trigger hormone for the generation of PMS. However, no differences have been identified in hormone levels following ovulation in women suffering with PMS, compared with asymptomatic controls. Therefore, it seems that women develop PMS because they are hypersensitive to their normal endogenous levels of progesterone produced after ovulation. The concept that women who are hypersensitive to natural progesterone are also hypersensitive to synthetic progestogens is discussed below in more detail.

Neurotransmitters and PMS

The role of serotonin in depression has been extended to PMS research. Low serotonin levels in red cells and platelets[11] have been demonstrated in PMS patients. This serotonin deficiency seems to enhance sensitivity to progesterone. Selective serotonin reuptake inhibitors (SSRIs) have been shown to be an extremely efficacious treatment for severe PMS/PMDD. A recent meta-analysis of 15 trials showed an overall odds ratio of 6.91 in favor of SSRIs[12]. Common adverse effects were headache, nervousness, insomnia, drowsiness/fatigue, sexual dysfunction and gastrointestinal disturbances. Unlike anxiolytics and non-SSRI antidepressants they do not cause dependence.

Fluoxetine (Prozac®) is now licensed for PMDD. Most of the above trials used continuous dosing regimens, but targeted luteal-phase regimens may offer minimal side-effects while maintaining efficacy.

Other neurotransmitters may have relevance to PMS, for example γ-aminobutyric acid (GABA), dopamine and acetylcholine, although research data are less convincing for these in comparison with serotonin. There are relatively new data suggesting that lack of allopregnanolone (a progesterone metabolite which acts as a neurotransmitter and has GABA-ergic activity) may be involved[13]. However, confirmatory data are awaited.

Based on the above observations, a plausible etiological theory, which allows some understanding of the proposed treatment methods for PMS, is as follows. Ovulation is the trigger through the release of progesterone into the circulation. However, there is no hormone excess or deficiency. Women with PMS are thought to be hypersensitive to their own, normal progesterone levels. This progesterone hypersensitivity seems to be secondary to a dysfunctional serotoninergic system.

HRT-INDUCED PREMENSTRUAL SYNDROME

HRT is prescribed to women whose ovarian cycles have ceased (due to the menopause or bilateral oophorectomy), or as part of 'add-back' therapy with GnRH analogs. The benefits of HRT for postmenopausal women are well known. The use of progesterone in HRT is essential to protect the endometrium from stimulation induced by estrogen use[14]. Progestogens prevent endometrial hyperplasia and cancer[15]. However, during the progesterone phase of therapy, a significant percentage of women develop physical and psychological symptoms that are indistinguishable from PMS.

Women known to suffer from PMS and who had undergone hysterectomy and bilateral salpingo-oophorectomy, and who were commenced on cyclical HRT, remained asymptomatic during the estrogen-only phase. However,

they started with PMS-like symptoms while on progestogen. This demonstrates fairly clearly that the patients remained sensitive to the effects of ovarian hormones and that the ovarian hormones were directly responsible for the PMS[16,17].

Magos and colleagues[18] demonstrated the influence of progestogens on mood and behavior. A total of 58 postmenopausal hysterectomized women were treated with subcutaneous estradiol and testosterone implants. There was a dose-dependent increase in depression, loss of energy, loss of libido and mastalgia when norethisterone was added. Severity of symptoms was related to duration of progestogen therapy. Moreover, different progestogens cause different adverse symptoms. Norethisterone is less likely to cause negative-affect complex symptoms, and is possibly more likely to cause pain complex symptoms than either medroxyprogesterone acetate or dydrogesterone[10].

HRT-induced premenstrual symptoms, or even PMS, seem to be a major cause of decreased compliance in HRT users. In studies looking at the reasons for not taking prescribed HRT among menopause clinic attendees, 35–39% of the women on HRT reported PMS-like symptoms. These symptoms were severe enough for some of them to discontinue the treatment[19,20]. The potential severity of the problem is highlighted by a long-term study in which such symptoms led to hysterectomy in 10% of the patients[10]. However, there are few clinical studies addressing this common and important issue.

There are many strategies that could be adopted to decrease the risk of HRT-induced PMS. These include the following:

(1) Continuous progestogen therapy was introduced in an attempt to improve compliance and acceptability of HRT[21,22]. The advantages of the continuous regimen include reduction of bleeding and the possible reduction of progestogen-related subjective and metabolic side effects. This is because of lower overall progestogen doses than those used in sequential regimens[22].

(2) Local progestogen delivery via a levonorgestrel-releasing intrauterine system (LNG-IUS) has been found to be effective in suppressing the endometrium and reversing hyperplasia, in addition to being well accepted by patients[23,24]. This effect is, most probably, secondary to the low serum concentration of levonorgestrel in women using the LNG-IUS, despite the high concentration in the endometrium[25]. Barrington and Bowen-Simpkins[26] found the device to be useful in avoiding PMS symptoms in 56% of the study population.

(3) If the patient is sufficiently beyond the menopause that bleeding will not be a problem, then tibolone may be a suitable option. There is evidence from randomized controlled trials of its benefit in PMS, particularly when used as add-back therapy with GnRH analogs[27,28]. However, the occasional patient complains of PMS symptoms continuously in the first few months of treatment.

(4) Three-monthly-bleed HRT could potentially decrease the frequency of occurrence of HRT-induced PMS, because this will only happen during the progestogenic phase of each 3-monthly cycle. However, this advantage should be balanced against the possibility of increased bleeding problems.

(5) Selective estrogen receptor modulators (SERMs) have virtually no effect on menopausal symptoms. However, if the aim of HRT is to protect bone, then SERMs can be used without development of PMS.

(6) Given the known beneficial response to SSRIs in PMS, a parallel effect may arise in the HRT scenario, although such an approach has not been published.

HRT-induced premenstrual symptoms remain difficult to treat. There have been no large randomized controlled trials to study their prevention or treatment. As this is a major cause of limited compliance in HRT users, attempts should be made to individualize HRT prescribing following careful assessment and counselling.

References

1. O'Brien PMS. *Premenstrual Syndrome*. London: Blackwell Science, 1987
2. DSM-IV, *Diagnostic and Statistical Manual of Mental Disorders*, 4th edn. Washington: American Psychiatric Association, 1994
3. Dalton K. *The Premenstrual Syndrome and Progesterone Therapy*. London: Heinemann, 1977
4. Wyatt K, Ismail KM, Dimmock P, Jones P, O'Brien PMS. GnRH analogues in PMS. Systematic review. *Fertil Steril* 2003; in press
5. Sarno APJ, Miller EJJ, Lundblad EG. Premenstrual syndrome: beneficial effects of periodic, low-dose danazol. *Obstet Gynecol* 1987; 70:33–6
6. Wyatt KM, Dimmock PW, O'Brien PMS. Premenstrual syndrome. In Barton S, ed. *Clinical Evidence*. London: Barton Publishing Group, 2000;1121–33
7. O'Brien PMS, Abukhalil IEH. Randomized controlled trial of the management of premenstrual syndrome and premenstrual mastalgia using luteal phase only danazol. *Am J Obstet Gynecol* 1999;180:18–23
8. Magos AL, Brincat M, Studd JW. Treatment of premenstrual syndrome by subcutaneous oestradiol implants and cyclical oral norethisterone: placebo-controlled study. *Br Med J* 1986;292: 1629–33
9. Wyatt KM, Dimmock PW, Jones PW, O'Brien PMS. Progesterones and progestogens in PMS. Systematic review. *Br Med J* 2001;323:776–80
10. Smith RNJ, Holland EFN, Studd JW. The symptomatology of progestogen intolerance. *Maturitas* 1994;18:87–91
11. Rapkin AJ. The role of serotonin in premenstrual syndrome. *Clin Obstet Gynecol* 1992;35:629–36

12. Dimmock PW, Wyatt KM, Jones PW, O'Brien PMS. Efficacy of selective serotonin-reuptake inhibitors in premenstrual syndrome. A systematic review. *Lancet* 2000;356:1131–6

13. Rapkin AJ, Morgan M, Goldman L, *et al.* Progesterone metabolite allopregnanolone in women with premenstrual syndrome. *Obstet Gynecol* 1997;90:709–14

14. Marsleu V, Riss B, Christiansen C. Progestogens: therapeutic and adverse effects in early post-menopausal women. *Maturitas* 1991;13:7–16

15. Gambrell RD. Prevention of endometrial cancer with progestogens. *Maturitas* 1986;8:159–68

16. Hammarback S, Backstrom T, Hoist J, von Schoultz B, Lyrenas S. Cyclical mood changes as in the premenstrual tension syndrome using sequential oestrogen–progestagen postmenopausal replacement therapy. *Acta Obstet Gynecol Scand* 1985;64:393–7

17. Henshaw C, Foreman D, Belcher J, Cox J, O'Brien PMS. Can one induce premenstrual symptomatology in women with prior hysterectomy and bilateral oophorectomy? *J Psychosom Obstet Gynaecol* 1996;17:21–8

18. Magos AL, Brewster E, Singh R, *et al.* The effects of norethisterone in postmenopausal women on oestrogen replacement therapy: a model of the premenstrual syndrome. *Br J Obstet Gynaecol* 1986; 93:1290–6

19. Mansour D. Management of HRT side effects update. *Menopause* 1999;6:57–8

20. McCleery JM, Gebbie AE. Compliance with hormone replacement therapy at a menopause clinic in a community setting. *Br J Fam Plann* 1994;20:73–5

21. Staland B. Continuous treatment with natural oestrogens and progestogens. A method to avoid endometrial stimulation. *Maturitas* 1981;3: 145–56

22. Mattsson LA, Cullberg G, Samsioe G. Evaluation of a continuous oestrogen – progestogen regimen for climacteric complaints. *Maturitas* 1982;4:95–102

23. Suhonen S, Holmstrom T, Lahteenmaki P. Three year follow up of the use of a levonorgestrel-releasing intrauterine system in hormone replacement therapy. *Acta Obstet Gynecol Scan* 1997;76:145–50

24. Wollter-Svensson LO, Stadberg E, Andersson K, *et al.* Intrauterine administration of levonorgestrel 5 and 10 µg/ 24 hrs in perimenopausal hormone replacement therapy. A randomized clinical study during 1 year. *Acta Obstet Gynecol Scand* 1997;76:449–54

25. Nilsson CG, Haukkamaa M, Vierola H, Luukkainen T. Tissue concentrations of levonorgestrel in women using a levonorgestrel-releasing IUD. *Clin Endocrinol* 1982;17:529–36

26. Barrington JW, Bowen-Simpkins P. The levonorgestrel intrauterine system in the management of menorrhagia. *Br J Obstet Gynaecol* 1997;104:614–16

27. Taskin O, Gokdeniz R, Yalcinoglu A, *et al.*, Placebo-controlled crossover study of effects of tibolone on premenstrual symptoms and peripheral β-endorphin concentrations in premenstrual syndrome. *Hum Reprod* 1998;13: 2402–5

28. Di Carlo C, Palomba S, Tommaselli GA, *et al.* Use of leuprolide acetate plus tibolone in the treatment of severe premenstrual syndrome. *Fertil Steril* 2001;75: 380–4

13

Women, hormones and depression

J. Studd

INTRODUCTION

On Boxing Day 1851, Charles Dickens attended the patients' Christmas dance at St Luke's Hospital for the Insane. On describing his visit in an article for *Household Words*, he commented that the experience of the asylum proved that insanity was more prevalent among women than men. Of the 18 759 inmates over the century, 11 162 had been women. He adds: 'It is well known that female servants are more frequently affected by lunacy than any other class of persons.'

Dickens was as great an observer as any Nobel Prize winner and indeed this passage is one of the very few references in Victorian literature that make the connection between gender and depression, but there are none to my knowledge relating reproductive function to depression. Jane Eyre's red room and Berthe Mason's monthly madness in the same novel may be coded examples of this from Charlotte Bronte's pen. Modern epidemiology confirms that depression is more common in women than men whether we look at hospital admissions, population studies, suicide attempts or the prescription of antidepressants[1]. The challenge remains to determine whether this increase in depression is environmental, reflecting women's perceived role in contemporary society, or whether it is due to hormonal changes.

It is clear that this excess of depression in women starts at puberty and is no longer present in the sixth and seventh decades. The peaks of depression occur at times of hormonal fluctuation in: (1) the premenstrual phase; (2) the postpartum phase; and (3) the climacteric perimenopausal phase, particularly in the 1 or 2 years before the periods cease. This triad of hormone responsive mood disorders (HRMD) often occur in the same vulnerable woman. The depression of these patients can be usually trreated effectively with estrogens, preferably by the transdermal route and in a moderately high dose. Transdermal estrogen patches of 200 µg have been used in our published placebo-controlled studies but the 100 µg dose is frequently effective.

The 45-year-old, depressed, perimenopausal woman who is still menstruating will often have a history of previous postnatal depression and depression before periods. She will often be in very good mood during pregnancy and also have systemic manifestations of hormonal fluctuation in the form of menstrual headaches or menstrual migraine. Such a woman will often say that she last felt well during her last pregnancy, but then developed postnatal depression for several months. When the periods returned, the depression became cyclical and as she approached the menopause the depression became more constant. The problem with this clear clinical history of a woman who will probably respond to estrogens is that psychatrists believe such patients are ideal for the use of antidepressants. This is because they would recognize that they would have had 'premorbid history' of depression and therefore they would have chronic relapsing depressive illness to be treated by psychiatrists. The fact that this depression is postnatal or premenstrual in timing usually escapes them. It is sad that both gynecologists and psychiatrists are products of their own training with too little overlap in knowledge. The patients thus become victims of this professional schism.

The clue to the use of estrogens came with the important and somewhat eccentric paper by Klaiber[2], who performed the placebo-controlled study of very-high-dose estrogens in patients with chronic relapsing depression. They had various diagnoses and were both premenopausal and postmenopausal. They were given Premarin® 5 mg daily with an increase in dose of 5 mg each week until a maximum of 30 mg/day was used. There was a huge improvement in depression with these high doses (Figure 1), but this work has not been repeated because of anxiety over high-dose estrogens.

PREMENSTRUAL SYNDROME

This condition is mentioned in the fourth century BC by Hippocrates but became a medical epidemic in the nineteenth century. Victorian physicians were aware of menstrual madness, hysteria, chlorosis, ovarian mania, as well as the commonplace neurasthenia. In the 1870s, Maudsley[3], the most distinguished psychiatrist of the time, wrote: '...The monthly

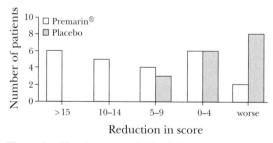

Figure 1 Placebo-controlled trial of women with chronic relapsing depression given large doses – up to 30 mg – of Premarin® per day, showing a significant improvement in the Hamilton Depression Score in women receiving the active preparation

activity of the ovaries which marks the advent of puberty in women has a notable effect upon the mind and body; wherefore it may become an important cause of mental and physical derangement. . .'. This and other female maladies were recognized, rightly or wrongly, to be due to the ovaries. As a consequence, bilateral oophorectomy – Battey's operation[4] – became fashionable, being performed in approximately 150 000 women in North America and Northern Europe in the 30 years from 1870. Longo[5], in his brilliant historical essay on the decline of Battey's operation, posed the question whether it worked or not. Of course they had no knowledge of osteoporosis and the devastation of long-term estrogen deficiency. Therefore, on balance the operation was not helpful as a long-term solution but it probably did, as was claimed, cure the 'menstrual/ovarian madness' which would be a quaint Victorian way of labeling severe premenstrual syndrome (PMS). The essential logic of this operation was to remove cyclical ovarian function but happily this can now effectively be achieved by simpler medical therapy.

Only in 1931 was the phrase 'premenstrual tension' introduced by Frank[6], who described 15 women with the typical symptoms of PMS as we know it. Greene and Dalton[7] extended the definition to 'premenstrual syndrome' in 1953, recognizing the wider range of symptoms. Severe PMS is a poorly understood collection of cyclical symptoms, which cause considerable psychologic and physical distress. The psychologic symptoms of depression, loss of energy, irritability, loss of libido, and abnormal behavior, and the physical symptoms of headaches, breast discomfort and abdominal bloating, may occur for up to 14 days each month. There may also be associated menstrual problems, pelvic pain, and menstrual headaches and the woman may only enjoy as few as seven good days per month. It is obvious that the symptoms mentioned can have a significant impact on the day-to-day functioning of women.

It is estimated that up to 95% of women have some form of PMS, but about 5% of women of reproductive age will be affected severely with disruption of their daily activities. Considering these figures, it is disturbing that many of the consultations at our specialist PMS clinics start with women saying that for many years they have been told that there are no treatments available and that they should simply 'live with it'. In addition, many commonly used treatments for PMS, particularly progesterone or progestogens, have been shown by many placebo-controlled trials not only to be ineffective, but to commonly make the symptoms worse as these women are progesterone- or progestogen intolerant.

The exact cause is uncertain but fundamentally it is due to the hormonal or biochemical changes (whatever they are) that occur with ovulation, and the resulting complex interaction between ovarian steroids, the complex GABA system in the brain, serotonin release, and other neuro-endocrine factors. These chemical fluctuations produce the varied symptoms in women who are somehow vulnerable to changes in their normal reproductive hormone levels. These cyclical chemical changes, probably due to progesterone or one of its metabolites, such as allopregnanalone, produce the cyclical symptoms of PMS.

ESTROGENS

PMS does not occur if there is no ovarian function[8]. Obviously, it does not occur before puberty or after the menopause, or after oophorectomy; it does not occur during pregnancy. However, it is important to realize that hysterectomy with conservation of the ovaries does not often cure PMS[9], as patients are left with the usual cyclical symptoms and cyclical headaches. This condition, best-called the 'ovarian cycle syndrome'[10], is usually not recognized to be hormonal in etiology, as there is no reference point of menstruation. The failure to make this diagnosis is regrettable because these monthly symptoms of depression, irritability, mood change, bloating, and headaches, which might affect the woman for most days in the month with only perhaps one good week each month, can easily be treated with transdermal estrogens which suppress ovarian function and thus remove the symptoms.

A medical Battey's operation can be achieved by the use of gonadotropin-releasing hormone (GnRH) analogs and Leather and co-workers[11] have demonstrated that 3 months of Zoladex® therapy cures all the symptom groups of PMS (Figure 2). The women do, of course, have hot flushes and sweats but these are usually far preferable to the cyclical depression, irritability and headaches. The long-term risk of Zoladex® therapy is bone demineralization, but the same group showed that add-back with a product containing 2 mg estradiol valerate and cyclical levonorgestrel (Nuvelle®) maintains the bone density at both the spine and the hip[12] (Figure 3). Most of the PMS symptoms remain improved with this add-back but bloating, tension and irritability recur – probably due to the cyclical progestogen. Livial® may be a better add-back preparation.

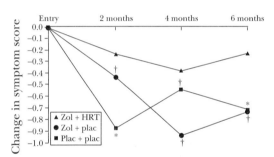

Figure 2 Improvement in depression in women with severe premenstrual syndrome, using Zoladex® (zol, control) and Zoladex® plus add-back estradiol/ progestogen (HRT), compared with placebo (plac); $*p < 0.05$ vs. baseline and plac + plac; $^\dagger p < 0.05$ vs. baseline

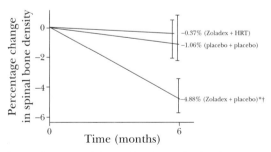

Figure 3 Loss of bone density at the lumbar spine after 6 months of Zoladex® treatment is prevented by add-back with Nuvelle® (HRT, 2 mg estradiol and norgestrel)

In a Scandinavian study, Sundstrom and colleagues[13] used low-dose GnRH analogs (100 µg buserelin) with good results on the symptoms of PMS, but the treatment still caused anovulation in as many as 56% of patients. Danazol is another method for treating PMS, by inhibiting pituitary gonadotropins, but it has side-effects including androgenic and virilizing effects. When used in the luteal phase alone it only relieved mastalgia but not the general symptoms of PMS, though side-effects were minimal[14].

Greenblatt and co-workers[15] showed the effects of an anovulatory dose of estrogen implants for the use of contraception. The first study of its use for PMS was by Magos and co-workers[16] using 100 mg estradiol implants – the dose that had been shown to inhibit ovulation by using ultrasound and day-21 progesterone measurements in earlier studies by the same group. This showed a huge 84% improvement with placebo implants but the improvements of every symptom cluster were greater in the active estradiol group. In addition, the placebo effect usually waned after a few months compared with a continued response to estradiol. These patients, of course, were also given oral progestogen 12 days per month to prevent endometrial hyperplasia and irregular bleeding[17]. It was clear that the addition of progestogen attenuated the beneficial effect of estrogen. Subsequently, a placebo-controlled trial of cyclical levonorgestrel in well-estrogenized hysterectomized women reproduced the typical symptoms of PMS[18]. This study of cyclical oral progestogen in the estrogen-primed woman is the model for PMS. It is also significant that progestogen intolerance is one of the principal reasons why older, postmenopausal women stop taking HRT[19], particularly if they have a past history of PMS or progesterone intolerance. It is common for progestogens to cause PMS-like symptoms in these women in the same way endogenous cyclical progesterone secretion is the probable fundamental cause of PMS.

Our group still uses estradiol implants – often with the addition of testosterone for loss of energy and loss of libido – in our PMS clinics but we have reduced the estradiol dose, never starting with 100 mg. We now insert pellets of estradiol, 50 or 75 mg, with 100 mg of testosterone. These women must have endometrial protection by oral progestogen or a Mirena® levonorgestrel-releasing intrauterine system (LNG IUS)[20]. As women with PMS respond well to estrogens but are often intolerant to progestogens, it is commonplace for us to reduce the orthodox 13-day course of progestogen to 10 or 7 days starting, for convenience, on the first day of every calendar month. Thus, the menstrual cycle is reset with the woman having the obvious additional advantage of 12 periods/year instead of 13. She can also easily plan her withdrawal bleeds to avoid holidays and other important functions.

The Mirena® IUS also plays a vital role in preventing PMS-like symptoms as it performs its function of protecting the endometrium without systemic absorption. A recent study has shown a 50% decrease in hysterectomies in our practice since the introduction of the Mirena® IUS in 1995[17]. With its profound effect on menorrhagia and fewer progestogenic side-effects, Mirena® looks a very promising component of PMS treatment in the future.

Hormone implants are not licensed in all countries and are unsuitable for women who may wish to easily discontinue treatment in order to become pregnant. Estradiol patches are an alternative and our original double-blind cross-over study used a 200 µg estradiol patch twice weekly[21]. This produced plasma estradiol levels of 800 pmol/l and suppressed luteal phase progesterone and ovulation. Once again this treatment was better than placebo in every symptom cluster of PMS. Figure 4 shows the response to estradiol treatment and placebo in a 6-month cross-over study. This is now our treatment of choice for severe PMS.

Subsequently, a randomized but uncontrolled observational study from our PMS clinic indicated that PMS sufferers could have the same beneficial response to 100 µg patches as they do with the 200 µg dose. They also have fewer symptoms of breast discomfort and bloating and there is less anxiety from the patient or general practitioner about high-dose estrogen

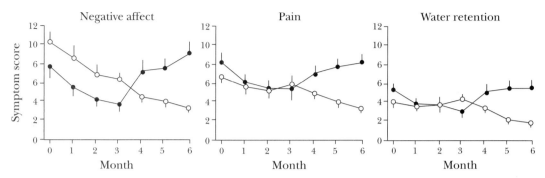

Figure 4   Results from a placebo-controlled crossover trial of 200 µg estradiol patch (Estraderm®) on the symptoms of severe premenstrual syndrome; ●, control; ○, treatment

therapy[22]. Twenty-one-day progesterone assays in the patients receiving 100 µg showed low anovulatory levels prompting the intriguing notion that even this moderate dose might reliably suppress ovulation and be contraceptive (Figure 5). Clearly, a great deal of work must be done before we can suggest that this treatment is effective for birth control, but it is of great importance because many young women using this therapy for PMS would be pleased if it was also an effective contraceptive. This is a study that needs to be conducted.

The original studies outlined in this paper are all scientifically valid placebo-controlled trials showing a considerable improvement of PMS symptoms with estrogens. Although this treatment is used by most gynecologists in the United Kingdom, its value has not been exploited by psychiatrists anywhere in the world. We believe that the benefit of this therapy in severe PMS is due to the inhibition of ovulation but there is probably also a central mental tonic effect. Klaiber and co-workers[2] in their study of high-dose Premarin® showed this, and our other psycho-endocrine studies of climacteric depression[23] and postnatal depression[24] have shown the benefit of high-dose transdermal estrogens for these conditions, which is not related to or dependent on suppression of ovulation.

Ultimately there are some women who, after treatment with estrogens and Mirena® coils will prefer to have a hysterectomy in order to remove all cycles with a virtual guarantee of improvement of symptoms. This should not be

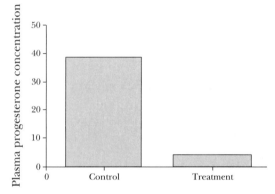

Figure 5   Twenty-one-day plasma progesterone levels in women with premenstrual syndrome receiving no treatment and those receiving 100 µg patches, indicating that such a dose suppresses ovulation in the majority of these women. However, it cannot be assumed that this treatment is contraceptive

seen as a failure or even the treatment of last resort as it does carry many other advantages[25].

It is important that those women who have had a hysterectomy and bilateral salpingo-oophorectomy have effective replacement therapy, ideally with replacement of the ovarian androgens. Implants of estradiol 50 mg and testosterone 100 mg are an ideal route and combination of hormones for this long-term therapy post-hysterectomy, with a continuation rate of 90% at 10 years[17]. We have a study of 47 such patients who have had a hysterectomy, bilateral salpingo-oophorectomy and implants of estradiol and testosterone for severe PMS, who have gone through many years of treatment with transdermal estrogens and cycle progestogens or Mirena® coil. The symptoms are removed in all patients and all but one was 'very satisfied' with the outcome.

POSTNATAL DEPRESSION

Postnatal depression is another example of depression being caused by fluctuations of sex hormones and having the potential to be effectively treated by hormones. It is a common condition that affects 10–15% of women following childbirth and may persist for over 1 year in 40% of those affected. There does seem to be a lack of any overall influence of psychosocial background factors in determining vulnerability to this postpartum disorder although it can be recurrent.

Although common, the disease is often not reported to the health care professional, particularly the general practitioner or the visiting midwife, as the exhaustion and depression is regarded as normal. Indeed the symptoms of postnatal depression may be confused with the normal sequelae of childbirth. The symptoms can consist of depressed mood with lack of pleasure with the baby or any interest in the surroundings. There may be sleep disturbance, either insomnia or hypersomnia. There may be loss of weight, loss of energy and certainly loss of libido together with agitation, retardation and feelings of worthlessness or guilt. Frequent thoughts of death and suicide are common.

Postnatal depression is not more common after a long labor, difficult labor, Cesarean section, or separation from the baby after birth, nor is it determined by education or socioeconomic group. The only environmental factor that seems to be important is the perceived amount of support given by the partner. There is no doubt that the first 6 or more months after delivery can be an exhausting time, full of anxiety and insecurity in mothers with the new responsibility of the baby. Even allowing for that, there does seem to be a clear hormonal aspect to this condition.

Postnatal depression is severe and more prolonged in women who are lactating. Lower estradiol levels are found in depressed women following delivery than in controls. It is probable that the low estradiol levels with breast feeding and the higher incidence of depression are related in a causative way.

We studied the effect of high-dose transdermal estrogens in this condition in an attempt to close the circle of studies treating this triad of hormone responsive depressions – premenstrual depression, climacteric depression and postnatal depression. This was a double-blind placebo-controlled trial of 60 women with major depression that began within 3 months of childbirth and persisted for up to 18 months postnatally[24]. They had all been resistant to antidepressants and the diagnosis of postnatal depression was made by two psychiatrists who are experts in the field. We excluded breast-feeding women from the study. The women were given either placebo patches or transdermal estradiol patches 200 µg daily for 3 months without any added progestogen. After 3 months, cyclical Duphaston® 10 mg daily was added for 12 days each month. The women were assessed monthly be a self-rating of depressive symptoms on the Edinburgh Postnatal Depression Score (EPDS) and by clinical psychiatric interview. Both groups were severely depressed with a mean EPDS score of 21.8 before treatment. During the first month of therapy the women who received estrogen improved rapidly and to a greater extent than controls. None of the other factors – age, psychiatric, obstetric or gynecologic history, severity and duration of current episode of depression, and concurrent antidepressant medication – influenced the response to treatment.

The study showed that the mean EPDS score was lower with the active group at 1 month and then maintained for 8 months, and that the percentage of women with EPDS scores over 14 (diagnostic of postnatal depression) was reduced by 50% at 1 month and 90% at 5 months. This was much better than the placebo response (Figure 6).

Not only did this study show that transdermal estrogens were effective for the treatment of postnatal depression, but a subsequent study by

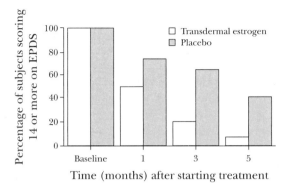

Figure 6 Improvement in Edinburgh Postnatal Depression Scores (EPDS) in women with postnatal depression using 200 μg estradiol patches, compared with placebo

Lawrie and co-workers[26] showed that depot progestogen was worse than placebo, causing increase in the severity of postnatal depression. Thus we have again the picture of the mood-elevating effect of estrogens and the depressing effect of progestogen.

An uncontrolled study showed similar improvements using sublingual estradiol in 23 women with major postnatal depression[27]. These women had plasma levels of 79 pmol/l before the treatment with sublingual estradiol. The estradiol levels were 342 pmol/l at 1 week and 480 pmol/l at 8 weeks.. There was improvement in 12 of the 23 patients at 1 week and recovery in 19 after 2 weeks.

The mean Montgomery Asberg Depression Rating Scale (MADRS) was 40.7 before treatment, 11 at 1 week and 2 at 8 weeks. At the end of the second week of treatment the MADRS scores were compatible with clinical recovery in 19 of 23 patients. This study stressed the rapidity of response to the estradiol therapy and this was our observation also. However, it must be stressed that this is an uncontrolled study in women with a very low, almost postmenopausal level of estradiol. Another placebo-controlled study is required, together with information about bleeding patterns, to support or refute our original paper[24].

It would support the hormonal pathogenesis of this condition if we could mimic postnatal depression by hormonal manipulation. This was done in a study by Bloch and co-workers[28],

who studied 16 women, eight with a history of postnatal depression. They induced hypogonadism with leuprolide acetate and simulated pregnancy by add-back supraphysiologic doses of estradiol and progesterone for 8 weeks, before withdrawing both steroids. Five of the eight women (62.5%) with a history of postnatal depression, and none of the women without a prior history, developed significant mood symptoms during the withdrawal period.

This study supported the view that there is an involvement of the reproductive hormones estrodiol and progesterone in the development of postnatal depression in a set group of women. Furthermore, the study showed that women with a history of postnatal depression are differentially sensitive to the mood-destabilizing effects of gonadal steroids.

CLIMACTERIC DEPRESSION

Like many aspects of depression in women, the diagnosis of climacteric depression and its treatment remains controversial. Whereas gynecologists who deal with the menopause have no difficulty in accepting the role of estrogens in the causation and the treatment of this common disorder, psychiatrists seem to be implacably opposed to it. This may be because there is no real evidence of an excess of depression occurring *after* the menopause, nor any evidence that estrogens help *post*menopausal depression or what used to be called 'involutional melancholia'. This is quite true and indeed many women with longstanding depression improve considerably when the periods stop. This is because the depression created by PMS, heavy painful periods, menstrual headaches and the exhaustion that attend excess blood loss disappears. Therefore, the longitudinal studies of depression carried out by many psychologists, particularly those as notable as Hunter[29], have shown no peak of depression in a large population of menopausal women. The depression that occurs in women around the time of the menopause is at its worst in the 2 or 3 years before the periods stop. This, of course, is perimenopausal depression and is, no doubt, related to premenstrual depression as it becomes worse with age and with falling estrogen levels.

The earliest placebo-controlled study that defined the precise menopausal syndrome showed that estrogens helped hot flushes, night sweats and vaginal dryness. They also had a mood-elevating effect[30]. This work was further supported by that of Campbell and Whitehead[31], who used Premarin®, and by the study of Montgomery and co-workers[23] using higher-dose estradiol- and estradiol-plus-testosterone implants. This study of 90 peri- and postmenopausal women with depression showed considerable improvement in the treatment group compared with placebo but only in the perimenopausal women (Figure 7). There was no improvement in depression in the postmenopausal women with this treatment when compared with placebo. This effect is not transient and we have shown that the improvement in depression is maintained even at 23 months. By this stage, the placebo patients had dropped out and there was no placebo group in the study. It was therefore decided not to publish this uncontrolled observational study, but Figure 8 shows this data and the reader can make whatever conclusions necessary.

At last, after 15 years, psychiatrists, particularly in the USA, are coming round to the view that transdermal estrogens are effective in the treatment of depressed perimenopausal women. Soares and colleagues[32] in 2001 studied

50 such women: 26 with major depressive disorder, 11 with dysthymic depression and 30 with minor depressive illness. They treated them with 100 μg estradiol patches in a 12-week placebo-controlled study. There was a remission of depression in 17 of 25 treatment patients (68%), and only five of the 25 placebo patients (20%). This improvement occurred regardless of the Diagnostic and Statistics Manual IV (DSM-IV) diagnosis.

Rasgon and co-workers[33] studied 16 perimenopausal women with unipolar major depressive disorder for an 8-week open protocol trial comparing low-dose 0.3 mg Premarin® plus fluoxetine daily. There was a greater response with estrogen alone. All but two of the total patients responded but the response was greater in the estrogen replacement therapy (ERT) patients, and it was significant that the reduction of depression scores began rapidly after the first week of treatment.

More recently, Harlow and co-workers[34] studied a large number (976) of perimenopausal women with a history of major depression and others without. Those with a history of depression had higher FSH levels and lower estradiol levels at enrolment to the study, and women with a history of antidepressant medication use had three times the rate of early menopause. A similar excess rate was found in perimenopausal women who had a history of severe depression.

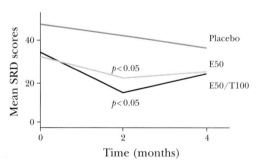

Figure 7 Improvement in depression and anxiety (SRD 30 score) at 2 months in women with perimenopausal depression treated with estradiol implants (E50) or estradiol/testosterone (E50/T100) implants, compared with placebo

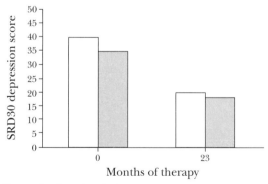

Figure 8 Sustained improvement in depression scores after 23 months of treatment with estradiol implants (□) or estradiol plus testosterone implants (■)

It is reassuring for those 'menopausologists' who have been trying to persuade the world of psychiatry that estrogens have a place in the treatment of depressed women, and pleasing to read at last the view that 'periods of intense hormonal fluctuations have been associated with the heightened prevalence and exacerbation of underlying psychiatric illness, particularly the occurrence of premenstrual dysphoria, puerperal depression and depressive treatment during the perimenopause. It is speculated that sex steroids such as estrogens, progestogens (sic), testosterone and dehydro-epiandrosterone (DHEA) have a significant modulatory effect on brain functioning. There are preliminary, but promising, data on the use of estradiol (particularly transdermal estradiol) to alleviate depression during the menopause'[34]. At last we are getting through!

PROGESTOGEN INTOLERANCE

Women having moderately-high-dose estrogen therapy must of course have cyclical progestogen if they still have a uterus, to prevent irregular bleeding and endometrial hyperplasia. The problem is that women with hormone responsive depression enjoy a mood elevating effect with estrogens but this is attenuated by the necessary progestogen[35]. This hormone can produce depression, tiredness, loss of libido, irritability, breast discomfort, and in fact all the symptoms of PMS, particularly in women with a history of PMS. A randomized trial of norethisterone versus placebo in estrogenized, hysterectomized women, already referred to, clearly showed this, and in fact the paper was subtitled a *A model for the premenstrual syndrome*[16].

If women become depressed with 10–12 days of progestogen, it may be necessary to halve the dose, decrease the duration or change the progestogen used[36]. It is our policy to routinely shorten the duration of progestogen administration in women with hormone responsive depression because adverse side-effects with any progestogen are almost invariable. We would therefore use transdermal estrogens, either a 100 or 200 μg estradiol patch or a 50 mg estradiol implant, and would then reset the menstrual bleeding by prescribing norethisterone 5 mg for the first 7 days of each calendar month. This will produce a regular bleed on about day 10 or 11 of each calendar month.

If heavy periods occur (they usually do not), extend the duration of progestogen to the more orthodox 12 days/month. At this stage many women prefer to have a Mirena® coil inserted so there will be no bleeding, no cycles, nor any need to take oral progestogen with its side-effects. It is not unusual for women at this stage who understand the benefits of estrogens and the problems of their menstrual cycles, to request hysterectomy and bilateral salpingo-oophorectomy and HRT with estradiol and testosterone[37]. This is a fact of medical life and patient choice but it will be at least another 15 years before psychiatrists attempt to leap over that hurdle.

SUMMARY

(1) Estrogen therapy is effective for the treatment of postnatal depression, premenstrual depression and perimenopausal depression – the triad of hormone responsive mood disorders.

(2) Transdermal estradiol 100 or 200 μg patches producing plasma levels of approximately 500 and 800 pmol/l respectively should be used.

(3) These patients often require plasma levels of more than 600 pmol/l for efficacy.

(4) Consider adding testosterone for depression, libido and energy.

(5) Patients who still have a uterus require a cyclical progestogen or Mirena® IUS.

(6) The most effective long-term medical therapy is estradiol patches or an implant of estradiol and testosterone with a Mirena® IUS *in situ*.

(7) Ultimately, a hysterectomy plus bilateral salpingo-oophorectomy and implants with testosterone may be requested.

References

1. Panay N, Studd JWW. The psychotherapeutic effects of estrogens. *Gynecol Endocrinol* 1998;12: 353–65

2. Klaiber EL, Broverman DM, Vogel W, Kobayashi Y. Estrogen therapy for severe persistent depressions in women. *Arch Gen Psychiatry* 1979;36: 550–4

3. Maudsley H. Sex in mind and education. *Fortnightly Review* 1874

4. Battey R. Battey's operation – its matured results. *Transactions of the Georgia Medical Association* 1873

5. Longo LD. The rise and fall of Battey's operation: a fashion in surgery. *Bull Hist Med* 1979;53:244–67

6. Frank RT. The hormonal basis of premenstrual tension. *Arch Neurol Psychiatry* 1931;26:1053–7

7. Greene R, Dalton K. The premenstrual syndrome. *Br Med J* 1953;1:1007–14

8. Studd JWW. Premenstrual tension syndrome. *Br Med J* 1979;1:410

9. Backstrom T, Boyle H, Baird DT. Persistence of symptoms of premenstrual tension in hysterectomized women. *Br J Obstet Gynaecol* 1981;88: 530–6

10. Studd JWW. Prophylactic oophorectomy at hysterectomy. *Br J Obstet Gynaecol* 1989;96:506–9

11. Leather AT, Studd JWW, Watson NR, Holland EFN. The treatment of severe premenstrual syndrome with goserelin with and without 'add-back' estrogen therapy: a placebo-controlled study. *Gynecol Endocrinol* 1999;13:48–55

12. Leather A T, Studd JWW, Watson NR, Holland EFN. The prevention of bone loss in young women treated with GnRH analogues with 'add back' estrogen therapy. *Obstet Gynecol* 1993; 81:104–7

13. Sundstrom I, Myberg S, Bixo M, Hammarback S, Backstrom T. Treatment of premenstrual syndrome with gonadotropin-releasing hormone agonist in a low-dose regimen. *Acta Obstet Gynecol Scand* 1999;78:891–9

14. O'Brien PM, Abukhalil IE. Randomized controlled trial of the management of premenstrual syndrome and premenstrual mastalgia using luteal phase-only danazol. *Am J Obstet Gynecol* 1999;180:18–23

15. Greenblatt RB, Asch RH, Mahesh VB, Bryner JR. Implantation of pure crystalline pellets of estradiol for conception control. *Am J Obstet Gynecol* 1977;127:520–7

16. Magos AL, Brincat M, Studd JWW. Treatment of the premenstrual syndrome by subcutaneous estradiol implants and cyclical oral norethisterone: placebo controlled study. *Br Med J (Clin Res Ed)* 1986;292:1629–33

17. Studd JWW, Domoney C, Khastgir G. The place of hysterectomy in the treatment of menstrual disorders. In: *Disorders of the Menstrual Cycle.* RCOG Press 2000;313–232

18. Magos AL, Brewster E, Studd JWW, *et al.* The effects of norethisterone in postmenopausal women on oestrogen replacement therapy: a model for the premenstrual syndrome. *Br J Obstet Gynaecol* 1986;93:1290–6

19. Bjorn I, Backstrom T. Drug related negative side-effects is a common reason for poor compliance in hormone replacement therapy. *Maturitas* 1999;32:77–86

20. Panay N, Studd JWW. Progestogen intolerance and compliance with hormone replacement therapy in menopausal women. *Hum Reprod Update* 1997;3:159–71

21. Watson NR, Studd JWW, Savvas M, Garnett T, Baber RJ. Treatment of severe premenstrual syndrome with oestradiol patches and cyclical oral norethisterone. *Lancet* 1989;23:730–2

22. Smith RNH, Studd JWW, Zambleera D, Holland EFN. A randomised comparison over 8 months of 100 micrograms and 200 micrograms twice weekly doses in the treatment of severe premenstrual syndrome. *Br J Obstet Gynaecol* 1995; 102; 6475–84

23. Montgomery JC, Brincat M, Studd JWW, *et al.* Effect of oestrogen and testosterone implants on psychological disorders in the climacteric. *Lancet* 1987;1:297–9

24. Gregoire AJP, Kumar R, Everitt B, Henderson A, Studd JWW. Transdermal oestrogen for treatment of severe postnatal depression. *Lancet* 1996;3347:930–3

25. Khastgir G, Studd JWW. Patients outlook, experience and satisfaction with hysterectomy, bilateral oophorectomy and subsequent continuation of hormone replacement therapy. *Am J Obstet Gynecol* 2000;183:1427–33

26. Lawrie TA, Hofmeyr GJ, De Jager M, *et al.* A double-blind randomised placebo controlled study of postnatal norethisterone enanthate: the effect on postnatal depression and hormones. *Br J Obstet Gynaecol* 1998;105:1082–90

27. Ahokas A, Kaukoranta J, Wahlbeck K, Aito M. Estrogen deficiency in severe postpartum depression: successful treatment with sublingual physiologic 17beta-estradiol: a preliminary study. *J Clin Psychiatry* 2001;62:332–6.

28. Bloch M, Schmidt PJ, Danaceau M, *et al.* Effects of denerbal steroids in women with a history of postpartum depression. *Am J Psychiatry* 2000;57: 924–30

29. Hunter MS. Depression and the menopause. *Br Med J* 1996;313:1217–8

30. Utian WH. The true clinical features of postmenopause and oophorectomy, and their response to oestrogen therapy. *S Afr Med J* 1972; 46:732–7

31. Campbell S, Whitehead M. Oestrogen therapy and the menopausal syndrome. *Clin Obstet Gynecol* 1977;1:31–47

32. Soares CN, Almeida OP, Joffe H, Cohen LS. Efficacy of estradiol for the treatment of depressive disorders in perimenopausal women: a double-blind randomized, placebo-controlled trial. *Arch Gen Psychiatry* 2001;58:529–34

33. Rasgon NL, Altshuler LL, Fairbanks LA, *et al.* Estrogen replacement therapy in the treatment of major depressive disorder in perimenopausal women. *J Clin Psychiatry* 2002;63(Suppl)7:545–8

34. Harlow BL, Wise LA, Otto MW, Soares CN, Cohen LS. Depression and its influence on reproductive endocrine and menstrual cycle markers associated with perimenopause: the Harvard Study of Moods and Cycles. *Arch Gen Psychiatry* 2003;60:29–36

35. Smith RN, Holland ES, Studd JWW. The symptomatology of progestogen intoleerance. *Maturitas* 1994;18:87–91

36. Panay N, Studd JWW. Progestogen intolerance and compliance with hormone replacement therapy in menopausal women. *Hum Reprod Update* 1997;3:159–71

37. Watson NR, Studd JWW, Savvas M, Bayber R. The long-term effects of estrogen implant therapy for the treatment of premenstrual syndrome. *Gynecol Endocrinol* 1990;4:99–107

14

The use of hormonal intrauterine systems in menopausal women

C. Ng, J. Hockey and N. Panay

INTRODUCTION

For many years hormone replacement therapy (HRT) has been a recognized and accepted treatment in ameliorating the unwelcome consequences of the menopause. Unfortunately, studies have shown that about 50% of women who start HRT discontinue within 1 year[1]. It has been reported that patients are more likely to discontinue therapy if they experience side-effects related to treatment, and are more likely to continue if side-effects are less common[2]. Women with an intact uterus need progestin administration whenever estrogen replacement therapy (ERT) is used; this avoids endometrial hyperplasia and neoplasia[3,4]. Cyclical administration of progestin causes withdrawal bleeding, which leads to decreased compliance[5]. In many studies, the dislike of the withdrawal bleed is a major factor in women avoiding or discontinuing HRT[6–8]. In addition to the scheduled bleed, women on cyclical HRT also have a higher incidence of abnormal vaginal bleeding compared with non-HRT users. This results in a greater number of gynecological investigations in these women, which further reduces compliance[9]. Other factors cited as reducing compliance include mastalgia, weight gain, fear of cancer, and symptoms of pre-menstrual syndrome[10].

Continuous combined (cc)HRT or 'period-free' HRT was first used 20 years ago in Scandinavia to overcome some of these problems and improve patient satisfaction and compliance[11]. In ccHRT, the estrogen and progestogen components are often combined in a single tablet or patch with a consistent daily dosage. The primary aim of ccHRT is to avoid the monthly withdrawal bleed, and is achieved by inducing endometrial atrophy through the antiproliferative effect on the endometrium of the continuously administered low-dose progestogen. Continuous combined regimens have proved to be as effective as cyclical regimens in preventing endometrial hyperplasia[3], and may even be more protective against endometrial cancer than cyclical regimens[12]. In addition, women on continuous combined regimens have a lower rate of abnormal vaginal bleeding than those on cyclical regimens and consequently undergo fewer gynecological investigations[13].

The use of continuous combined regimens is however reserved for women who report more than 12 months amenorrhea and are thought to be menopausal. If ccHRT is administered to perimenopausal women, erratic vaginal breakthrough bleeding may be experienced due to inconsistent endogenous hormone levels being produced by the ovaries[10].

Progesterone and its derivatives in the systemic circulation have an essentially anti-estrogenic effect and could potentially counteract the beneficial effects of estrogens, depending on the type and dosage used. Progestogen may also compromise the cardioprotective action of estrogen by increasing the pulsatility index, which results in a decrease in vascular compliance[14].

To minimize the problems associated with systemic progestogenic side-effects, and to increase the suitability of continuous combined therapy in the perimenopausal woman, a novel approach using an intrauterine system to deliver the necessary progestin has been introduced.

An impregnated intrauterine system can deliver the progestogens directly to the endometrium, where it is needed, with only minimal levels systemically. Currently in the UK, Mirena® 20 µg is the only levonorgestrel intrauterine system available for use. It is licensed for contraception and the treatment of menorrhagia but not for progestogenic opposition in HRT. There are clinical trials currently taking place with other intrauterine systems and at different dosages. The intrauterine delivery of progestogens has been introduced in both perimenopausal[15] and postmenopausal[16] women using oral, transdermal and sustained-release subdermal implanted ERT[17]. This chapter will describe the use of intrauterine systems in menopausal women, particularly in relation to their use in HRT.

STRUCTURE AND MECHANISM OF ACTION OF INTRAUTERINE SYSTEMS

Structure

The intrauterine system available in the UK is the Mirena® levonorgestrel intrauterine system (Figure 1). It is currently licensed in the UK for contraception and the treatment of menorrhagia, and consists of a white or almost white hormone–elastomer core, mounted on a T-body and covered with opaque polydimethylsiloxane tubing that regulates the release of levonorgestrel. The Mirena® has horizontal arms of 32 mm and a vertical arm of 32 mm in length and 3.2 mm diameter. The reservoir contains 52 mg of levonorgestrel, the levoisomer of norgestrel, derived from the 19-nortestosterone progestogens, which is released at a rate of 20 µg/day.

Other intrauterine systems, not yet licensed in the UK, include Progestasert® (Figure 1), Fibroplant® and a 10 µg menopausal levonorgestrel intrauterine system (MLS). All three products are currently undergoing clinical trials.

The Progestasert® intrauterine progesterone system consists of a polymeric T-shaped platform with a reservoir containing 38 mg of progesterone, which is released at a rate of 65 µg/day. The total quantity of progesterone contained in one Progestasert® system is less than the amount produced in 1 day by the

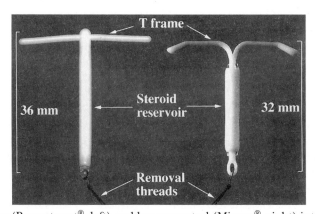

Figure 1 Progesterone (Progestasert®, left) and levonorgestrel (Minera®, right) intrauterine systems

corpus luteum during the latter part of the menstrual cycle. The drug is distributed in silicone (polydimethylsiloxane) fluid. The Progestasert® is licensed in the USA for 1 year's usage with up to 2 years' bioavailability.

Fibroplant® and the 10 μg MLS are both intra-uterine systems developed specifically for use in postmenopausal women receiving ERT. Both are currently in the initial stages of clinical trials.

The Fibroplant® levonorgestrel intrauterine system consists of the standard GyneFix® anchoring device without the copper tubes attached to the thread. Instead of copper tubes, a pilot study has described a 3 or 4 cm-long, 1.2 mm-wide fibrous delivery system. These were capable of delivering 10 and 14 μg levonor-gestrel/day, respectively[18]. The Fibroplant® levonorgestrel intrauterine system is fixed to the anchoring thread by means of a metal clip 1 cm from the anchoring knot. The anchoring knot is implanted into the myometrium of the uterine fundus using the GyneFix® insertion instrument, permanently securing the implant in the uterine cavity. The metal clip ensures visibility of the system on ultrasound and X-ray, enabling proper location of the system in the uterine cavity at insertion and at follow-up. The fibrous delivery system is also visible on ultrasound. The advantage of the Fibroplant® levonorgestrel intrauterine system is that, being frameless and completely flexible, it is able to adapt to uterine cavities of various sizes and shapes[18].

The MLS has a white plastic body, in a modified T shape, with a cylinder around the vertical arm and removal threads tied to the loop at the end of the vertical arm. The flexible, curved horizontal arms have an overall length of 28 mm. The length of the vertical arm is 28 mm and the diameter is 2.3 mm. The polydimethyl-siloxane cylinder contains 11 mg of homogen-eously dispersed levonorgestrel and is covered by a polydimethylsiloxane membrane for a controlled-release rate of 10 μg every 24 hours[19].

The rationale for the development of a smaller system with the same structure as Mirena® is to both increase the ease of fitting (by decreasing its diameter) and to adapt it to the smaller-sized uterus found in the post-menopausal woman. Encouraging results of the MLS have recently been published that highlight a greater ease of fitting and similar efficacy compared with the 20 μg levonorgestrel system[19].

Endometrial effects

The progestogen effect on the endometrium is mediated via a decrease in estrogen receptors and an increase in 17-α-oxoreductase activity that converts estradiol to estrone. Progestogens inhibit mitotic activity, as shown by the decrease in the number of mitoses in both the glandular epithelium and stroma. They also induce secretory transformation, with production of stromal edema, pseudo-decidualization, and glandular suppression[14]. In a woman using estrogen treatment, the effect of progestogens is protective to the endometrium in a dose- and duration-dependent manner[20].

The levonorgestrel released locally from an intrauterine system has been found to inhibit the expression of both estrogen and progester-one receptors in the human endometrium[21]. The levonorgestrel also causes atrophy of the endometrial glands and decidualization of the stroma. The mucosa becomes thin and the stroma becomes swollen. There is also evidence of a decline in proliferative activity associated with an increase in apoptosis, in both the endometrial glands and stroma. Spiral arteriole suppression has been reported with capillary thrombosis and a local inflammatory response after levonorgestrel intrauterine system insertion[22]. The endometrium becomes unresponsive to estrogen, with no menstrual shedding, as a result of the suppression caused by the local release of hormone, mediated by the regulatory action of high local levels of pro-gestogen on endometrial estrogen receptors[23].

Endometrial suppression with decidual transformation is also the main mechanism of action with Progestasert®. The Progestasert® has been shown to be effective at controlling endometrial hypertrophy by suppressing endo-metrial growth[24] and at treating endometrial hypertrophy[25]. Endometrial biopsy studies indicate that the continuous application of progesterone to the uterus results in changes indicative of an inactive endometrium. No cellular abnormalities were attributed to the use of the system[26].

Pharmacokinetics

The bioavailability of oral levonorgestrel is almost 90%. A half-life of 20 hours is considered the best estimate, although some studies have reported values as short as 9 hours and others as long as 80 hours. Levonorgestrel is extensively bound to proteins (mainly sex-hormone-binding globulin) and extensively metabolized to a large number of inactive metabolites[7].

Serum levonorgestrel concentrations have been shown to stabilize within a few weeks after the insertion of a levonorgestrel intrauterine system in fertile women of reproductive age. These steady levels are lower than the mean serum concentrations during daily intake of the progestogen-only pill containing 30 µg of levonorgestrel[27,28]. The plasma concentration achieved by the levonorgestrel intrauterine system is also lower than those seen in women using the levonorgestrel implant for contraception. In spite of the lower serum levonorgestrel concentrations in women using levonorgestrel intrauterine systems, high tissue concentrations are achieved locally in the uterus[29].

Serum and endometrial levonorgestrel levels remain stable for 6–7 years, though there is marked interindividual variation in serum levonorgestrel levels (1–200 pg/ml). Endometrial concentrations after 6 years are still in excess of the capacity of local progesterone receptors. The typical histologic characteristics in the endometrium induced by the levonorgestrel intrauterine system are maintained for at least 7 years[30].

BENEFITS OF INTRAUTERINE SYSTEMS IN MENOPAUSAL WOMEN

Endometrial suppression during estrogen replacement therapy

Women with an intact uterus need progestogen administration with ERT, to protect the endo-metrium from endometrial hyperplasia and neoplasia[31]. A sufficient local effect on the endometrium with minimal systemic effect is the most important characteristic of the progestogen component in HRT[32]. Cyclic administration of progestogen causes withdrawal bleeding and premenstrual syndrome-like symptoms, which decreases compliance. Oral progestogens can have significant negative effects on mood[14], and adverse androgenic effects both on the skin and cardiovascular risk markers. About 20% of women will have a significant progestogen intolerance, with about half this number having serious effects that will prevent them from continuing with treatment[20]. This intolerance of progestogenic effects is one of the reasons for poor compliance with HRT leading to high discontinuation rates of prescribed HRT[33].

The levonorgestrel intrauterine system has been shown in studies to be effective in providing progestogenic opposition in perimenopausal and postmenopausal women using oral[15], transdermal gel[18], and implanted estrogen[34,35]. Transvaginal ultrasound and endometrial biopsies were used in the studies to confirm atrophy. There were no cases of endometrial hyperplasia in any of the levonorgestrel intrauterine system users. The proportion of women with amenorrhea using the intrauterine system after 1 year was up to 80% in one study[34].

Endometrial suppression is also achieved by using an intrauterine system delivering only 5 µg of levonorgestrel to the uterus. Both a 5 µg and 10 µg system produced histologically nonproliferative endometrium after 12 months with similar bleeding patterns in both groups of women[36].

Clinical trials are currently ongoing in the development of intrauterine systems specifically for the purpose of endometrial suppression in women using ERT. The lower doses of the 10 µg levonorgestrel intrauterine system and Fibroplant® delivering either 10 or 14 µg have been shown to be a safe and effective method for suppressing the endometrium during ERT in perimenopausal and postmenopausal women. Atrophy of the endometrium and amenorrhea are induced in the majority of women[18,19]. No difference in the endometrial effect between the two Fibroplant® dosage forms was reported following ultrasound examination. Scanty bloody discharge can occur, mainly in perimenopausal women, but is found to be infrequent and of little significance.

The other advantage of the locally delivered levonorgestrel intrauterine system is its strong contraceptive effect and although the fertility of perimenopausal woman is lower than that of younger women, the risk of pregnancy can still exist.

Tamoxifen induced endometrial hyperplasia

Tamoxifen is currently one of the most commonly used hormonal treatments for breast cancer. Tamoxifen is not a pure antiestrogen, as it has estrogenic effects in the skeletal system, in lipid metabolism[37] and in the uterus[38]. This unopposed estrogenic effect promotes occult uterine lesions to develop into polyps, fibroids and endometrial hyperplasia and is responsible for a two to three-fold increase in endometrial cancer. These lesions commonly cause unscheduled bleeding episodes. The use of systemic progestogens may blunt the efficacy of tamoxifen in preventing recurrence of breast cancer. Levonorgestrel-releasing intrauterine systems have shown a protective action against the uterine effects of tamoxifen with uniform decidualization of the endometrium[39].

Effects on lipid and lipoprotein metabolism

Postmenopausal women have a different lipid profile to women of fertile age. The levels of serum cholesterol, low-density lipoprotein (LDL) cholesterol, and triglycerides increase and levels of high-density lipoprotein (HDL) cholesterol may decrease after the menopause[40]. High serum cholesterol and LDL cholesterol levels are associated with a high risk of cardiovascular disease.

ERT reduces cholesterol and LDL cholesterol levels in the serum and increases the HDL cholesterol fraction[41]. When a progestogen is added to ERT, either as sequential or as a continuous combined therapy, the lipid and lipopotein profile may be adversely altered in a dose- and duration-dependent manner[42].

A recent study by Raudaskoski and co-workers[19], using 2 mg estradiol valerate and the Mirena® intrauterine system, showed HDL cholesterol remaining at baseline level after 12 months of treatment. This result is similar in the group of patients using 2 mg estradiol valerate and oral medroxyprogesterone acetate. However, an increase in mean concentration of HDL cholesterol was shown in the group using the lower-dose 10 μg MLS. Similar results were shown in the study by Wollter-Svensson and co-workers[43] where 5 μg and 10 μg levonorgestrel intrauterine systems were used. The increase in HDL cholesterol levels must be considered to be an estrogenic effect that was not opposed by the lower doses of levonorgestrel. This strongly indicates that the influence of levonorgestrel on HDL cholesterol is dose dependent. The LDL cholesterol levels were reduced by all the levonorgestrel intrauterine system doses[19,43].

These results show that ccHRT with an intrauterine administration of levonorgestrel in low doses does not abolish the beneficial lipid metabolic effects seen after estrogen administration. These changes might be favorable in cardioprotection.

PROBLEMS ASSOCIATED WITH INTRAUTERINE HORMONE-RELEASING SYSTEMS

Unscheduled vaginal bleeding

A universal problem with all intrauterine systems is the occurrence of menstrual-like bleeding and spotting during the first few months of use. This occurs in combination with various types of continuous estrogen therapy. In the study by Raudaskoski and co-workers[19], bleeding was described as 'spotting' mainly and did not reduce blood hemoglobin values. Perimenopausal women experienced more episodes of spotting and bleeding[20]. The majority of bleeding episodes settled after 6 months[15,32]. This finding concurs with that seen in premenopausal women who use the device for contraception. Whether this is simply because of a foreign body or as a consequence of a hormonal effect remains to be elucidated, although a hormonal effect appears more likely because women fitted with a standard intrauterine contraceptive device rarely have such long-term bleeding.

Fitting the system

The intrauterine system should only be fitted by doctors trained in fitting and inserting the intrauterine system. As a consequence of the steroid reservoir, the intrauterine system has a slightly wider-diameter vertical stem than the copper intrauterine contraceptive device. This has necessitated a wider insertion tube in the case of the Mirena®. The insertion diameter is greater with Progestasert® due to the arms initially being folded down against the stem. These wider diameters may lead to difficulty fitting the systems and may require some gentle cervical dilatation prior to insertion.

The smaller, lower-dose MLS and the frameless Fibroplant® try to address this issue. The initial trial results showed that the insertion of the smaller MLS was often easier than Mirena®. The diameter of the MLS is 2.3 mm, whereas the diameter of Mirena® is 3.2 mm. A smaller intrauterine system did not result in increased expulsion rate[19]. In another study by Wollter-Svensson and co-workers[36], a much smaller intrauterine system (delivering 5 or 10 μg/day of levonorgestrel) with horizontal arms of only 14 mm length, combined with oral estradiol valerate, was expelled in five of 108 perimenopausal women during 1 year of study. It seems that the length of the horizontal arms of 28 mm in the smaller MLS maybe the ideal size to eliminate the risk of expulsion. Fibroplant® also seems to be fitted without discomfort or causing abdominal pains. Fibroplant® has a diameter of 1.2 mm[18].

Adequate analgesia required prior to cervical dilatation (if needed) can usually be achieved either by the administration of a non-steroidal anti-inflammatory drug, given 1 hour before insertion or by the use of a paracervical block using a fine dental syringe or a 1% lignocaine or xylocaine cervical spray.

Adequate attention and care to achieving asepsis must be observed to avoid infection when inserting the intrauterine system, particularly as complications such as perforation, embedment and expulsion can occur.

Adverse progestogenic effects

The serum level of progestogen achieved using the intrauterine system is much lower than when using the oral or transdermal route. After the insertion of the levonorgestrel intrauterine system in fertile women, serum levonorgestrel concentration will stabilize in a few weeks to a level of 94–188 pg/ml (300–575 pmol/l)[27]. However, despite the low serum levels of progestogen, some women still seem to experience adverse progestogenic effects. These can be both physical – such as edema, headache, breast tenderness, acne and hirsutism – and metabolic, such as decreased LDL cholesterol levels[20]. The most probable explanation for the above is that the progestogen within the levonorgestrel intrauterine system is derived from the 19-nortestosterone group of progestogens, which have more physical and metabolic side-effects than the C21 progesterone group of progestogens. There are no significant effects on carbohydrate metabolism, coagulation parameters or liver enzymes.

The physical effects have been shown to subside after the first few months of usage. It is therefore extremely important that patients are counseled adequately and constant reassurance given that the side-effects are usually transient. It may be worth pointing out that the levonorgestrel intrauterine system achieves much lower constant serum levels of progestogen than that achieved in other routes of administration. Converting to other forms of progestogens may result in higher serum levels and thus more side-effects.

Studies on Progestasert®, which uses progesterone, have shown no significant systemic effects. It may therefore be a suitable choice for women who are severely progestogen intolerant.

CONCLUSION

The addition of progestogen is essential in non-hysterectomized women using ERT. There are currently a variety of methods available for this purpose. Intolerance of progestogenic side-effects and the wish to avoid vaginal bleeding remain a major obstacle to the maximization of patient compliance with HRT. The relatively novel approach of using an intra-uterine system appears to be a good alternative for the delivery of progestogen. There is good evidence to show that this method is an effective, safe and practical way of counteracting the endometrial proliferative effect of ERT, thus eliminating the risk of endometrial hyperplasia and potential neoplasm. The insertion difficulties of the Mirena® may pose a minor problem with this method. However, the smaller MLS and Fibroplant® will become available in the near future and will have an even greater impact on women's health in long-term HRT use.

References

1. Ryan P, Harrison R, Blake G, Fogelman I. Compliance with hormone replacement therapy after screening for postmenopausal osteoporosis. *Br J Obstet Gynaecol* 1992;99:325–8

2. Schneider H, Gallagher J. Moderation of the daily dose of HRT: benefits for patients. *Maturitas* 1999;33:S25–9

3. Grady D, Gebretsadik, Kerlikowske K, *et al.* Hormone replacement therapy and endometrial cancer risk: a meta-analysis. *Obstet Gynecol* 1995; 85:304–12

4. Lobo RA, Archer DF, Ettinger B, *et al.* Role of progestogen in hormone replacement therapy in women: position statement of the North American Menopause Society. *Menopause* 2003; 10:113–32

5. Smith RN, Holland EF, Studd JW. The symptomatology of progestogen intolerance. *Maturitas* 1994;18:87–91

6. Hope S, Rees MCP. Why do British women start and stop hormone replacement therapy? *J Br Meno Soc* 1995;1:26–7

7. Electronic Medicine Compendium. Mirena. Available from: http://www.medicine.org.uk

8. Karakoc B, Erenus M. Compliance considerations with hormone replacement therapy. *Menopause* 1998;5:102–6

9. Ettinger B, Selby JV, Citron JT, *et al.* Gynecologic complications of cyclic estrogen–progestin therapy. *Maturitas* 1993;17: 197–204

10. Ng C, Cloke B, Panay N. Low-dose hormone replacement therapy and phyto-oestrogens. In Barter J, Hampton N, eds. *The Year in Gynaecology 2001.* Oxford: Clinical Publishing Services, 2001;193–214

11. Staland B. Continuous treatment with natural estrogens and progestogens: a method to avoid endometrial stimulation. *Maturitas* 1981;3: 145–56

12. Weiderpass E, Adami HD, Baron JA. Risk of endometrial cancer following estrogen replacement with and without progestins. *J Nat Cancer Institute* 1999;91:1131–7

13. Ettinger B, Li DK, Klein R. Unexpected vaginal bleeding and associated gynecologic care in post-menopausal women using hormone replacement therapy: a comparison of cyclic versus continuous combined schedules. *Fertil Steril* 1998;69:865–9

14. Panay N, Studd J. Progestogen intolerance and compliance with hormone replacement therapy in menopausal women. *Hum Reprod Update* 1997;3:159–71

15. Andersson K, Mattsson LA, Rybo G, Stadberg E. Intrauterine release of levonorgestrel: a new way of adding progestogen in hormone replacement therapy. *Obstet Gynecol* 1992;79:963–7

16. Raudaskoski T, Lahti E, Kauppila A, *et al.* Transdermal estrogen with a levonorgestrel-releasing intrauterine device for climacteric complaints: clinical and endometrial responses. *Am J Obstet Gynecol* 1995;172:114–19

17. Suhonen SP, Allonen H, Lahteenmaki P. Sustained release estradiol implants and a

levonorgestrel releasing intrauterine device in hormone replacement therapy. *Am J Obstet Gynecol* 1995;172:562–7

18. Wildemeersch D, Schacht E. Endometrial suppression with a new 'frameless' levonorgestrel releasing intrauterine system in perimenopausal and postmenopausal women. *Maturitas* 2000;36:63–8

19. Raudaskoski T, Tapanainen E, Tomas E, *et al.* Intrauterine 10 and 20 μg levonorgestrel systems in postmenopausal women receiving oral oestrogen replacement therapy: clinical, endometrial and metabolic response. *Br J Obstet Gynaecol* 2002;109:136–44

20. Panay N, Studd J. Non-contraceptive uses of the hormone-releasing intrauterine systems. In Studd J, ed. *Progress in Obstetrics and Gynaecology 13.* Edinburgh: Churchill Livingstone, 1998

21. Zhu P, Liu X, Luo H, *et al.* The effect of the levonorgestrel-releasing intrauterine device on human endometrial estrogen and progesterone receptors after 1 year of use. *Hum Reprod* 1999; 14:970–5

22. Zhu P, Hongzhi, Ruhua X, *et al.* The effect of intrauterine devices, the stainless steel ring, the copper T220 and releasing levonorgestrel, on the bleeding profile and the morphological structure of the human endometrium: a comparative study of three IUDs. *Contraception* 1989; 40:425–38

23. Luukkainen T, Allonen H, Haukkamaa M, *et al.* Five years' experience with levonorgestrel-releasing IUDs. *Contraception* 1986;33:139–48

24. Marthez-Manautou J, Maqueo M, Aznar R, *et al.* Endometrial morphology in women exposed to uterine systems releasing progesterone. *Am J Obstet Gynecol* 1975; 121:175–9

25. Volpe A, Botticelli A, Abrate M, *et al.* An intrauterine progesterone contraceptive system (52 mg) used in pre- and perimenopausal patients with endometrial hyperplasia. *Maturitas* 1982;4:73–9

26. Erickson RE, Mitchell C, Pharris BB, Place VA. The intrauterine progesterone contraceptive system. In *Advances in Planned Parenthood.* Princeton: Excerpta Medica 1976;167–74

27. Nilsson CG, Lahteenmaki PLA, Luukkainen T, Robertson DN. Sustained intrauterine release of levonorgestrel over five years. *Fertil Steril* 1986; 45:805–7

28. Weiner E, Victor A, Johansson EDB. Plasma levels of d-norgestrel after oral administration. *Contraception* 1976;14:563–70

29. Nilsson CG, Haukkamaa M, Vierola H, Luukkainen T. Tissue concentrations of levonorgestrel in women using a levonorgestrel releasing IUD. *Clin Endocrinol* 1982;17:529–36

30. Silverberg SG, Haukkamaa M, Arko H, *et al.* Endometrial morphology during long-term use

of levonorgestrel-releasing intrauterine devices. *Int J Gynecol Pathol* 1986; 5:235–41

31. Whitehead M, Lobo RA. Progestagen use in postmenopausal women. Consus Conference. *Lancet* 1988;2:1243–4

32. Suhonen S, Holmstrom T, Allonen, *et al.* Intrauterine and subdermal progestin administration in postmenopausal hormone replacement therapy. *Fertil Steril* 1995;63:336–42

33. Studd J. Complications of hormone replacement therapy in postmenopausal women. *J R Soc Med* 1992;85:376–8

34. Raudaskoski T, Tytti H, Lahti, *et al.* Transdermal estrogen with a levonorgestrel-releasing intrauterine device for climacteric complaints: clinical and endometrial responses. *Am J Obstet Gynecol* 1995;172:114–19

35. Suhonen S, Holmstrom T, Lahteenmaki P. Three-year follow-up of the use of a levonorgestrel-releasing intrauterine system in hormone replacement therapy. *Acta Obstet Gynecol Scand* 1997;76:145–50

36. Wollter-Svensson LO, Stadberg E, Andersson K, *et al.* Intrauterine administration of levonorgestrel 5 and 10 μg/24 hours in perimenopausal hormone replacement therapy. *Acta Obstet Gynecol Scand* 1997;76:449–54

37. Love RR, Wieve DA, Newcomb PA, *et al.* Effects of tamoxifen on cardiovascular risk factors in postmenopausal women. *Ann Intern Med* 1991; 115:860–4

38. Kedar RP, Bourne TH, Powles TJ, *et al.* Effects of tamoxifen on uterus and ovaries of postmenopausal women in a randomised breast cancer prevention trial. *Lancet* 1994;343:1318–21

39. Gardner FJ, Konje JC, Abrams KR, *et al.* Endometrial protection from tamoxifen stimulated changes by a levonorgestrel releasing intrauterine system: a randomised controlled trial. *Lancet* 2000; 356:1711–17

40. Matthews KA, Meilahn E, Kuller LH, *et al.* Menopause and risk factors for coronary heart disease. *N Engl J Med* 1989;321:641–6

41. Barnes RB, Roy S, Lobo RA. Comparison of lipid and androgen levels after conjugated estrogen or depo medroxyprogesterone acetate treatment in postmenopausal women. *Obstet Gynecol* 1985;66: 216–9

42. Jensen J, Nilas l, Christiansen C. Cyclic changes in serum cholesterol and lipoproteins following different doses of combined postmenopausal hormone replacement therapy. *Br J Obstet Gynaecol* 1986;93:613–18

43. Wollter-SvenssonL, Stadberg E, Andersson K, *et al.* Intrauterine administration of levonorgestrel in two low doses in HRT. A randomized clinical trial during one year: effects on lipid and lipoprotein metabolism. *Maturitas* 1995;22: 199–205

15

Clinical use of bone density measurements

J. A. Kanis

INTRODUCTION

Increased awareness of the problem of osteoporotic fractures together with the recent development of effective treatments has increased demands on physicians to manage patients with the disease. This in turn will demand increasing reliance on, and facilities for, the assessment of skeletal status. Bone mineral measurements provide the cornerstone of patient assessment, since osteoporosis is defined in terms of bone mass[1]. Indeed, bone mineral measurements are used to diagnose the disorder, assess prognosis and monitor the natural history of the treated or untreated disease. The field is complicated by the increasing number of sites that can be measured with an ever increasing number of technologies. No one technology or site subserves optimally all the functions demanded of these assessments. This chapter reviews briefly the use of such measurements in clinical practice.

TECHNIQUES AND MEASUREMENT

There are many techniques utilized to assess bone mass (Table 1). They variously assess mineral content of regional sites, particularly those sites at risk of osteoporotic fracture such as the wrist, spine and hip, but also the whole skeleton[2]. The two most widely used techniques are single energy absorptiometry and dual energy absorptiometry.

Table 1 Performance characteristics of various techniques of bone mass measurement at various sites. Reproduced with permission from World Health Organization. *Assessment of fracture risk and its application to screening for postmenopausal osteoporosis.* WHO Technical Report Series 843. Geneva: WHO, 1994[2]

Technique	Site	Percentage cancellous bone	Precision error in vivo (%)	Accuracy error in vivo (%)	Scan time (min)	Effective dose equivalent (μSv)
SPA	forearm – distal	5	1–2	2–5	10	< 1
	forearm – ultradistal	40	1–2	2–5	10	< 1
	heel	95	1–2	2–5	10	< 1
DEXA	lumbar – AP	50	1	5–8	10	1
	lumbar – lateral	90	3	5–10	20	5
	proximal – femur	40	1–2	5–8	10	1
	total body	20	1	1–2	20	3
QCT	spine – single energy	100	2–4	5–10	15	60
	spine – dual energy	100	4–5	3–6	20	90

SPA, single photon absorptiometry; DEXA, dual energy X-ray absorptiometry; QCT, quantitative computerized tomography; AP, anteroposterior

Single energy absorptiometry measures bone mineral at a peripheral (appendicular) site such as the heel or the forearm. Single photon absorptiometry (SPA) utilizes a photon emitting source such as iodine-125; the bone mineral in traversed tissue attenuates the photons, from which the mineral content is calculated. Single energy X-ray absorptiometry (SEXA) has now supplanted SPA as a single energy technique for scanning the wrist. It is more precise and avoids the need for isotopes. Sites such as the spine and hip cannot be measured accurately by SPA or SEXA. Dual energy absorptiometry utilizing photons (DPA) or X-rays (DEXA) permits bone mineral to be measured at these sites.

The amount of calcium present at a specific site of a scan is termed bone mineral content. When the bone mineral content is divided by the area or volume assessed (the region of interest), a value for bone mineral density is provided. With single and dual energy absorptiometry the bone mineral content is divided by the area assessed (because of the two dimensional scan) and is not, therefore, a true volumetric density but an areal density.

Quantitative ultrasound (QUS) methods have been introduced in recent years for the assessment of skeletal status in osteoporosis. The most widely evaluated assessments are broad-band ultrasound attenuation (BUA) and speed of sound (SOS) (or ultrasound velocity) at the heel and finger. The interest in their use lies in their low cost and portability, and in the fact that they do not involve ionizing radiation and may provide some information concerning the structural organization of bone in addition to bone mass.

The performance of QUS techniques has been evaluated in a large number of studies[3]. Current evidence supports the use of QUS techniques for the assessment of fracture risk in elderly women, where the prognostic value for future fracture is nearly as good as that of DEXA[4,5]. Additional clinical applications of QUS, specifically the assessment of rates of change in bone mineral for monitoring disease progression or response to treatment, require further investigation.

Computerized tomography (CT) has been applied both to the appendicular skeleton and to the spine[6]. The major advantage of CT in the assessment of cancellous bone density is that the result provides a measure of true volumetric density, rather than an areally adjusted result (as is the case with DEXA). Cancellous bone is more responsive to many interventions than is cortical bone, so the technique is suitable for monitoring of treatment. It also avoids the influence of degenerative disease that is a particular problem with DEXA at the spine. Although the technique also gives information on the shape and architecture of bone, the resolution of cancellous structure is not optimal. The major disadvantages are radiation exposure and cost.

Magnetic resonance imaging (MRI) provides no direct information on density but, with the positive background given by all types of bone marrow, it is able to provide exceptional resolution of the internal structure of cancellous bone, down to the connections of individual trabeculae[6]. Limitations arise owing to the need for patients to keep still for long periods of time. At present, MRI investigation of the skeleton remains a research procedure.

Of the many techniques that have been developed to assess bone mass, bone mineral or other related aspects of skeletal mass or structure, the technique that has had the greatest attention in terms of technical development and biological validation is DEXA, which, for now, is the 'gold standard'[7]. Although DEXA neglects the very many other techniques that are available, it provides a platform against which the performance characteristics of less well established methodologies can be compared in terms of the uses demanded of these techniques.

APPLICATION OF TECHNIQUES

There are broadly three uses for bone mass measurements in the context of osteoporosis. They may be used for diagnosis, to assess prognosis and to monitor the natural history of the treated or untreated disorder.

Diagnostic use

In 1994, an expert panel of the World Health Organization (WHO) recommended thresholds of bone mineral density in women to define osteoporosis[2,8] that have been widely but not universally accepted by the international scientific community and by regulatory agencies[9,10]. Osteoporosis in postmenopausal Caucasian women is defined as a value for bone mineral density (BMD) more than 2.5 standard deviations below the young average value. Severe osteoporosis (established osteoporosis) uses the same threshold, but in the presence of one or more fragility fractures.

The diagnostic threshold identifies approximately 15–20% of postmenopausal women as having osteoporosis when measurements using DEXA are made at the spine or the hip (Table 2). Given an approximately linear loss of BMD with age, and because of the Gaussian distribution of BMD values, the incidence of osteoporosis increases exponentially after the age of 50 years, as is also the case for many osteoporosis-related fractures. When measurements are made at the three sites most vulnerable to fracture (the hip, spine and wrist), about 30% of postmenopausal women would have osteoporosis (Table 2). This approximates the average lifetime risk for any one of these fractures.

The aim of diagnostic assessment is to stratify individuals within this distribution[2]. The ability of techniques to do this depends upon their accuracy errors, which range from 2 to 10% for absorptiometric techniques and are greatest at the lumbar spine (Table 1)[11]. In addition, osteoarthrosis, vascular calcification and fractures confound measurements at this site (Table 3).

A further source of error relates to biological variability. Bone is not a homogeneous structure, and different sites have variable proportions of cancellous and cortical bone. The problem is compounded by variable rates of bone loss at different sites with advancing age. This represents the 'biological' inaccuracy in predicting BMD at one site from measurements made at another site.

These factors compound the problem that individuals deemed to be osteoporotic at one skeletal site may not be found to be osteoporotic at another[13,14]. Correlations between sites or between technologies at the same site are sufficiently poor (r^2 less than 80% in young healthy individuals and generally less than 50% in patients) to be of very low predictive value. Even within the hip, correlation coefficients between regions are too low to be predictive. It is thus clear that the T-score cannot be used as a diagnostic criterion interchangeably with different techniques and at different sites. Even within the hip, there is variation in the degree with which the T-score changes with age. Indeed, were the T-score to be used with differ-

Table 2 Proportion (%) of White women with osteoporosis by age, adjusted to 1990 US White women, defined as a bone mass below 2.5 standard deviations of the young adult reference range at the spine, hip or midradius. Reproduced with permission from World Health Organization. *Assessment of fracture risk and its application to screening for postmenopausal osteoporosis.* WHO Technical Report Series 843. Geneva: WHO, 1994[2]

Age range (years)	Any site	Hip alone
30–39	0	0
40–49	0	0
50–59	14.8	3.9
60–69	21.6	8.0
70–79	38.5	24.5
80 +	70.0	47.5
≥ 50	30.3	16.2

Table 3 Sources of diagnostic inaccuracies in the measurement of bone mineral by dual energy X-ray absorptiometry (DEXA). Reproduced with permission from Kanis JA, Delmas P, Burckhardt P, *et al.*, on behalf of the European Foundation for Osteoporosis and Bone Disease. Guidelines for diagnosis and management of osteoporosis. *Osteoporosis Int* 1997;7:390–406[12]

Osteomalacia
Osteoarthritis (spine but also the hip)
Vascular calcification (especially the spine)
Overlying metal objects
Contrast media (spine)
Previous fracture (spine, hip and wrist)
Severe scoliosis
Vertebral deformities due to osteoarthrosis, Scheuermann's disease
Inadequate reference ranges
Inadequate machine calibration

ent techniques, the prevalence of osteoporosis and proportion of individuals allocated to any diagnostic category would vary so much[14] as to devalue totally the credibility of the field of osteoporosis (Table 4).

The same holds true in principle for hypertension, where measurements made at the leg may differ substantially from measurements made at the arm. One solution would be to designate individuals with osteoporosis at the spine but not at the hip as having osteoporosis of the spine, rather than using the term osteoporosis alone. This seems unsatisfactory for a systemic disease, and confuses the field still further in much the same way as hypertension of the leg would do. It appears more appropriate, therefore, to select a standardized site for the purpose of diagnosis, but not necessarily for risk assessment.

The hip as a reference site

The foregoing considerations suggest that a gold standard should be adopted in terms of site and technology for diagnostic purposes. No one technique or site subserves all the demands of densitometry, but if one site is to be chosen for diagnosis and prognostic purposes, the total hip or femoral neck is a strong candidate. Measurements at the hip have the highest predictive value for hip fracture, which has been well established in many prospective studies[15]. Moreover, it is the site of greatest biological relevance,

since hip fracture is the dominant complication of osteoporosis in terms of morbidity and cost. Several studies have shown that BMD of the femoral neck best predicts cervical fractures, whereas the trochanteric site best predicts trochanteric fractures, but the total hip best reflects the risk of any hip fracture[16,17].

The WHO criteria were established largely with DEXA in mind, since this was the dominant technology at the time. The available evidence suggests that the diagnostic use of T-scores should be reserved for DEXA at the hip, a view recently endorsed by the International Osteoporosis Foundation[7]. In the case of other sites and techniques, it may be preferable to express deviations of measurements from normal in units of measurement or units of risk. Examples of the latter include 5- or 10-year fracture probability, or an age-standardized relative risk of hip fracture or any fracture. This enfranchises the use of other techniques and sites for risk assessment. Indeed, where techniques give information on the likelihood of fracture, they can all be used in combination perhaps with other risk factors, to determine further investigation or treatment.

Reference ranges

The choice of a reference range is important for the accurate categorization of patients, as too is the estimate of the variance around the mean value. In choosing a cut-off value of -2.5

Table 4 Estimates of T-scores and prevalence of osteoporosis according to site and technique in women aged 60 years with an average bone mineral density. Reproduced with permission from Kanis JA, Gluer C-C, for the Committee of Scientific Advisers, International Osteoporosis Foundation. An update on the diagnosis and assessment of osteoporosis with densitometry. *Osteoporosis Int* 2000;11:192–202[7]

Measurement site	Technique	T-score at 60 years	WHO classification	Prevalence of osteoporosis (%)
Spine	QCT	− 2.5	OP	50
Spine	lateral DEXA	− 2.2	LBM	38
Spine	DEXA	− 1.3	LBM	14
Forearm	DEXA	− 1.4	LBM	12
Heel	Achilles	− 1.5	LBM	11
Total hip	DEXA	− 0.9	N	6
Heel	Sahara	− 0.7	N	3

QCT, quantitative computerized tomography; DEXA, dual energy X-ray absorptiometry; WHO, World Health Organization; OP, osteoporosis; LBM, low bone mass; N, normal

standard deviations (SD), the intention of the WHO group was to make osteoporosis a rarity in healthy women before the menopause. Assuming a Gaussian distribution of bone mineral density, 0.7% of the young adult population would be characterized as having osteoporosis.

Recently, US reference data for the hip have been generated from the National Health and Nutrition Examination Survey (NHANES) III study, and could serve as a standardization platform[18,19]. The use of NHANES III reference ranges derived from women aged 20–29 years and applied to the total hip decreases the apparent prevalence of osteoporosis in a reference population in the USA from 49% using the femoral neck and laboratory reference ranges of Hologic to 28%[20], more in line with the thresholds envisaged by the WHO.

Should different countries or different races utilize their own reference ranges or would a common gold standard be sufficient? Normal ranges for DEXA are available from many countries where the difference in mean BMD and the standard deviations used are relatively small. The use of reference ranges in Whites in the USA accommodates the higher bone mass and lower fracture risk in Blacks[18].

Variations in BMD between populations appear to be substantially less than variations in fracture risk. Age- and sex-specific risk of hip fracture differs more than ten-fold, even in Europe[21–23]. These differences are very much larger than can be accounted for by any differences in BMD between these communities. Indeed, in Asia, hip fracture risk is lower than in Northern Europe or the USA, but bone mineral density is lower. In view of the disparity between population fracture risks and BMD, it is uncertain whether reference ranges should be drawn from local populations. There is a case, therefore, particularly for simplicity, to adopt an international reference range and standard deviations, such as the NHANES material, until further work tempers this view[7]. The same holds true for other diagnostic methods, in that reference ranges should be derived from large population bases appropriate for international use.

Diagnosis in men

The reference ranges utilized for the diagnosis of osteoporosis are suggested for women. Cut-off values for men have variously used values derived from female or male populations. Not surprisingly, the prevalence of osteoporosis is greater using male-specific ranges at the hip[18]. In men, the risk of fracture is substantially lower for a bone mineral measurement within their own reference range, so that a more stringent criterion is appropriate to yield the same risk as in women[2,18]. The use of the same absolute value of BMD as a cut-off in men as that used in women gives approximately the same absolute risk of vertebral and of hip fracture[24–26]. For this reason, it may be appropriate from both a scientific and pragmatic view to utilize the same absolute threshold in both men and women[7,27], but it is important to recognize that the data on men are scanty, and not all studies show comparable gradients of fracture risk with BMD in men[28].

It is also important to recognize that the use of T-scores for diagnostic assessment has some limitations, even though the presence of osteoporosis over the age of 50 years is a strong reason for considering treatment. However, the T-score of − 2.5 SD in Swedish women aged 50 carries a 10-year hip fracture probability of 1.8%. The hip fracture probability with the same T-score but at the age of 80 years is 11.3%[27]. These probabilities require adjustment for countries other than Sweden, where the incidence of fracture and mortality rates may differ.

Thus, although a T-score of less than − 2.5 SD is an appropriate diagnostic threshold for osteoporosis[8], this threshold does not necessarily provide an intervention threshold. This will depend upon other factors such as age, history and the medication to be used.

Prognostic use

The use of bone mass measurements for prognosis also depends upon accuracy. Accuracy in this context, however, is the ability of the measurement to predict fracture. In general, all absorptiometric techniques have high specificity but low sensitivity (i.e. detection rate), which varies with the cut-off chosen to designate high risk. Many prospective studies indicate that the relative risk for fracture increases by a factor of 1.5–3.0 for each standard deviation decrease in bone mineral density[15] (Table 5). The performance depends on the type of fracture. For example, bone mineral density assessments by DEXA to predict hip fracture are better where measurements are made at the hip rather than the spine or forearm (Table 5).An individual with a T-score of − 3 SD at the hip would have a 2.6^3 or greater than 15-fold higher risk of hip fracture than an individual with a T-score of 0 SD. The same T-score at the spine (T = − 3 SD) would carry only a four-fold increase in hip fracture risk (1.6^3). Where the intention is to predict any osteoporotic fracture, the commonly used techniques are comparable. The risk of fracture increases approximately 1.5-fold for each SD decrement in measurement. Thus, an individual with a measurement 3 SD below the average value for age would have a 1.5^3 or greater than three-fold higher risk than an individual with an average BMD.

The ability of BMD to predict fracture is comparable to the use of blood pressure to predict stroke, and significantly better than the ability of serum cholesterol to predict myocardial infarction. Prognostic accuracy is considerably enhanced by the concurrent use of other risk factors. These include biochemical estimates of resorption and/or formation, historical information such as prior fragility fractures, and factors contributing to risk independent of bone density (such as postural stability). In the immediately postmenopausal population, measurements at any site (hip, spine and wrist) predict any osteoporotic fracture equally well. The choice of site depends, therefore, upon the clinical context in which prognostic evaluation is made. In the elderly the hip is likely to be the most favorable site. The measurement of more than one site by absorptiometric techniques provides little added value.

Enhancing prognostic information

The consideration of other risk factors in conjunction with BMD assessments improves the predictive value of the test[29,30]. Examples are given in Table 6 of factors that contribute significantly to fracture risk over and above that provided by bone density measurements or age. Thus, the presence of multiple risk factors can be used to enhance a case-finding strategy in osteoporosis, and has been incorporated into practice guidelines in the USA[31]. So, the presence, say, of low ultrasound attenuation or velocity, together with independent risk factors, might qualify individuals for treatment, without the need for BMD assessment at the hip. In other words, it is the probability of fracture that is important rather than the fulfilment of a diagnostic criterion. A caveat is that the risk identified by some risk factors is not amenable to particular treatments, so the relationship between total risk and reversible risk is important. Liability to falls is an appropriate example where the risk of fracture is high, but treatment with agents affecting bone metabolism may have little effect to reduce that risk. Other risk factors, particularly a prior fragility fracture, contribute to a risk that is responsive to interventions.

Table 5 Relative risk (with 95% confidence interval) of fracture for 1 standard deviation decrease in bone mineral density (absorptiometry) below age-adjusted mean. Adapted with permission of the BMJ Publishing Group from Marshall D, Johnell O, Wedel H. Meta-analysis of how well measurements of bone mineral density predict occurrence of osteoporotic fractures. *Br Med J* 1996;312:1254–9[15]

Site of measurement	Forearm fracture	Hip fracture	Vertebral fracture	All fractures
Distal radius	1.7 (1.4–2.0)	1.8 (1.4–2.2)	1.7 (1.4–2.1)	1.4 (1.3–1.6)
Hip	1.4 (1.4–1.6)	2.6 (2.0–3.5)	1.8 (1.1–2.7)	1.6 (1.4–1.8)
Lumbar spine	1.5 (1.3–1.8)	1.6 (1.2–2.2)	2.3 (1.9–2.8)	1.5 (1.4–1.7)

Table 6 Examples of relative risks of hip fracture in women with and without adjustment for bone mineral density (BMD). Reproduced with permission from Kanis JA, Johnell O, Oden A, *et al.* Risk of hip fracture derived from relative risk. An analysis applied to the population of Sweden. *Osteoporosis Int* 2000;11:120–7[30]

| | *Relative risk* | |
Risk assessment	Crude	Adjusted*
Hip BMD 1 SD below mean population value	2.6	
Non carboxylated osteocalcin above normal	2.0	1.8
Biochemical index of bone resorption (CTX) above premenopausal range	2.2	2.0
Prior fragility fracture after the age of 50 years	1.4	1.3
Body weight below 57.8 kg	1.8	1.4
First degree relative with a history of fragility fractures aged 50 years or more	1.7	1.5
Maternal family history of hip fracture	2.0	1.9
Current cigarette smoking	1.9	1.2
Poor visual acuity (< 2/10)	2.0	2.0
Low gait speed (/1 SD decrease)	1.4	1.3
Increase in body sway (/1 SD)	1.9	1.7

*Adjusted for BMD; SD, standard deviation; CTX, C-telopeptide fragments of collagen I

In countries such as the UK and other European nations, a more conservative view is taken in that only patients with osteoporosis are offered treatment[12,32]. The presence of risk factors provides only the opportunity to direct individuals for assessment by DEXA. Whereas clinical risk factors (e.g. low body mass index, premature menopause, corticosteroid use) are traditionally used to trigger investigation by DEXA, the wide availability and proliferation of peripheral densitometry and QUS devices suggest that, where low values are found, these might be used to trigger the more formal assessment with DEXA at the hip. A middle road between these approaches is a strategy of triage in which individuals at very high risk would qualify for treatment, those at very low risk would not be further evaluated, and only those at intermediate risk would have further assessment by DEXA at the hip.

Assessment and treatment thresholds

Thresholds of risk used to characterize multi-factorial diseases are often arbitrarily defined. In the case of osteoporosis, fracture risk increases continuously with decreasing BMD, so there is no biological break-point to distinguish absolutely an individual who will fracture from one who will not. Nevertheless, thresholds are useful in a clinical setting, where they give information on prognosis or treatment. In the case of BMD assessment both types of information are given, but need to be cautiously interpreted.

In the case of diagnostic thresholds, it is relevant to recall that a positive (or negative) test may be spurious. The finding of a low BMD should raise the question of why this is so, and other causes of low BMD (technical, confounding and clinical) should be excluded to fulfil a diagnostic criterion. Also, because the same diagnostic threshold in one country will not identify individuals with the same fracture risk in another country with an identical T-score, it is important not to confuse diagnostic thresholds with treatment thresholds. This was not the intention of the WHO, but the diagnostic criterion is interpreted by many practitioners and health-care agencies as an intervention threshold. But intervention thresholds depend not only on risk, which varies with age, but also on the benefits and costs of interventions.

The notion that intervention thresholds may differ from diagnostic thresholds requires the elucidation of intervention thresholds for osteoporosis in much the same way as for cardio-vascular disease[33]. This will demand the conversion of BMD results into absolute fracture probabilities. An example of absolute probabilities is given in Table 7. This clearly illustrates that a diagnostic threshold for osteoporosis (T-score = – 2.5 SD) has quite different implications at different ages. At the age of 50 years, the 10-year probability of hip fracture in women is 1.7%, but is > 10% at the age of 75 years or more. Thus, intervention thresholds are more logically set by threshold probabilities[34]. If an intervention threshold were set (for example) as a 10-year probability of hip fracture that exceeded 10%, this threshold would be attained in women with osteoporosis at the age of 65 years or more. The same threshold of risk is attained in an average population of women aged 75 years or more. The use of absolute risk preserves the utility of the T-score for diagnosis with DXA at the hip, and enhances the value of all technologies to characterize the populations most at risk from fractures.

Evolution of risk assessment

The appreciation that several clinical risk factors contribute to fracture probability independently of age and BMD means that these factors can be used to enhance a case-finding strategy. Consider, for example, a 70-year-old woman. From Table 7 it is seen that, with a T-score of − 2.5, her 10-year probability of hip fracture is 8.8%, which lies below the (hypothetical) intervention threshold of 10%. The same individual with a family history of hip fracture has a risk 90% higher (relative risk = 1.9; Table 6). Thus, her 10-year hip fracture probability is substantially greater than the 10% threshold. Thus, the combination of BMD and independent risk factor enhances the number of individuals detected and improves a case-

finding strategy. The general relationship between relative risk and fracture probability is given in Table 8[35,36]. Before multiple clinical risk factors can be used (e.g. family history plus fragility fracture), the independence of each of these factors needs to be incorporated into suitable models. It will also demand that clinicians and regulatory agencies accept the notion that a given probability of osteoporotic fracture provides an intervention threshold.

Monitoring

In contrast to the diagnostic and prognostic use of bone mineral measurements, the use of bone density measurements to monitor changes in bone mass depends upon precision. The long-term errors of the most precise techniques (DEXA and SEXA) are in the order of 1–2% (Table 1), a change of 3–6% being required in a single patient to assess treatment effectiveness[2]. Treatment-induced changes are generally most marked at sites of cancellous bone such as the lumbar spine. In most instances, repeating bone mass measurements at an interval shorter than 1 or 2 years after initiating therapy is not helpful for making decisions about treatment. More frequent measurements may, however, aid compliance, but the optimum interval has not been elucidated.

Table 7 Ten-year probability (%) of hip fracture in Swedish men and women according to age and bone mineral density (BMD) at the femoral neck. Adapted with permissioon from Kanis JA, Johnell O, Oden J, *et al.* Ten-year probabilities of osteoporotic fractures according to BMD and diagnostic thresholds. *Osteoporosis Int* 2001;12:989–95[34]

Age (years)	Men				Women			
	Population	T-score −1	T-score −2.5	T-score ≤ −2.5	Population	T-score −1	T-score −2.5	T-score ≤ −2.5
45	0.5	0.7	2.2	3.4	0.4	0.4	1.4	2.2
50	0.8	1.1	3.4	5.1	0.6	0.5	1.7	2.9
55	0.8	0.9	3.1	4.9	1.2	0.7	2.9	4.9
60	1.2	1.2	3.7	6.0	2.3	1.1	4.4	7.8
65	2.1	1.9	5.3	8.8	3.9	1.5	5.9	11.3
70	3.4	2.7	8.5	14.3	7.3	2.0	8.8	18.3
75	5.9	4.1	14.2	24.2	11.7	2.3	11.1	24.6
80	7.6	4.6	13.7	24.3	15.5	2.5	11.5	27.9
85	7.1	7.6	10.5	19.9	16.1	2.1	10.0	25.8

Table 8 Ten-year probability (%) of fracture in men and women from Sweden according to age and the risk (RR) relative to the average population. Reproduced with permission from Kanis JA, Johnell O, Oden A, *et al.* Ten-year risk of osteoporotic fracture and the effect of risk factors on screening strategies. *Bone* 2002;30:251–8[35]

	Age (years)			
RR	50	60	70	80
Hip fracture				
Men				
1	0.84	1.26	3.68	9.53
2	1.68	2.50	7.21	17.89
3	2.51	3.73	10.59	25.26
4	3.33	4.94	13.83	31.75
Women				
1	0.57	2.40	7.87	18.0
2	1.14	4.75	15.1	32.0
3	1.71	7.04	21.7	42.9
4	2.27	9.27	27.7	51.6
Hip, clinical spine, humeral or Colles' fracture				
Men				
1	3.3	4.7	7.0	12.6
2	6.5	9.1	13.5	23.1
3	9.6	13.3	19.4	13.9
4	12.6	17.3	24.9	39.3
Women				
1	5.8	9.6	16.1	21.5
2	11.3	18.2	29.4	37.4
3	16.5	26.0	40.0	49.2
4	21.4	33.1	49.5	58.1

CONCLUSION

The clinical uses of bone mineral measurements are in diagnosis, prognosis (risk assessment) and monitoring disease progression. For diagnostic purposes, osteoporosis should be diagnosed using DEXA at the proximal femur. For men, the same threshold for osteoporosis can be used as that computed for women. The T-score is best reserved for diagnostic use. For risk assessment, all validated techniques can provide useful clinical information, although the use of T-scores for this purpose is inappropriate. Rather, measurement results should be converted to fracture probabilities. Risk assessment by BMD can be enhanced by the knowledge of BMD-independent risk factors, again expressed as absolute risk. More work is required to delineate accurately the level of risk that should be used as an intervention threshold.

References

1. Anonymous. Consensus development conference: diagnosis, prophylaxis and treatment of osteoporosis. *Am J Med* 1993;94:646–50

2. World Health Organization. *Assessment of fracture risk and its application to screening for postmenopausal osteoporosis.* WHO Technical Report Series 843. Geneva: WHO, 1994

3. Gluer C-C, for the International Quantitative Ultrasound Consensus Group. Quantitative ultrasound techniques for the assessment of osteoporosis: expert agreement on current status. *J Bone Miner Res* 1997;12:1280–8

4. Porter RW, Miller CG, Granger D, Palmer SB. Prediction of hip fractures in elderly women; a prospective study. *Br Med J* 1990;301:638–41

5. Hans D, Dargent-Molina P, Schott AM, *et al.* Ultrasonographic heel measurements to predict hip fracture in elderly women: the EPIDOS prospective study. *Lancet* 1996;348:511–14

6. Lang T, Augat P, Majumdar S, *et al.* Non-invasive assessment of bone density and structure using computed tomography and magnetic resonance. *Bone* 1998;22(Suppl 1):149S–53S

7. Kanis JA, Gluer C-C, for the Committee of Scientific Advisors, International Osteoporosis Foundation. An update on the diagnosis and assessment of osteoporosis with densitometry. *Osteoporosis Int* 2000;11:192–202

8. Kanis JA, Melton LJ, Christiansen C, *et al.* The diagnosis of osteoporosis. *J Bone Miner Res* 1994; 9:1137–41

9. Committee for Proprietary Medicinal Products (CPMP). *Note for guidance on involutional osteoporosis in women.* CPMP/EWP/552/95. London: European Agency for the Evaluation of Medicinal Products, 1997

10. World Health Organization. *Guidelines for pre-clinical evaluation and clinical trials in osteoporosis.* Geneva: WHO, 1998

11. Svendsen OL, Hassager C, Skodt V, Christiansen C. Impact of soft tissue on *in vivo* accuracy of bone mineral measurement in the spine, hip and forearm: a human cadaver study. *J Bone Miner Res* 1995;10:864–73

12. Kanis JA, Delmas P, Burckhardt P, *et al.*, on behalf of the European Foundation for Osteoporosis and Bone Disease. Guidelines for diagnosis and management of osteoporosis. *Osteoporosis Int* 1997;7:390–406

13. Arlot ME, Sornay-Rendu E, Garnero P, *et al.* Apparent pre- and postmenopausal bone loss evaluated by DEXA at different skeletal sites in women: the OFELY cohort. *J Bone Miner Res* 1997;12:683–90

14. Faulkner KG, von Stetten E, Miller P. Discordance in patient classification using T-scores. *J Clin Densitometry* 1999;2:343–50

15. Marshall D, Johnell O, Wedel H. Meta-analysis of how well measurements of bone mineral density predict occurrence of osteoporotic fractures. *Br Med J* 1996;312:1254–9

16. Nevitt MC. Bone mineral density predicts non-spine fracture in very elderly women. *Osteoporosis Int* 1994;4:235–1

17. Schott AM, Cormier C, Hans D, *et al.*, for the EPIDOS group. How hip and whole body bone mineral density predict hip fracture in elderly women: the EPIDOS prospective study. *Osteoporosis Int* 1998;8:247–54

18. Looker AC, Orwoll ES, Johnston CC, *et al.* Prevalence of low femoral bone density in older US adults from NHANES III. *J Bone Miner Res* 1997;12:1761–8

19. Looker AC, Wahner HW, Dunn WL, *et al.* Updated data on proximal femur bone mineral levels of US adults. *Osteoporosis Int* 1998;8:468–89

20. Chen Z, Maricic M, Lund P, *et al.* How the new Hologic hip normal reference values affect the densitometric diagnosis of osteoporosis. *Osteoporosis Int* 1998;8:423–7

21. Elffors L, Allander E, Kanis JA, *et al.* The variable incidence of hip fracture in Southern Europe: the MEDOS study. *Osteoporosis Int* 1994; 4:253–63

22. Bacon WE, Maggi S, Looker A, *et al.* International comparison of hip fracture rates in 1988–1989. *Osteoporosis Int* 1996;6;69–75

23. Johnell O, Gullberg B, Allander E, Kanis JA. The apparent incidence of hip fracture in Europe: a study of national register sources. *Osteoporosis Int* 1992;2:298–302

24. Wasnich RD, Ross PD, Heilbrun LK, Vogel JM. Prediction of postmenopausal fracture risk with use of bone mineral measurements. *Am J Obstet Gynecol* 1985;153:745–51

25. DeLaet CEDH, Van Hout BA, Burger H, *et al.* Bone density and risk of hip fracture in men and women: cross sectional analysis. *Br Med J* 1997; 315:221–5

26. DeLaet CEDH, Van Hout BA, Burger H, *et al.* Hip fracture prediction in elderly men and women: validation in the Rotterdam Study. *J Bone Miner Res* 1998;13:1587–93

27. Kanis JA, Johnell O, Oden A, *et al.* Diagnosis of osteoporosis and fracture threshold in men. *Calcif Tissue Int* 2001;69:218–21

28. Melton LJ, Atkinson EJ, O'Connor MK, *et al.* Bone density and fracture risk in men. *J Bone Miner Res* 1998;12:1915–23

29. Hui SL, Slemenda CW, Johnston CC. Age and bone mass as predictors of fracture in a prospective study. *J Clin Invest* 1988;81:1804–9

30. Kanis JA, Johnell O, Oden A, *et al.* Risk of hip fracture derived from relative risk. An analysis applied to the population of Sweden. *Osteoporosis Int* 2000;11:120–7

31. National Osteoporosis Foundation. Analyses of the effectiveness and cost of screening and treatment strategies for osteoporosis: a basis for development of practice guidelines. *Osteoporosis Int* 1998;8(Suppl 4):1–88

32. Royal College of Physicians. *Clinical guidelines for the prevention and treatment of osteoporosis.* London: RCP, 1999

33. Dyslipidaemia Advisory Group on behalf of the Scientific Committee of the National Heart Foundation of New Zealand. National Heart Foundation Clinical Guidelines for the assessment and management of dyslipidaemia. *NZ Med J* 1996;109:224–32

34. Kanis JA, Johnell O, Oden A, *et al.* Ten-year probabilities of osteoporotic fractures according to BMD and diagnostic thresholds. *Osteoporosis Int* 2001;12:989–95

35. Kanis JA, Johnell O, Oden A, *et al.* Ten-year risk of osteoporotic fracture and the effect of risk factors on screening strategies. *Bone* 2002;30: 251–8

16

Prevention and correction of osteoporosis

D. I. Crosbie and D. M. Reid

DEFINITION OF OSTEOPOROSIS

In the most recent National Institutes of Health consensus statement, osteoporosis is defined as 'a skeletal disorder characterized by compromised bone strength predisposing a person to an increased risk of fracture. Bone strength primarily reflects the integration of bone density and bone quality'[1]. What is clear is that osteoporosis is an asymptomatic condition until fragility fracture occurs, but, unfortunately, the consequences of fracture have great significance both to the individual and to public health.

ETIOLOGY

Osteoporosis is a multi-factorial condition with etiologic contributions from both genetic and environmental factors. The importance of genetic factors is demonstrated by the fact that a family history of fracture is an independent predictor of fracture with a relative risk of 1.5–3.0, with the greatest risk seen with maternal hip fracture[2]. There are several genetic polymorphisms of interest including the vitamin D receptor gene, the estrogen receptor gene, the collagen 1A1 gene and genes for various cytokines including interleukin-6 and tumor growth factor-β[3]. The environmental factors will be discussed in the section on prevention of osteoporosis.

OUTCOME

It is estimated that one in three women and one in 12 men over the age of 50 will develop osteoporosis[4]. The financial cost to the UK Exchequer for the acute and social care of males and females following a fracture has been estimated as £1.7 billion per annum[5]. As the prevalence of osteoporosis rises as the population ages it can be anticipated that these cost will continue to rise.

In addition to the financial costs of osteoporotic fracture there are significant personal costs. The 1-year mortality rate following hip fracture is reported as 21% for women and 36% for men[6]. Survivors of hip fracture experience significant morbidity with on-going pain, impairment in mobility and increased dependence. One year post hip-fracture, 40% of survivors are unable to walk unaided while 60% require assistance in at least one essential activity of daily living[6].

In view of these personal and financial costs there is an imperative to identify those at risk of fragility fracture and initiate measures to reduce their risk.

DIAGNOSIS

Bone mineral density (BMD) accounts for between 75 and 90% of the variance in bone strength. The association between BMD and fracture is superior to the association between serum lipids and risk of coronary artery disease[7]. It is possible to estimate BMD by a number of techniques and on this basis assess fracture risk.

Dual energy X-ray absorptiometry (DEXA)

DEXA involves measuring the attenuation of X-rays of two different energies to estimate BMD. Axial DEXA scanners allow estimation of BMD at the spine and hip which are important sites of fracture. Measurement of BMD at sites where the risk of morbidity and mortality are greatest allows axial DEXA to be the most useful tool in the assessment of osteoporosis. Axial DEXA involves the patient lying on a table whilst a radiation source and detector assembly moves over the area being scanned. Conventional pencil-beam scanners take 10–15 minutes to complete a scan, while more modern scanners using a fan beam take only a few minutes. The scan is painless and the patient is not enclosed.

Peripheral DEXA scanners have been produced that have the advantage of being less expensive and more portable. They can scan sites such as the distal radius, hand and heel. While these scans give useful information about the site measured, they are slightly less predictive of fracture risk at clinically more significant sites[8]. The rate of bone loss is lower at the os calcis than at the lumbar spine or hip and it may be inappropriate to use the current thresholds for diagnosis of osteoporosis at this site. Furthermore, the effect of therapies on peripheral sites is less predictable and of lesser magnitude, so monitoring response to treatment with peripheral devices is problematic. Thus the ideal role of peripheral DEXA scans in the diagnosis, assessment, and monitoring of intervention in osteoporosis is yet to be fully elucidated.

Quantitative computed tomography (QCT)

While DEXA produces an estimate of BMD in g/cm^2, QCT is able to make a true volumetric estimate of BMD in mg/cm^3. This has advan-

tages as it allows assessment of both cancellous and cortical bone and can assess the cancellous bone structure. The use of this technique to assess the lumbar spine or hip is limited as the radiation dose is 12-fold greater than a DEXA scan[9]. QCT can be used to assess peripheral sites such as the distal radius. This involves lower doses of radiation but also gives a less useful prediction of fracture risks at sites other than that directly measured.

Quantitative ultrasound (QUS)

It is possible to measure several peripheral sites by QUS. At present it is not entirely clear what parameters of the bone are being assessed. How the changes detected by ultrasound are influenced by therapy is also unclear. It is possible to measure the speed of travel of ultrasound through the tissue or the speed of a reflected wave (speed of sound) and the degree of attenuation (broadband ultrasound attenuation), or a combination of these values, to estimate BMD and fracture risk. The technique is portable and free from radiation and may have some role to play in population screening, although there remain some technical issues to resolve. However, not all QUS scanners have the same precision or modus operandi[10].

Interpretation of results

The World Health Organization (WHO) has defined categories for the diagnosis of osteoporosis in women based on the young adult mean BMD as follows:

Normal: within 1 standard deviation (SD) of the young adult mean;

Osteopenia: > 1 SD below the young adult mean but < 2.5 SD below this value;

Osteoporosis: > 2.5 SD below the young adult mean; and

Severe osteoporosis: > 2.5 SD below the young adult mean in the presence of one or more fragility fractures[11].

This allows fracture risk to be estimated and has come to provide a threshold for initiation of therapy although the latter was not the initial aim. UK guidelines have recommended that individuals with a T-score ≤ −2.5, that is, more than 2.5 SD below the young adult mean, should be considered for therapeutic intervention to reduce their risk of fracture[12]. The proposed threshold for initiation of therapy is lower for patients on glucocorticoid therapy, where a T-score ≤ −1.5 has recently been proposed for subjects less than 65 years of age[13].

PREVENTION

As reduction in bone mass is an inevitable consequence of aging, achieving peak bone mass in the young adult years is important in delaying the development of bone density that would fall within the osteoporotic range. Strategies to ensure the achievement of peak bone mass begin *in utero*; evidence suggests the skeletal growth trajectory is established during intrauterine development or early (first 2 years) postnatally[14]. Maternal nutrition and lifestyle factors thus appear to influence skeletal development of the child with consequences that may manifest several decades later.

Nutrition

Sustained optimal intakes of calcium and vitamin D are important to allow an individual to attain their peak BMD during their young adult years. Several studies have demonstrated increases in BMD in children given calcium supplementation[15-17]. The benefit of supplementation began to fade once the supplements were discontinued, demonstrating the importance of sustained intake[15,18]. However, calcium and vitamin D are not the only nutritional factors important in bone development, with other trace elements such as potassium and magnesium, and food groups such as fruit and vegetables, having a potential role[19].

Exercise

Exercise during the growth years of childhood has been shown to increase the accumulation of bone in the young skeleton[20]. Similar positive effects have been demonstrated in young adults[21]. In older individuals there is some evidence to suggest exercise may constrain the rate of bone loss[22]. The beneficial effect of exercise on falls-prevention in older people has a greater benefit in reducing their fracture risks than the change in BMD[23].

Lifestyle

Cigarette smoking lowers BMD with current smokers having a lower BMD than former smokers, who have a lower BMD than individuals who have never smoked[24].

Excessive alcohol consumption may induce osteopenia and increase fracture risk[25]; it also predisposes to falls resulting in a further increase in fracture risk. However, moderate doses of alcohol may have a beneficial effect on bone health.

TREATMENT

Once osteoporosis is established there are a number of therapeutic strategies that have been shown to increase BMD and reduce fracture risk (Table 1).

Hormonal therapies

As rapid loss of bone density occurs as a result of estrogen deficiency in the early postmenopausal years, the use of hormone replacement therapy (HRT) is a rational approach to delaying this bone loss.

Estrogens act on receptors present on both osteoclasts and osteoblasts to suppress osteoclast formation, recruitment and activation. Estrogen deficiency also results in an increased level of cytokines, many of which have adverse effects on bone. Unfortunately the benefits of HRT are lost soon after withdrawal of treatment and the popularity of prolonged treatment with these agents is diminishing in light of recent evidence about long term safety[26]. Nevertheless the recent Women's Health Initiative (WHI) trial demonstrated a significant 24% reduction in the risk of osteoporotic fractures as a whole,

Table 1 Currently available evidence for interventions in osteoporosis

| | Postmenopausal bone loss | Fracture risk reduction | | |
Drug		Spine	Hip	Other
Alendronate	A	A	A	A
Calcitonin	A	A	B	B
Calcium and vitamin D	A	ND	A	A
Etidronate	A	A	B	B
HRT	A	A	A	B
Raloxifene	A	A	ND	ND
Risedronate	A	A	A	A

A, meta-analysis of at least one randomized controlled trial or well-designed controlled study without randomization; B, at least one well-designed other trial type (cohort, case–control or quasi-experimental study); HRT, hormone replacement therapy; ND, not determined. Adapted with permission from the Royal College of Physicians and Bone and Tooth Society Guidelines[48]

and specifically a 34% reduction in the risk of hip fracture and a 34% reduction in the risk of spinal fracture. It also showed that HRT can be used cost-effectively in perimenopausal women to reduce fracture rates[27].

The selective estrogen receptor modulators (SERMs), of which raloxifene is the only agent currently available in the UK, have been shown to reduce the rate of vertebral fracture in postmenopausal women with osteoporosis. As yet there is no evidence of any reduction in fracture rate at non-vertebral sites. While raloxifene has been shown to significantly reduce the rate of estrogen-receptor-positive breast cancer during therapy of up to 4 years duration, it does increase the relative risk of venous thromboembolism by the same two- to three-fold as conventional HRT[28].

Bisphosphonates

Chemical analogs of pyrophosphate bisphosphonates are potent antiresorptive agents. The first agents to be used clinically were the non-nitrogen-containing bisphosphonates etidronate and clodronate. These compounds act by forming a toxic analog of adenosine triphosphate within osteoclasts, reducing the resorptive capacity of the cell and under some circumstances causing cell death[29]. Both agents are effective in the treatment of osteoporosis[30,31] but are considerably less effective than the newer nitrogen containing bisphosphonates such as alendronate and risedronate.

The nitrogen-containing bisphosphonates act on the 3-hydroxy-3-methylglutaryl coenzyme A (HMG-CoA) mevalonate pathway, inhibiting prenylation of specific guanosine triphosphates resulting in osteoclast apoptosis[32].

Alendronate

Alendronate is available as a 70 mg once weekly dose and daily doses of 10 mg or 5 mg. It has been shown to increase BMD in postmenopausal females and also in males. Anti-fracture efficacy has been demonstrated at the hip, spine and other sites[33]. The magnitude of risk reduction is consistently around 50%[34]. Alendronate has been studied in combination with HRT with greater increases in BMD demonstrated with the combination than with either agent as monotherapy[35].

Risedronate

Risedronate is now available as a 35 mg once weekly dose and daily doses of 5 mg. It has similar anti-fracture efficacy to alendronate and has been shown to significantly reduce the risk of vertebral fracture within 1 year[36].

Other bisphosphonates

Numerous other bisphosphonates are currently under development including intravenous zolendronate which has been shown to be effective with infusions at 3, 6 and 12-monthly intervals[37]. Oral and intravenous ibandronate has been shown to reduce fracture risk at various dosing schedules, including an intermittent oral dose of 2.5 mg on alternate days for 12 doses every 3 months[38]. The efficacy of bisphosphonates in increasing BMD and reducing fracture risk is clear; continued developments strive to increase the ease of administration and acceptability of treatment.

Calcitonin

Calcitonin is a 32-amino-acid peptide produced by the C cells of the thyroid. It is secreted in response to elevated serum calcium levels and binds to osteoclast receptors resulting in inhibition of bone resorption. In addition to its limited role in the management of osteoporosis it is a useful agent in the management of hypercalcemia of malignancy. Calcitonin administered by subcutaneous injection has been shown to increase lumbar spine BMD in late postmenopausal women and reduce the risk of further vertebral fracture in a small study of women who had already sustained more than one vertebral fracture[39]. The use of injectable calcitonin is limited by side-effects including nausea and flushing and reactions at the injection site. Nasal calcitonin has been shown to have some anti-fracture efficacy[40], but this major study had a discontinuation rate of 59% at 5 years and failed to identify any reduction in fracture risk in the higher-dose treatment arm of the study. Although it is likely that calcitonin reduces vertebral fractures, its effect on non-vertebral fractures remains more uncertain[41].

Calcium and vitamin D supplementation

As previously discussed, maintaining adequate intake of both calcium and vitamin D through-out life is important in achieving and subsequently maintaining skeletal integrity.

There is some evidence that supplementation of dietary intake with additional calcium (1200 mg per day) and vitamin D (800 IU per day) results in an increase in BMD and a reduction in non-vertebral fracture rate in a population of elderly institutionalized women[42]. A Cochrane review, however, concluded that there was uncertainty as to whether it was calcium, vitamin D or the combination that had a beneficial effect on fracture rates[43] and this has been compounded by a very recent study showing a modest effect of 4-monthly oral vitamin D on fracture rates[44].

New agents for the treatment of osteoporosis

Parathyroid hormone

Parathyroid hormone (PTH) is the principal hormone in calcium homeostasis in humans. In response to low serum calcium levels PTH secretion is increased, enhancing bone resorption and liberating calcium from the skeleton, thus elevating serum calcium. PTH induces 1-α-hydroxylase activity in the kidney, increasing the levels of 1,25-dihydroxy vitamin D3 which increases calcium uptake from the gut and enhances renal tubular reabsorption of filtered calcium. Although persistently elevated levels of PTH result in a loss of BMD, there is evidence that pulsed therapy administered subcutaneously on a daily basis has a marked anabolic effect with significant increases in BMD and reduction in fracture risk. In a recent study in women with previous vertebral fracture comparing placebo with either 20 or 40 μg of PTH daily, 14% of the placebo group experienced a further fracture while only 5% of those receiving 20 μg PTH daily and 4% receiving 40 μg daily sustained further fracture, giving a relative risk of 0.35 and 0.31, respectively[45]. The use of PTH is likely to be hindered by the considerable cost of treatment and, to a lesser extent, by the inconvenience of subcutaneous administration.

Strontium ranelate

Strontium is a trace element that occurs in small amounts in human tissue. When combined with ranelic acid it inhibits bone resorption and stimulates bone formation by uncoupling the remodeling process. Initial results suggest strontium ranelate is effective at reducing both vertebral[46] and non-vertebral fractures[47].

CONCLUSIONS

Osteoporosis is a major public health issue for the twenty-first century. It has the potential to cause significant morbidity and mortality and result in huge financial cost. Osteoporosis is a treatable condition with increasingly effective and well-tolerated therapies emerging. These therapies also come at considerable expense. Population strategies to ensure that every individual maximizes their peak bone density, combined with appropriate investigation and management of those at risk of osteoporosis and thus fragility fracture, should enable us to reduce the burden of this disease.

References

1. NIH Consensus Development Panel on Osteoporosis Prevention, Diagnosis and Therapy. Osteoporosis prevention, diagnosis, and therapy. *J Am Med Assoc* 2001;285:785–95
2. Torgerson DJ, Campbell MK, Thomas RE, Reid DM. Prediction of perimenopausal fractures by bone mineral density and other risk factors. *J Bone Miner Res* 1996;11:293–7
3. Ralston SH. Genetic control of susceptibility to osteoporosis. *J Clin Endocrinol Metab* 2002;87:2460–6
4. National Osteoporosis Society. http://www.nos.org.uk
5. Torgerson DJ, Iglesias CP, Reid DM. The economics of fracture prevention. In Barlow DH, Francis RM, Miles A, eds. *The Effective Management of Osteoporosis*. London: Aesculapius Medical Press, 2001;111–21
6. Walker-Bone K, Dennison E, Cooper C. Epidemiology of osteoporosis. *Rheum Dis Clin North Am* 2001;27:1–18
7. The WHO Study Group. *Assessment of Fracture Risk and its Application to Screening for Postmenopausal Osteoporosis*. Geneva: World Health Organization, 1994
8. Marshall D, Johnell O, Wedel H. Meta-analysis of how well measures of bone mineral density predict occurrence of osteoporotic fractures. *Br Med J* 1996;312:1254–9
9. Kalender WA. Effective dose values in bone mineral measurements by photon absorptiometry and computed tomography. *Osteoporos Int* 1992;2:82–7
10. Stewart A, Reid DM. Precision of quantitative ultrasound: comparison of three commercial scanners. *Bone* 2000;27:139–43
11. Assessment of fracture risk and its application to screening for postmenopausal osteoporosis. Report of a WHO Study Group. *World Health Organ Tech Rep Ser* 1994;843:1–129
12. Royal College of Physicians. *Osteoporosis: Clinical Guidelines for Prevention and Treatment*. London: Royal College of Physicians, 1999
13. *Glucocorticoid Induced Osteoporosis: Guidelines for Prevention and Treatment*. London: Royal College of Physicians, 2002
14. Barker DJP. Programming the baby. In *Mothers, Babies and Disease: Later Life*. London: BMJ Publishing Group, 1994;14–36
15. Johnston CC, Miller JZ, Slemenda CW, *et al.* Calcium supplementation and increases in bone mineral density in children. *N Engl J Med* 1992;327:82–7
16. Lloyd T, Andon MB, Rollings N, *et al.* Calcium supplementation and bone mineral density in adolescent girls. *J Am Med Assoc* 1993;270:841–4
17. Lee WTK, Leung SSF, Leung DMY, *et al.* A randomized double-blind controlled calcium supplementation trial and bone and height acquisition in children. *Br J Nutr* 1995;74:125–39
18. Slemenda CW, Reister TK, Peacock M, *et al.* Bone growth in children following the cessation of

calcium supplementation. *J Bone Miner Res* 1993; 8(Suppl):154–9

19. Reid DM, Macdonald HM. Nutrition and bone: is there more to it than just calcium and vitamin D? *Q J Med* 2001;94:53–6

20. Bradney M, Pearce G, Naughton G, *et al.* Moderate exercise during growth in prepubertal boys: changes in bone mass, size, volumetric density, and bone strength: a controlled prospective trial. *J Bone Miner Res* 1998;13: 1814–21

21. Friedlander AL, Genant HK, Sadowsky S, *et al.* A two year program of aerobics and weight training enhances bone mineral density of young women. *J Bone Miner Res* 1995;10:574–85

22. Prince RL, Devine A, Dick I, *et al.* The effects of calcium supplementation (milk powder or tablets) and exercise on bone density in post-menopausal women. *J Bone Miner Res* 1995;10: 1068–75

23. Province MA, Hadley EC, Hornbrook MC, *et al.* The effects of exercise on falls in elderly patients. A preplanned meta-analysis of the FICSIT trials. Frailty and Injuries: Cooperative Studies of Intervention Techniques. *J Am Med Assoc* 1995; 273:1341–7

24. Kiel DP, Zhang Y, Hannan MT, *et al.* The effect of smoking at different life stages on bone mineral density in elderly men and women. *Osteoporos Int* 1996;6:240–8

25. Johnell O, Nilsson BE, Wiklund PE. Bone morphomety of alcoholics. *Clin Orthop* 1982;165: 253–8

26. Writing Group for the Women's Health Initiative Investigators. Risks and benefits of estrogen plus progestin in healthy postmenopausal women. *J Am Med Assoc* 2002;288:321–33

27. Fleurence R, Torgerson DJ, Reid DM. Cost-effectiveness of hormone replacement therapy for fracture prevention in young postmeno-pausal women: an economic analysis based on a prospective cohort study. *Osteoporos Int* 2002; 13:637–43

28. Cranney A, Tugwell P, Zytaruk N, *et al.* Meta-analyses of therapies for postmenopausal osteo-porosis IV. Meta-analysis of raloxifene for the prevention and treatment of postmenopausal osteoporosis. *Endocr Rev* 2002;23:524–8

29. Frith JC, Monkkonen J, Blackburn GM, *et al.* Clodronate and liposome-encapsulated clod-ronate are metabolized to a toxic ATP analogue, adenoside 5′ (β,γ-dichloromethylene) triphos-phate, by mammalian cells *in vitro. J Bone Miner Res* 1997;12:1358–67

30. Filipponi P, Critallini S, Rizzello E, *et al.* Cyclical intravenous clodronate in postmenopausal osteoporosis: results of a long-term clinical trial. *Bone* 1996;18:179–84

31. Heaney RP, Saville PD. Etidronate disodium in postmenopausal osteoporosis. *Clin Pharmacol Ther* 1976;20:593–604

32. Russell RGG, Rogers MJ, Frith JC, *et al.* The pharmacology of bisphosphonates and new insights into their mechanisms of action. *J Bone Miner Res* 1999;14:53–65

33. Black DM, Thompson DE, Bauer DC, *et al.* Fracture risk reduction with Alendronate in women with osteoporosis: The Fracture Intervention Trial. *J Clin Endocrinol Metab* 2000; 85:4118–24

34. Cranney A, Wells G, Willan A, *et al.* Meta-analyses of therapies for postmenopausal osteoporosis. II. Meta- analysis of alendronate for the treatment of postmenopausal women. *Endocr Rev* 2002;23: 508–16

35. Lindsay R, Cosman F, Lobo RA, *et al.* Addition of alendronate to ongoing hormone replacement therapy in the treatment of osteoporosis. A randomized, controlled clinical trial. *J Clin Endocrinol Metab* 1999;84:3076–81

36. Cranney A, Tugwell P, Adachi J, *et al.* Meta-analyses of therapies for postmenopausal osteo-porosis III. Meta-analysis of risedronate for the treatment of postmenopausal osteoporosis. *Endocr Rev* 2002;23:517–23

37. Reid IR, Brown JP, Burckhardt P, *et al.* Intra-venous zolendronic acid in postmenopausal women with low bone density. *N Engl J Med* 2002;346:653–61

38. Delmas P, Recker R, Stakkestad JA, *et al.* Oral ibandronate significantly reduces fracture risk in postmenopausal women with osteoporosis when administered daily or with a unique drug-free interval: results from a pivotal phase III study. *Osteoporos Int* 2002;13:S15

39. Rico H, Revilla M, Hernandez ER, *et al.* Total and regional bone mineral content and fracture rate in postmenopausal osteoporosis treated with salmon calcitonin: a prospective study. *Calcif Tissue Int* 1995;56:181–5

40. Chestnut CH, Silverman SL, Adrianio K, *et al.* A randomized trial of nasal spray salmon calcitonin in postmenopausal women with established osteoporosis: the Prevent Recurrence of Osteoporotic Fracture Study. *Am J Med* 2000; 109:267–76

41. Cranney A, Tugwell P, Zytaruk N, *et al.* Meta-analyses of therapies for postmenopausal osteo-porosis. VI. Meta-analysis of calcitonin for the treatment of postmenopausal osteoporosis. *Endocr Rev* 2002;23:540–51

42. Chapuy MC, Arlot ME, Duboeuf F, *et al.* Vitamin D3 and calcium to prevent hip fractures in the elderly women. *N Engl J Med* 1992;327:1637–43

43. Gillespie WJ, Avenell A, Henry DA, *et al.* Vitamin D and vitamin D analogues for preventing

fractures associated with involutional and post-menopausal osteoporosis. *Cochrane Database Syst Rev* 2001;1: CD000227

44. Trivedi DP, Doll R, Khaw KT. Effect of four-monthly oral vitamin D3 (cholecalciferol) supplementation on fractures and mortality in men and women living in the community: randomised double blind controlled trial. *Br Med J* 2003;326:469–72

45. Neer RM, Arnaud CD, Zanchetta JR, *et al.* Effect of parathyroid hormone (1-34) on fractures and bone mineral density in postmenopausal women with osteoporosis. *N Engl J Med* 2001;344:1434–41

46. Meunier PJ, Roux C, Ortolani S, *et al.* Strontium ranelate reduces the vertebral fracture risk in women with postmenopausal osteoporosis. *Osteoporos Int* 2002;13(Suppl 1):45

47. Reginster JY, Sawicki A, Devogelaer JP, *et al.* Strontium ranelate reduces the risk of hip fracture in women with postmenopausal osteoporosis. *Osteoporosis Int* 2002;13(Suppl 3):14

48. Royal College of Physicians, Bone and Tooth Society. *Osteoporosis. Clinical Guidelines for Prevention and Treatment. Update on Pharmacological Interventions and an Algorithm for Management.* London: Royal College of Physicians, 2000

17

Bleeding patterns and hormone replacement therapy

F. Al-Azzawi and M. Wahab

NEED FOR WITHDRAWAL BLEEDING

The benefits of estrogen replacement therapy in estrogen-deficient women have been widely documented. Such treatment relieves vasomotor symptoms, improves mental functions, prevents bone loss and reduces the risk of cardiovascular disease. Administered to women with an intact uterus, unopposed estrogen can stimulate endometrial growth, resulting in a high incidence of endometrial hyperplasia and endometrial carcinoma[1,2]; this can lead, in turn, to a high incidence of gynecological intervention[3]. It has been established that the administration of a progestogen for 10–12 days every 28 days may protect the endometrium against hyperplasia and diminish the risk for developing endometrial carcinoma. The addition of a progestogen in a cyclical manner results in the reinitiation of cyclical bleeding, which for the majority of postmenopausal women is not a welcome event, is regarded as a burden that serves little purpose, and becomes tolerable only as a price to be paid for the relief of symptoms. To promote long-term continuation with postmenopausal hormone replacement therapy (HRT), the regulation of menstrual episodes, in terms of cycle length, duration and amount of bleeding, becomes an essential clinical skill to facilitate the care of postmenopausal women. The alternative would be the administration of an amenorrheic regimen, but this is not a straightforward solution.

RELATIVE SAFETY OF HRT PREPARATIONS

Down-regulation of estrogen receptor expression is the intended action in the uterus of continuous progestogen administration, but given the ubiquitous distribution of the estrogen receptors throughout the body, the issue of long-term safety adds further concerns about the suitability of available combinations and their potential attenuation of bone sparing, or cardiovascular benefits.

The long-term safety of one type of continuous combined HRT (ccHRT) regimen has been addressed in two reported randomized placebo- controlled trials in the primary (Women's Health Initiative, WHI)[4] and secondary (Heart and Estrogen/progestin Replacement Study, HERS)[5] prevention of ischemic heart disease (IHD), which used conjugated equine estrogens and medroxyprogesterone acetate (MPA). Unopposed by a progestogen, conjugated equine estrogens have been in use for about 50 years in hysterectomized women, as well as in those with an intact uterus, and the majority of observational studies point to its preventive effects against IHD[6,7]. Indeed, the estrogen–placebo-controlled arm of the WHI study has been allowed to continue, since no increased incidence of coronary events or breast cancer has been noted. The adverse coronary artery constrictive effect of MPA has been elegantly described in primates[8]. Sequential HRT regimens have not yet been subjected to a randomized controlled trial for the primary or secondary prevention of IHD. However, shorter tissue exposure to the progestogen may be rectified by the subsequent, longer, estrogen-only phase.

REGULARITY OF THE NATURAL MENSTRUAL CYCLE AND BLEEDING INTERVALS

Endometrial growth, differentiation and subsequent shedding represent a highly integrated cascade of events in response to cyclical ovarian function. Therefore, natural menstruation is an expression of failure of potential implantation during the previous cycle, and represents in itself the start of another series of preparative steps in anticipation of hormonal changes in the following ovarian cycle. For the woman, menstruation is perceived evidence of potential fertility and health, and by inference is a feature of the young female. Consequently, menstruation is a significant event in a woman's life, and, irrespective of their sociocultural background, most women are clearly aware of their menstrual rhythm, especially the 'regularity' of the event.

The published literature maintain that only 13–16% of women have a range of cycle length of less than 6 days, i.e. the difference between the longest and the shortest cycle recorded. These studies confirm the wide variability of the natural cycle in the individual woman. Furthermore, these studies show a steady decline in average cycle length from the youngest to the oldest age groups, being highest for women aged 15–19 years and lowest for 20–39-year-old women[9–14]. This notion forms the basis for education and counselling of women using HRT, when variability of bleeding intervals raises health concerns in these women.

ASSESSMENT OF BLEEDING PATTERNS

Menstrual dates and patterns, as collected through interviews or questionnaires, are subject to problems of recall, and such data are less accurate the longer is the interval between the occurrence of the event and its reporting. Therefore, for more accurate data collection, prospective recording is favored, and is best achieved by conscientious noting of bleeding episodes or spotting (blood loss that does not require sanitary protection) in a menstrual diary, as well as the noting of bleed-free days. Analysis of menstrual data can be based on the conventional perception of '28-day' menstrual cycles, and this is useful when evaluating menstrual rhythms in conjunction with a 28-day gonadal steroid regimen.

The clinically important parameters of menstrual assessment are centered on the number of bleeding/spotting episodes, mean lengths of episodes and range of lengths of bleed-free intervals[15]; hence, the following definitions have been introduced:

(1) Bleeding episode: bleeding per vaginam for 1 or more days with at least 2 bleed-free days before and after;

(2) Progestogen-associated bleed (PAB): bleeding per vaginam starting between day 8 of progestogen administration of one cycle and day 7 after its discontinuation, inclusive; all other bleeding is defined as intermenstrual bleeding (IMB);

(3) Bleeding interval: the number of days between the first days of bleeding of two consecutive PABs.

It is interesting to note that sequential HRT regimens have been marketed as 28-day treatment cycles, when one might be able to argue for a calendar month-based cyclical progestogen administration, instead. To reduce the frequency of bleeding episodes, a regimen was devised to administer the progestogen once every 3 months, but the amount of blood loss was excessive, and these women frequently experienced progestogenic adverse effects due to the high dose of the progestogen used. In 15% of endometrial samples obtained at the end of the estrogen phase, endometrial hyperplasia was detected, but all were reversed after the progestogen phase[16]. The long-term endometrial safety of such regimens, therefore, remains questionable.

Interpretation of menstrual diaries

In clinical studies involving postmenopausal women treated with a sequential combined HRT regimen, for example, the summary statistics of mean and standard deviation used for the description of the day of onset of bleeding, its duration and the amount of blood loss can give an idea of the overall efficacy of that regimen. However, summary statistics tend to be dominated by data obtained from women with frequent, short cycles, and may give a falsely optimistic impression of the efficacy of a given regimen in the management of the individual woman[17].

A menstrual diary completed by the woman represents individual responses to a particular treatment, and can be used for comparison with the natural physiological cycles or with other treatment regimens without forcing the data into an artificial method of analysis, the summary statistics, to which neither the woman nor the clinician is able to relate. Analysis of individual women's diaries and stratifying them by the mean day of onset of bleeding has identified two groups of women: early bleeders and late bleeders. Early bleeders, whose mean day of onset of bleeding commenced before the end of the progestogen phase, had a wide variability of the day of onset of bleeding (i.e. poor predictability), with longer and heavier episodes of withdrawal bleeding compared with those women whose mean day of onset of bleeding occurred after the end of the progestogen phase, or late bleeders[18]. This method was prospectively applied to a dose-ranging study of a new progestogen, trimegestone, in which the bleeding characteristics of early and late bleeders were confirmed and the dose of progestogen was the main determinant for being an early or a late bleeder[19]. Indeed, the clinical applicability of this method of evaluation of the individual woman's experience of bleeding was further documented when the dose of trimegestone was changed[20], and in comparative studies with other progestogens[21]. Therefore, in clinical practice, we recommend analysis of the individual woman's diary, collected during a treatment phase, to adjust the dose of treatment or mode of administration of HRT regimens.

Severity of bleeding

The amount of blood loss is difficult to document, since it is difficult to evaluate between individual women, in whom the perceived amount of loss depends on myriad factors related to personal hygiene and social and cultural attributes. A method for measurement of blood loss by alkaline elution of hematin from collected sanitary towels has been established. The improved accuracy of measurement of blood loss is countered by the laborious nature of the technique, which requires stringent precautions against transmission of blood-borne diseases and is certainly not practical for large-scale studies[22]. A surrogate measure was suggested by Higham and colleagues[23], based on a pictorial chart (Figure 1). The woman completes her menstrual diary on a daily basis, and refers to the degree of soiling of sanitary towels or tampons. However, the reproducibility of this method has recently been questioned when applied to a group of women[24]; nonetheless, within-subject reproducibility is much more important in the management of the individual woman.

Intermenstrual bleeding

In analysing menstrual diaries, problems arise when trying to include episodes of spotting during the main menstrual phase, or the occurrence of truncated events, i.e. bleeding or spotting that occurs 1 or 2 days before or after the main menstrual event. Statistically presented summaries of menstrual data, particularly those collected over long observation periods, may not be seriously affected by such episodes in naturally menstruating women who are not using contraceptives. In these women, they are largely accepted as part of the physiological phenomenon, but not in postmenopausal women using HRT.

First day of menstruation

-- / -- / --

→

	1	2	3	4	5	6	7	8	9	10	11	12	13	14	15	16	17	18	19	20	21	22	23	24	25	26	27	28	29	30	31
None																															
Spotting																															
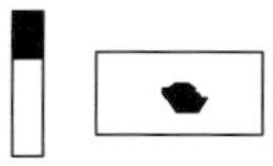																															
Clot-flooding																															
Pain																															

Figure 1 Menstrual calendar. This pictorial chart helps understanding of a woman's symptoms, and facilitates comparison of response to treatment. Adapted with permission from Higham JM, *et al.* Assessment of menstrual blood using a pictorial chart. *Br J Obstet Gynecol* 1990;97:734–9[23]

ASSESSMENT OF BLEEDING PATTERNS IN AMENORRHEIC REGIMENS

Since the re-establishment of uterine bleeding dissuades women from long-term use of HRT, an amenorrheic regimen was devised by providing continuously administered estrogen and a progestogen (ccHRT). The expectation in this case is that the progestogen will act significantly only on the uterus to induce atrophic endometrium that will not be shed.

The induction of an amenorrheic state is the most important feature for the increasing popularity of this type of HRT regimen. However, as many as 50% of women who commence ccHRT will experience bleeding episodes during the first 3–6 months, although for those who continue the treatment, amenorrhea is achieved in about 70–90%, with high continuation rates[25,26]. Other than the bleeding problems, women discontinue ccHRT owing to the adverse effects of progestogens, such as bloatedness, fluid retention and dysphoria.

A reference-period method of observation based on multiples of 30 days has been suggested[27], since menstruation occurs as a 'monthly event'. The reference-period method is particularly useful when assessing bleeding events associated with an intrauterine contraceptive device, long-acting injectable contraceptive steroids and the progestogen-only pill, on the 'mini pill'. Therefore, this method is more applicable for the evaluation of bleeding episodes associated with ccHRT regimens. With this method, the bleeding events are assessed as they happen during the observation period, but many such events will overlap the boundaries of the reference period. Regardless of the length of the reference period, the recording must start with the commencement of treatment, which permits uniformity of assessment between subjects. Data obtained through the reference-period method may not be easily assimilated in a clinical situation, particularly from the woman's viewpoint, since amenorrhea is the goal of ccHRT and any bleeding episode represents, in principle, treatment failure.

We recommend the use of 90-day reference-period diaries for practical reasons. First, it is implicit in this practice that bleeding events, should they occur with ccHRT, are assessed over a longer period and that the woman should not panic when such episodes occur. Second, this approach enables the woman who bleeds initially with ccHRT to evaluate the change in the pattern of bleeding during the second 3–6 months, and reassure herself of the progressive subsidence of these episodes; thus, in the majority of instances it helps to promote perseverance with treatment. Third, such an approach will reduce the frequency of unnecessary clinic visits. Finally, these diaries may also prompt uterine investigation should bleeding persist or become heavier, particularly after the first 3 months of treatment. In clinical studies, the 90-day reference period simplifies the assessment of bleeding episodes, and reduces the frequency of statistical handling of truncated bleeding events that overlap the boundaries of the reference periods.

HISTOLOGY OF THE ENDOMETRIUM

Changes in endometrial histology in response to the combined oral contraceptive (COC) pill are frequently described as 'retarded', and similarly the endometria of postmenopausal women treated with HRT[28]. These descriptions are largely related to poorer glandular development and stromal changes, compared with the luteal-phase endometrium of the natural cycle. This can be explained by the fact that the ovaries produce many intermediary steroid metabolites, all of which may contribute to gonadal steroid receptor activation. Consequently, these metabolites may influence the enzyme systems responsible for metabolic clearance of these steroids and their cognate receptors from the cell machinery. The metabolic handling and bioavailability of the constituting steroids used in COC and in HRT preparations result in different intermediary metabolites[29] and, as such, may not be adequate to sustain the physiological growth and integrity of the endometrium, as is the case with the natural cycle.

Another collective description commonly used by histopathologists is that of 'dyssynchronous endometrium', which denotes the out-of-phase changes in this tissue. This was well illustrated by Good and Moyer's approach to the adequacy of estrogen or progestogen contained in a particular treatment regimen[30], and was further documented in a mathematical model using a linear discriminant analysis technique[31]. Different progestogens, for example, induce different vascular patterns in the endometrium, with androgenic types resulting in smaller and a higher number of vascular spaces compared with the non-androgenic trimegestone or progesterone[32,33].

FACTORS THAT INFLUENCE BLEEDING PATTERNS WITH HRT

Ethnicity and geographical location

These may play an important role in the pattern of menstruation. European women tend to have more bleeding/spotting days, while women from Latin America have shorter bleeding episodes and longer bleed-free intervals. These features of menstrual loss have been observed in those using oral contraceptive pills, as well as in those menstruating spontaneously. Furthermore, only 25% of European women treated with depot MPA experienced amenorrhea by their fourth injection, compared with 72% of women in North Africa[34]. However, there are no comparative data on the influence of ethnicity or geographical location on menstrual events associated with the use of HRT.

Nature of the hormones used

Compared with the COC pill, orally administered HRT consists of a relatively low dose of estrogen and a high dose of progestogen. One of the main pathophysiological processes responsible for unscheduled bleeding in postmenopausal women taking HRT is the bioavailability of the estrogen used. In particular, the susceptibility of estradiol for inactivation by 17β-hydroxysteroid dehydrogenase and subsequent metabolic clearance to the weaker estrone and its conjugates is higher than that of the resistant ethinylestradiol, or of its 3-methyl ether, mestranol. In addition, the bioavailable dose of the sequential progestogen to the uterus may be inadequate to sustain endometrial stability until the end of the progestogen phase.

Increasing the dose of the progestogen may overcome this problem in some cases, but this is counterbalanced by a higher incidence of bloatedness, fluid retention and mastalgia. Furthermore, one should be mindful of the potential metabolic effect of long-term administration of high doses of progestogens, and therefore such regimens should be reviewed regularly. Alternatively, a higher dose of ethinylestradiol (20–30 µg) may be required, but there is general concern about prescribing higher doses of estrogen to older women.

Various progestogens have been used in combination with estrogen. Norethisterone (NET) is one of the most widely used progestogens in cyclical sequential regimens. However, in 50% of instances, withdrawal bleeding occurs before the end of the progestogen phase of treatment (Figure 2)[18]. MPA has been used in preference to NET because of its lesser androgenic adverse effect; however, it results in a less favorable bleeding pattern compared with other progestogens[35]. Women taking MPA bleed earlier in the progestogen phase, compared with levonorgestrel (LNG) or desogestrel[36,37].

Endometrial polyps

Endometrial polyps are localized outgrowths of endometrial tissue covered by epithelium, and contain a variable amount of glands, stroma and blood vessels. They are encountered most commonly during the fifth decade of life. In premenopausal women they may present clinically as intermenstrual bleeding or as heavy periods, but sometimes the clinical presentation is that of excessive vaginal discharge.

Endometrial polyps vary in size, from 1 mm to a large fleshy mass that may protrude through the cervix. They can be broad-based and sessile, or attached to the endometrium by a slender stalk. They are usually solitary, but multiple

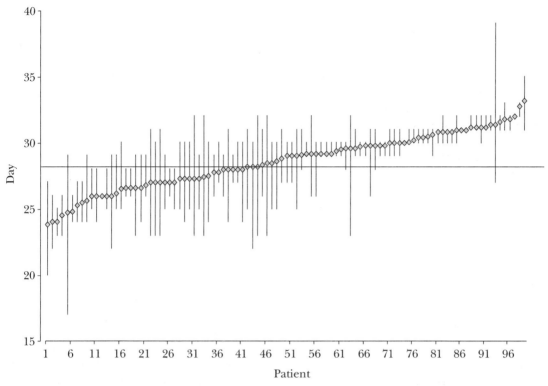

Figure 2 Mean day of onset of bleeding (± range) in women taking estradiol valerate 2 mg + cyclical norethisterone 1 mg. Reproduced with permission from Habiba MA, *et al.* Endometrial responses to hormone replacement therapy: the bleeding pattern. *Hun Reprod* 1996;11:503–8[18]

polyps can be found as well. The glandular element of a polyp is characteristically out of phase with the rest of endometrial development, and secretory changes in these glands are seldom found. Occasionally, hyperplasia or early carcinoma may develop exclusively in the polyp. There are indications for an increased incidence of endometrial hyperplasia and carcinoma in women found to have endometrial polyps[38], but this may be due to the increased propensity of such endometria to develop neoplasia rather than an inherent feature of the polyps.

In a prospective cohort study involving 248 women who underwent out-patient hysteroscopy and endometrial biopsy, 62 had endometrial polyps. These were compared with 186 endometrial samples that did not have polyps, taken as control. The incidence of hyperplasia in polyps was 11.3% compared with 4.3% in control samples, while the incidence of carcinoma was identical in both groups (3.2%)[39].

Removal of the polyp with endometrial curettage may be all that is required, but a check hysteroscopy is necessary, since the consistency of these polyps may be so pliable that they are missed by the curettage (Figure 3). Where hyperplastic changes are found localized to the polyp in premenopausal women, then polypectomy with curettage may be adequate. However, in postmenopausal women hysterectomy will be the appropriate choice if atypia is also present.

Submucous fibroids

The presence of submucous fibroids has been linked to the development of abnormal uterine bleeding. We documented a two-fold increase in the risk of having submucous fibroids in premenopausal women who presented with heavy and irregular menses, and a three-fold increase for the presence of these fibroids in postmenopausal women who presented with heavy and irregular bleeding with HRT, compared with asymptomatic controls[40]. Furthermore, the presence of submucous fibroids has been associated with heavy and prolonged bleeding in addition to a higher incidence of IMB in postmenopausal women taking HRT[41].

The identification of polyps and submucous fibroids may help to predict a woman's response to sex steroid therapy[42], and aids the planning of local surgical management if deemed necessary[43]. Moreover, 87% of postmenopausal women with heavy and unscheduled bleeding with HRT, who had their submucous fibroids removed by hysteroscopic laser myomectomy, improved and experienced regular bleeding when they resumed their HRT[44,45]. The result of this intervention, however, was less successful in premenopausal women, and adds further evidence that abnormal uterine bleeding in the presence of submucous fibroids in this group of women forms only part of the abnormal hormonal responsiveness of the endometrium. In women who present with spontaneous postmenopausal bleeding, the presence of submucous fibroids or polyps was not found to be more frequent than in controls[40]. It has long been recognized that the development of the endometrium overlying submucuos fibroids is less advanced, and shows a mixed picture of proliferative, secretory and poorly developed patches compared with the rest of the adjacent endometrium[28,46]. Whether such endometrial defects are due to the altered vascular pattern that supplies these fibroids, or due to paracrine factors induced as a result of the development of the fibroids, is not known.

Poor compliance with HRT

Irregular use of HRT regimens is an important issue that deserves thorough consideration in the clinical assessment of women presenting with heavy or unscheduled bleeding, since missing tablets, for example, may alter the bioavailability of gonadal steroids, render the endometrium unstable and cause bleeding. Where progestogenic adverse effects are experienced, women try to stop using part or the whole of the progestogen phase of the HRT regimen, to avoid these symptoms. It is estimated that about 30% of women who are prescribed sequential combined HRT regimens stop taking the progestogen component owing to symptoms of fluid retention, bloatedness, mastalgia and mood swings; consequently, the endometrial changes will be similar to those on unopposed estrogen. In the Postmenopausal Estrogen/Progestin Interventions (PEPI) trial[47], 62.5% of women with an intact uterus who used unopposed estrogen for 3 years developed abnormal bleeding or had an abnormal Papanicolaou test, which necessitated further investigation. Eighty per cent of unopposed estrogen users had endometrial abnormalities, of which 80.5% were simple hyperplasia, 18.8% atypical hyperplasia and 0.7% endometrial carcinoma.

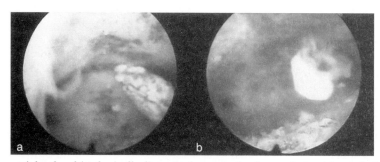

Figure 3 Endometrial polyp, histologically diagnosed as complex hyperplasia with atypia (a). The erythema in (b) is the result of sharp and thorough curettage. The endometrial cavity was re-hysteroscoped, which showed that only minimal damage was inflicted on the polyp

ENDOMETRIAL NEOPLASIA

The incidence of endometrial carcinoma varies with race and geographical location. Adjusted for age, the rate of endometrial cancer in the USA is reported to be from 17.6 to 22.2 per 100 000 in white women and 10.4 for Afro-Caribbean women, while that among Chinese women is 10–15 times lower[48]. Endometrial cancer is associated with one of the highest survival rates for all cancer sites; 74% of uterine cancer cases are diagnosed at a localized stage, and a great majority of women under the age of 50 have their cancer diagnosed at an early stage[49].

Hormonal treatment and endometrial cancer

Chronic unopposed estrogen administration induces a proliferative endometrium, which progresses to a well-differentiated endometrial adenocarcinoma in a significant number of women. Such progress is thought to pass through several intermediary stages of proliferation of increasing complexity, collectively termed 'endometrial hyperplasia'. The duration of use of unopposed estrogen in postmenopausal women remains the strongest predictor for the development of endometrial cancer. The relative risk increases exponentially from 1.4 (95% confidence interval (CI) 1.0–1.8) for less than 1 year of use to 9.5 (95% CI 7.4–12.3) among users for 10 years or more[50].

The effect of unopposed estrogen use on the risk of endometrial cancer is also directly related to the dose of estrogen[50–52], although a consistent dose–response relationship is lacking. Cessation of therapy results in a rapid decline of the risk within about 2 years, but may remain higher than in the non-user population for up to 10–15 years[53,54]. The cyclical addition of progestogen for 10–14 days each month to continuously administered estrogen has been shown to confer reduction in the risk of endometrial hyperplasia and cancer[55–57]. However, this addition of a progestogen does not eliminate the increased risk: 1.9 (95% CI 0.9–3.8), compared with 6.5 (95% CI 3.1–13.3) for unopposed estrogen users[51,58].

Indeed, Weiderpass and colleagues showed that sequential regimens with the progestogen being administered for fewer than 16 days in a 28-day treatment cycle were associated with increased risk of endometrial cancer: odds ratio (OR) 2.9 (95% CI 1.8–4.6) for 5 or more years of use[59]. In the same report, users of ccHRT enjoyed significant protection against endometrial hyperplasia and cancer: OR 0.2 (95% CI 1.1–1.8) for 5 or more years of use. The increased risk of endometrial cancer was dependent on the type and duration (days per treatment cycle) of the progestogen used. For example, 19-nortestosterone derivatives conferred higher protection than the progesterone-derived progestins.

INVESTIGATION OF ABNORMAL BLEEDING WITH HRT

The clinical principles that govern the management of abnormal bleeding associated with HRT are those of the management of spontaneous postmenopausal bleeding.

A detailed clinical history to include systems review and drug history is essential to exclude conditions that may be the underlying cause of bleeding, or which may influence subsequent management. A general physical examination including the breasts is required to establish normality, in particular a thorough abdominal examination to detect areas of tenderness, possible masses or ascites. Pelvic examination must be systematically conducted to exclude local vulvar, vaginal or cervical lesions. A cervical smear for cytological assessment is obtained, since the detection of abnormal squamous or glandular cells will be a clear indication for colposcopic assessment of the cervix and endometrial evaluation in this group of women. A bimanual examination is performed to assess overall uterine size, mobility of the uterus, characteristics of the supportive tissue and existence of adnexal masses.

ULTRASOUND SCAN

Pelvic organ imaging using ultrasound is a fundamental investigative tool in modern gynecologic practice. Ultrasound scanning of the pelvic organs helps to define the uterine silhouette, uterine cervix and maximum endometrial thickness, corresponding to the apposed endometrial surfaces, in the sagittal plane[60,61]. It may also identify the contrasting echoes of uterine fibroids or any fluid collection within the endometrial cavity. This imaging technology is invaluable in excluding ovarian cystic lesions.

Attempts at color Doppler imaging in conjunction with vaginal ultrasound scan to evaluate endometrial neovascularization did not fulfil the initial promise of adding further information obtained by ultrasound scan alone, and the technique did not discriminate between benign and malignant disease[62,63].

SALINE INSTILLATION SONOHYSTEROGRAPHY

The instillation of a contrast medium into the uterine cavity using normal saline helps to separate the anterior and posterior walls of the endometrial cavity[64–67] and delineate the presence of endometrial polyps, and sometimes submucous fibroids, as they distort the endometrial surface. Recently, a prospective comparison of the accuracy of the saline instillation sonohysterography (SIS) technique with that of panoramic hysteroscopy has documented its shortcomings[68].

HYSTEROSCOPY

Earlier reports described the use of the hysteroscope under general anesthesia; however, it is widely accepted that out-patient hysteroscopy with or without local anesthesia is a very well-tolerated procedure[69,70], and in experienced hands is just as accurate. Moreover, it is easier to repeat when required, for example, in cases of recurrence of postmenopausal bleeding.

The use of CO_2 gas or fluid distension for panoramic hysteroscopy offers a direct visual examination of the whole of the endometrial cavity. It helps to identify endometrial abnormalities such as polyps and submucous fibroids, and regional differences in endometrial thickness and its background color, as well as the endometrial vascular pattern. The outer diameter of the instruments in common use ranges from 3.5 to 6 mm and, therefore, the need for cervical dilatation is limited. The disadvantages of using a gas distension medium include bubble formation, but, by waiting for 30–60 s without manipulating the hysteroscope, these bubbles will burst, and the view of the cavity will become clearer. Note that the escape of gas through the Fallopian tubes may cause diaphragmatic irritation with a typical shoulder-tip referred pain. Alternatively, and especially in the event of bleeding, distension of the uterus with normal saline can be used.

Endometrial sampling

Having assessed the uterine cavity by ultrasound scan and/or by office-based hysteroscopy, an endometrial biopsy is essential to establish a definitive histologic diagnosis. The endometrial biopsy is obtained using a pipelle de Cornier sampler or the Vabra aspirator. Should there be a localized lesion deemed not to have been adequately sampled, hysteroscopically directed biopsy with a biopsy forceps or with the LENS device (Leicester endometrial needle sampler) will help[71].

CHOICE OF METHOD OF INVESTIGATION

The choice of method(s) of investigating the endometrium should be based on the objectives of that clinical encounter. If the question is purely whether the patient has endometrial neoplasia, then an adequate endometrial biopsy should suffice. If clinical evaluation of postmenopausal bleeding is required, then the clinician is obliged to provide a thorough clinical assessment and full investigation of the reproductive system.

The number of menopausal women is increasing, with the 'baby boomers' entering their sixth decade of life, and the problem of functional bleeding disorders may be encountered more often with the increase in HRT use. These functional bleeding disorders mandate effective methods in identifying endometrial polyps and submucous fibroids, since their removal is highly successful in rectifying abnormal bleeding while using HRT[44,45]. Moreover, appropriate and detailed evaluation of the endometrial histology may guide corresponding adjustment in the dose of estrogen or progestogen (see above).

The enthusiasm for ultrasound evaluation of the endometrium prompted many investigators to test how safe it would be to forgo the need for endometrial biopsy. Cut-off points in endometrial thickness have been tested, and the 5-mm limit has been widely adopted[72,73]. A prerequisite of a clear symmetrical endometrial echo of less than 5 mm encouraged Briley and Lindsell to omit endometrial biopsy[73].

Many reports, however, have shown that cancer cannot be excluded when endometrial thickness is below 5 mm, and have suggested 4- and 3-mm cut-off points instead[74–78]. Schramm and colleagues showed that the median endometrial thickness among uterine cancer patients was 4 mm, as opposed to 5.5 mm for those with an atrophic endometrium, in a prospective evaluation of transvaginal ultrasound (TVU) compared with dilatation and curettage (D&C) as an independent procedure in 195 women presenting with spontaneous postmenopausal bleeding[79]. Endometrial cancer was detected in 29 women (15%). By adopting a cut-off point of ≥ 4 mm for endometrial thickness, the sensitivity and specificity of TVU was 62 and 50%, respectively. Similar concerns were reported from a series of 54 women who presented with spontaneous postmenopausal bleeding, in which median endometrial thickness as measured by TVU was 5, 8.6 and 6 mm for histologically documented endometrial atrophy, hyperplasia and adenocarcinoma, respectively. Moreover, of the nine malignant samples, three cases had an endometrial thickness of 3 mm[80].

The SIS technique is claimed to provide accurate diagnosis of atrophic endometrium and endometrial polyps with a sensitivity of 87.8 and 89.6%, and specificity of 90.7 and 95%, respectively[81]. However, in this study, SIS diagnosed only 40% of endometrial cancers, confirming the fundamental requirement for histologic examination of the endometrium in all cases. Soares and colleagues equated the accuracy of SIS to that of the 'gold standard' hysteroscopy and endometrial biopsy in the diagnosis of benign lesions, i.e. polyps, submucous fibroids and endometrial hyperplasia in premenopausal infertile women, but it failed to diagnose accurately intrauterine adhesions[82]. A more cautious approach was suggested by O'Connell and co-workers, who concluded that an office-based SIS with endometrial biopsy would be reliable enough in the management of postmenopausal bleeding when no endometrial abnormality was detected[83]. Where intrauterine luminal masses are suspected, then the patient should be referred for hysteroscopy and fractional curettage.

In a series of 1398 women, 43% of whom were postmenopausal, diagnostic hysteroscopy and subsequent curettage confirmed that, in addition to being a basic tool in gynecological practice, the sensitivity, specificity and global diagnostic precision of hysteroscopic evaluation of the endometrium was 100, 99.4 and 99.5%, respectively[84]. A similar experience was recorded in 980 women presenting with menstrual disorders[85], and in another series of 106 women who presented with postmenopausal bleeding[72], confirming the accuracy, safety and simplicity of out-patient hysteroscopy and endometrial sampling.

MANAGEMENT OF IRREGULAR BLEEDING WITH HRT

The occurrence of an unscheduled or abnormal bleeding pattern in women using a sequential combined hormone replacement regimen is an indication for ultrasound assessment of the pelvic organs, and for endometrial evaluation by hysteroscopy and curettage. In women using ccHRT, the occurrence of irregular bleeding during the first 3 months of treatment is quite common. Full investigations will be required if such bleeding lasts for more than 6 months, or earlier in women with higher risks of developing endometrial neoplasia such as those with obesity, diabetes mellitus, nulliparity[86] or a family history of endometrial or colonic carcinoma[87]. In a population-based study, the incidence of adenomatous and atypical hyperplasia was estimated at 44 per 100 000 per year, and one of the characteristics of these women was overall obesity, rather than specific regional fat distribution[88]. Despite the identification of risk factors, investigation of the endometrium cannot be safely withheld from women who do not have these risks[86]. Where malignant disease is excluded, and in the absence of endometrial polyps or submucous fibroids, adjustment of the HRT regimen is attempted. A common approach is change of the progestogen to a more androgenic type, but this may cause bloatedness, fluid retention and mood swings. The use of a levonorgestrel-laiden intrauterine device (Mirena® coil) has been advocated, but this is not without drawbacks. Prolonged bleeding and spotting can be anticipated for up to 1 year, and the systemic absorption of levonorgestrel may result in androgenic adverse effects. Furthermore, long-term safety as a result of its systemic absorption with regard to the cardiovascular system and bone resorption has not been evaluated. Another approach involves reducing the dose of estrogen, but this may risk a recurrence of vasomotor symptoms or may not be adequate to control bone loss. A non-oral route of administration is generally associated with less bleeding, and this may be related to lesser amounts of estrone generated. In women treated with ccHRT a lower-dose formulation may be adequate. However, the view of the present authors is to offer a change to a sequential combined HRT regimen as the treatment of choice. This may improve endometrial thickness and thus result in more predictable withdrawal bleeding, which may be acceptable to the woman especially if these bleeding episodes are short and light.

CONCLUSIONS

Abnormal bleeding in women treated with HRT is an important cause of discontinuation of treatment. A woman's ability to predict the day of onset of bleeding in the following cycle, for example, helps her to plan various life events, and increases her confidence to continue with treatment in the long term. Understanding the bleeding phenomenon and accurate prediction of which woman is likely to have an abnormal bleeding pattern may enhance the clinical management of these women, and enable the clinician to adjust the HRT regimen appropriately. In postmenopausal women presenting with abnormal or unscheduled bleeding while receiving gonadal steroid treatment, thorough endometrial evaluation is mandatory. In the absence of neoplasia or structural abnormalities of the endometrial cavity, tailoring the treatment regimen to the individual woman's situation facilitates the administration of very effective health-promoting therapeutics. Such endeavor should be guided by the clinical presentation, information gleaned from menstrual diaries and detailed evaluation of the functional aspects of endometrial histology. Incomplete assessment can lead to inappropriate treatment, which eventually frustrates patients and prompts many of them to opt for cessation of treatment or for probably an unnecessary hysterectomy.

RECOMMENDED FURTHER READING

Al-Azzawi F, Wahab M. *Hormone Replacement Therapy and the Endometrium*. Lancaster, UK: Parthenon Publishing, 2001

References

1. Smith D, Prentice R, Thompson D, Herman W. Association of exogenous estrogen and endometrial carcinoma. *N Engl J Med* 1975;293: 1164–7

2. Weiss NS, Szekely DR, Austin DF. Increasing incidence of endometrial cancer in the United States. *N Engl J. Med* 1976;294:1259–62

3. Ettinger B, Selby JV, Citron JT, Ettinger VM, Zhang D. Gynecologic complications of cyclic estrogen–progestin therapy. *Maturitas* 1993;17: 197–204

4. Investigators, Working Group for the Women's Health Initiative Risks and benefits of estrogen plus progestin in healthy postmenopausal women: principal results from the Women's Health Initiative randomized controlled trial. *J Am Med Assoc* 2002;288:321–33

5. Hulley S, Grady D, Bush T, *et al.* Randomized trial of estrogen plus progestin for secondary prevention of coronary heart disease in post-menopausal women. Heart and Estrogen/progestin Replacement Study (HERS) Research Group. *J Am Med Assoc* 1998;280:605–13

6. Stampfer MJ, Colditz GA. Estrogen replacement therapy and coronary heart disease: a quantitative assessment of the epidemiologic evidence. *Prev Med* 1991;20: 47–63

7. Grady D, Rubin SM, Petitti DB, *et al.* Hormone therapy to prevent disease and prolong life in postmenopausal women [see Comments]. *Ann Intern Med* 1992;117:1016–37

8. Miyagawa K, Rösch J, Stanczyk F, Hermsmeyer K. Medroxyprogesterone interferes with ovarian steroid protection against coronary vasospasm [see Comments]. *Nature Med* 1997;3:324–7

9. Geist SH. The variability of menstrual rhythm and character. *Am J Obstet Gynecol* 1930;20:320–3

10. Gunn DL, Jenkin PM, Gunn AL. Menstrual periodicity; statistical observations on a large sample of normal cases. *J Obstet Gynaecol Br Emp* 1937;44:839–79

11. Goldzieher J, Henkin A, Hamblen E, Durham N. Characteristics of the normal menstrual cycle. *Am J Obstet Gynecol* 1947;54:668–75

12. Matsumoto S, Nogami Y, Ohkuri S. Statistical studies on menstruation; a criticism on the definition of normal menstruation. *Gunma J Med Sci* 1962;11:294–318

13. Chiazze L, Brayer FT, Macisco JJ, Parker MP, Duffy BJ. The length and variability of the human menstrual cycle. *J Am Med Assoc* 1968;203:377–80

14. Treloar A, Boynton R, Behn B, Brown B. Variation of the human menstrual cycle through reproductive life. *Int J Fertil* 1967;12:77–126

15. Belsey EM, Carlson N. The description of menstrual bleeding patterns: towards fewer measures. *Stat Med* 1991;10:267–84

16. Boerrigter PJ, van de Weijer PH, Baak JP, *et al.* Endometrial response in estrogen replacement therapy quarterly combined with a progestogen. *Maturitas* 1996; 24:63–71

17. Thompson JR. Analysis of menstrual cycle bleeding diary data. In Al-Azzawi F, Wahab M, eds. *Hormone Replacement Therapy and the Endometrium.* Lancaster, UK: Parthenon Publishing, 2001: 35–47

18. Habiba MA, Bell SC, Abrams K, Al-Azzawi F. Endometrial responses to hormone replacement therapy: the bleeding pattern. *Hum Reprod* 1996;11:503–8

19. Al-Azzawi F, Wahab M, Thompson J, Whitehead M, Thompson W. Acceptability and patterns of uterine bleeding in sequential trimegestone-based hormone replacement therapy: a dose-ranging study. *Hum Reprod* 1999;14:636–41

20. Wahab M, Thompson J, Whitehead M, Al-Azzawi F. The effect of a change in the dose of trimegestone on the pattern of bleeding in estrogen-treated post-menopausal women: 6 month extension of a dose-ranging study. *Hum Reprod* 2002;17:1386–90

21. Al-Azzawi F, Wahab M, Thompson J, *et al.* Acceptability and patterns of endometrial bleeding in estradiol-based HRT regimens: a comparative study of cyclical sequential combinations of trimegestone or norethisterone acetate. *Climacteric* 2001;4:343–54

22. Hallberg I, Nilsson I. Determination of menstrual blood loss. *Scand J Clin Lab Invest* 1964;16:244–8

23. Higham JM, O'Brien PM, Shaw RW. Assessment of menstrual blood loss using a pictorial chart. *Br J Obstet Gynaecol* 1990;97:734–9

24. Reid PC, Coker A, Coltart R. Assessment of menstrual blood loss using a pictorial chart: a validation study. *Br J Obstet Gynaecol* 2000;107: 320–2

25. Al-Azzawi F, Wahab M, Habiba M, Akkad A, Mason T. Continuous combined hormone replacement therapy compared with tibolone. *Obstet Gynecol* 1999;93:258–64

26. Doren M. Hormonal replacement regimens and bleeding. *Maturitas* 2000;34:S17–23

27. Rodriguez G, Faundes-Latham A, Atkinson LE. An approach to the analysis of menstrual patterns in the critical evaluation of contraceptives. *Stud Fam Plann* 1976;7:42–51

28. Dallenbach-Hellweg G, Poulsen H, eds. *Histopathology of the Endometrium*. New York: Springer, 1996;105–9.

29. Goldzieher JW. Pharmacokinetics and metabolism of ethynyl estrogens. In Goldzieher JW, Fotherby K, eds. *Pharmacology of the Contraceptive Steroids*. New York: Raven, 1994;127–53

30. Good RG, Moyer DL. Estrogen–progesterone relationships in the development of secretory endometrium. *Fertil Steril* 1968;19:37–49

31. Wahab M, Thompson J, Hamid B, Deen S, Al-Azzawi F. Endometrial histomorphometry of trimegestone-based sequential hormone replacement therapy: a weighted comparison with the endometrium of the natural cycle. *Hum Reprod* 1999;14:2609–18

32. Rogers PA, Au CL, Affandi B. Endometrial microvascular density during the normal menstrual cycle and following exposure to long-term levonorgestrel. *Hum Reprod* 1993;8:1396–404

33. Wahab M, Thompson J, Al-Azzawi F. Effect of different cyclical sequential progestins on endometrial vascularity in postmenopausal women compared with the natural cycle: a morphometric analysis [in Process Citation]. *Hum Reprod* 2000;15:2075–81

34. Belsey EM, d'Arcangues C, Carlson N. Determinants of menstrual bleeding patterns among women using natural and hormonal methods of contraception. II. The influence of individual characteristics. *Contraception* 1988;38:243–57

35. Marslew U, Munk-Nielsen N, Nilas L, Riis BJ, Christiansen C. Bleeding pattern and climacteric symptoms during different sequential combined HRT regimens in current use. *Maturitas* 1994;19:225–37

36. Byrjalsen I, Thormann L, Meinecke B, Riis BJ, Christiansen C. Sequential estrogen and progestogen therapy: assessment of progestational effects on the postmenopausal endometrium. *Obstet Gynecol* 1992;79:523–8

37. Sporrong T, Rybo G, Mattsson LA, Vilbergson G, Crona N. An objective and subjective assessment of uterine blood loss in postmenopausal women on hormone replacement therapy. *Br J Obstet Gynaecol* 1992;99:399–401

38. Armenia CS. Sequential relationship between endometrial polyps and carcinoma of the endometrium. *Obstet Gynecol* 1967;30:524–9

39. Bakour SH, Khan KS, Gupta JK. The risk of premalignant and malignant pathology in endometrial polyps. *Acta Obstet Gynecol Scand* 2000;79:317–20

40. Akkad AA, Habiba MA, Ismail N, Abrams K, Al-Azzawi F. Abnormal uterine bleeding on hormone replacement: the importance of intrauterine structural abnormalities. *Obstet Gynecol* 1995;86:330–4

41. Wahab M, Thompson J, Al-Azzawi F. The effect of submucous fibroids on the dose-dependent modulation of uterine bleeding by trimegestone in postmenopausal women treated with hormone replacement therapy. *Br J Obstet Gynaecol* 2000;107:329–34

42. Downes E, Al-Azzawi F. The predictive value of outpatient hysteroscopy in a menopause clinic – a prospective study of 254 patients. *Br J Obstet Gynaecol* 1993;100:1148–9

43. Neuwirth RS. Hysteroscopic submucous myomectomy. *Obstet Gynecol Clin North Am* 1995;22:541–58

44. Cravello L, de Montgolfier R, D'Ercole C, Boubli L, Blanc B. Hysteroscopic surgery in postmenopausal women. *Acta Obstet Gynecol Scand* 1996;75:563–6

45. Al-Azzawi F. Prediction of successful outcome following hysteroscopic laser myomectomy in women with heavy and unscheduled bleeding. *Climacteric* 1992;2:289

46. Mazur MM, Kurman RJ. *Diagnosis of Endometrial Biopsies and Curettage: a Practical Approach*. New York: Springer, 1995:8, 23, 234

47. The Writing Group for the Postmenopausal Estrogen/Progestin Interventions Trial. Effects of hormone replacement therapy on endometrial histology in postmenopausal women. The Postmenopausal Estrogen/Progestin Interventions (PEPI) Trial. The Writing Group for the PEPI Trial [see Comments]. *J Am Med Assoc* 1996;275:370–5

48. Parkin DM. Studies of cancer in migrant populations: methods and interpretation. *Rev Epidemiol Santé Publique* 1992;40:410–24

49. Miller BA, Ries LAG, Hankey BF eds. *SEER Cancer Statistics Review: 1973–1990*. Bethesda, MD: US Department of Health and Human Services, 1993

50. Grady D, Gebretsadik T, Kerlikowske K, Ernster V, Petitti D. Hormone replacement therapy and endometrial cancer risk: a meta-analysis. *Obstet Gynecol* 1995;85:304–13

51. Jick SS, Walker AM, Jick H. Estrogens, progesterone, and endometrial cancer. *Epidemiology* 1993;4:20–4

52. Brinton LA, Berman ML, Mortel R *et al.* Reproductive, menstrual, and medical risk factors for endometrial cancer: results from a case–control study. *Am J Obstet Gynecol* 1992;167:1317–25

53. Ferenczy A. Studies on the cytodynamics of human endometrial regeneration. I. Scanning electron microscopy. *Am J Obstet Gynecol* 1976;124:64–74

54. Finkle WD, Greenland S, Miettinen OS, Ziel HK. Endometrial cancer risk after discontinuing use of unopposed conjugated estrogens (California, United States). *Cancer Causes Control* 1995;6:99–102

55. Persson I, Adami HO, Bergkvist L et al. Risk of endometrial cancer after treatment with oestrogens alone or in conjunction with progestogens: results of a prospective study. Br Med J 1989; 298:147–51

56. Voigt LF, Weiss NS, Chu J, et al. Progestagen supplementation of exogenous oestrogens and risk of endometrial cancer. Lancet 1991;338: 274–7

57. Woodruff JD, Pickar JH. Incidence of endometrial hyperplasia in postmenopausal women taking conjugated estrogens (Premarin) with medroxyprogesterone acetate or conjugated estrogens alone. The Menopause Study Group [see Comments]. Am J Obstet Gynecol 1994;170: 1213–23

58. Brinton LA, Hoover RN. Estrogen replacement therapy and endometrial cancer risk: unresolved issues. The Endometrial Cancer Collaborative Group. Obstet Gynecol 1993;81: 265–71

59. Weiderpass E, Adami HO, Baron JA, et al. Risk of endometrial cancer following estrogen replacement with and without progestins. J Nat Cancer Inst 1999;91:1131–7

60. Green B. Pelvic ultrasonography. In Sarti DA, Sample WF, eds. Diagnostic Ultrasound Text and Cases. Boston: GK Hall, 1980:502–89

61. Fleischer AC, Kalemeris GC, Machin JE, Entman SS, James AE Jr. Sonographic depiction of normal and abnormal endometrium with histopathologic correlation. J Ultrasound Med 1986;5:445–52

62. Chan FY, Chau MT, Pun TC, et al. Limitations of transvaginal sonography and color Doppler imaging in the differentiation of endometrial carcinoma from benign lesions. J Ultrasound Med 1994;13:623–8

63. Vuento MH, Pirhonen JP, Makinen JI, et al. Screening for endometrial cancer in asymptomatic postmenopausal women with conventional and colour Doppler sonography [see Comments]. Br J Obstet Gynaecol 1999;106:14–20

64. Goldstein SR, Nachtigall M, Snyder JR, Nachtigall L. Endometrial assessment by vaginal ultrasonography before endometrial sampling in patients with postmenopausal bleeding. Am J Obstet Gynecol 1990;163:119–23

65. Parsons AK, Lense JJ. Sonohysterography for endometrial abnormalities: preliminary results. J Clin Ultrasound 1993;21:87–95

66. Dubinsky TJ, Parvey HR, Gormaz G, Makland N. Transvaginal hysterosonography in the evaluation of small endoluminal masses. J Ultrasound Med 1995;14:1–6

67. Cicinelli E, Romano F, Anastasio PS, Blasi N, Parisi C. Sonohysterography versus hysteroscopy in the diagnosis of endouterine polyps. Gynecol Obstet Invest 1994;38:266–71

68. Rogerson L, Bates J, Weston M, Duffy S. A comparison of outpatient hysteroscopy with saline infusion hysterosonography. Br J Obstet Gynaecol 2002;109:800–4

69. Broadbent JA, Hill NC, Molnar BG, Rolfe KJ, Magos AL. Randomized placebo controlled trial to assess the role of intracervical lignocaine in outpatient hysteroscopy [see Comments]. Br J Obstet Gynaecol 1992;99:777–9

70. Downes E, Al-Azzawi F. How well do perimenopausal patients accept outpatient hysteroscopy? Visual analogue scoring of acceptability and pain in 100 women. Eur J Obstet Gynecol Reprod Biol 1993;48:37–41

71. Al-Azzawi F, Habiba M, Bell SC. The Leicester endometrial needle sampler: a novel device for endometrial and myometrial junctional zone biopsy. Obstet Gynecol 1997;90:470–2

72. Loverro G, Bettocchi S, Cormio G, et al. Transvaginal sonography and hysteroscopy in postmenopausal uterine bleeding [in Process Citation]. Maturitas 1999;33:139–44

73. Briley M, Lindsell DR. The role of transvaginal ultrasound in the investigation of women with post-menopausal bleeding. Clin Radiol 1998;53: 502–5

74. Karlsson B, Granberg S, Wikland M, et al. Transvaginal ultrasonography of the endometrium in women with postmenopausal bleeding – a Nordic multicenter study [see Comments]. Am J Obstet Gynecol 1995;172: 1488–94

75. Guner H, Tiras MB, Karabacak O, et al. Endometrial assessment by vaginal ultrasonography might reduce endometrial sampling in patients with postmenopausal bleeding: a prospective study. Aust NZ J Obstet Gynaecol 1996;36:175–8

76. Kekre AN, Jose R, Seshadri L. Transvaginal sonography of the endometrium in south Indian postmenopausal women [see Comments]. Aust NZ J Obstet Gynaecol 1997;37:449–51

77. Granberg S, Ylostalo P, Wikland M, Karlsson B. Endometrial sonographic and histologic findings in women with and without hormonal replacement therapy suffering from postmenopausal bleeding. Maturitas 1997;27:35–40

78. Bakour SH, Dwarakanath LS, Khan KS, Newton JR, Gupta JK. The diagnostic accuracy of ultrasound scan in predicting endometrial hyperplasia and cancer in postmenopausal bleeding. Acta Obstet Gynecol Scand 1999;78: 447–51

79. Schramm T, Kurzl R, Schweighart C, Stuckert-Klein AC. [Endometrial carcinoma and vaginal ultrasound: studies of the diagnostic validity.] Geburtshilfe Frauenheilkd 1995;55:65–72

80. Buyuk E, Durmusoglu F, Erenus M, Karakoc B. Endometrial disease diagnosed by transvaginal ultrasound and dilatation and curettage. Acta Obstet Gynecol Scand 1999;78:419–22

81. Bernard JP, Lecuru F, Darles C, *et al.* Saline contrast sonohysterography as first-line investigation for women with uterine bleeding. *Ultrasound Obstet Gynecol* 1997; 10:121–5

82. Soares SR, Barbosa dos Reis MM, Camargos AF. Diagnostic accuracy of sonohysterography, transvaginal sonography, and hysterosalpingography in patients with uterine cavity diseases. *Fertil Steril* 2000;73:406–11

83. O'Connell LP, Fries MH, Zeringue E, Brehm W. Triage of abnormal postmenopausal bleeding: a comparison of endometrial biopsy and transvaginal sonohysterography versus fractional curettage with hysteroscopy. *Am J Obstet Gynecol* 1998;178:956–61

84. Torrejon R, Fernandez-Alba JJ, Carnicer I, *et al.* The value of hysteroscopic exploration for abnormal uterine bleeding. *J Am Assoc Gynecol Laparosc* 1997;4:453–6

85. Loverro G, Bettocchi S, Cormio G, *et al.* Diagnostic accuracy of hysteroscopy in endometrial hyperplasia. *Maturitas* 1996;25:187–91

86. Weber AM, Belinson JL, Piedmonte MR. Risk factors for endometrial hyperplasia and cancer among women with abnormal bleeding. *Obstet Gynecol* 1999;93:594–8

87. Farquhar CM, Lethaby A, Sowter M, Verry J, Baranyai J. An evaluation of risk factors for endometrial hyperplasia in premenopausal women with abnormal menstrual bleeding. *Am J Obstet Gynecol* 1999;181:525–9

88. Gredmark T, Kvint S, Havel G, Mattsson L. Adipose tissue distribution in postmenopausal women with adenomatous hyperplasia of the endometrium. *Gynecol Oncol* 1999;72:138–42

18

Immunological changes after the menopause and estrogen replacement therapy

S. Ocampo de Ruiz

BACKGROUND

The study of the immune system in the menopause is a relatively new field of research, and only few data are available on some key components of the immune system and hormonal ovarian deficiency in the menopause. In fact, only recently has this subject captured relevant attention in literature reviews.

The immune system is a function of the body affected profoundly by aging, and since the immune system interacts with every organ and tissue in the body, and the neuroendocrine system is affected by the menopause, numerous studies suggest that hormonal gonadal deficiency could also affect immune function. Thus, hormones can affect immune cells and, consequently, immune system activities.

Table 1 Age-related changes in the immune system. Reproduced with permission from Kamel HK, *et al.* Biological theories of aging. In Morley JE, van den Berg L, eds. *Endocrinology of Aging.* Humana Press, 1999[1]

Thymic gland involution
Reduced T-helper and T-suppressor cells
Decreased cell-mediated cytotoxicity
Increased circulating autoantibodies
Increase in circulating immune complexes
Decreased levels of specific antibody response
Diminished delayed hypersensitivity
Diminished production of interleukin-2
Increased production of interleukin-6

None the less, it is difficult to determine whether immunological differences observed in the menopause result from hormonal deficiency of ovarian steroids or instead are the results of age-related changes in immune function[1] (Table 1).

In addition, it is well documented that immunocompetence declines with age, and the immune system begins to lose some of its functions and cannot respond as quickly or as efficiently to stimuli. Age-related changes of the immune system have been observed at all levels, ranging from chemical changes within cells to differences in the kinds of proteins found on the cell surface, and even to alterations of entire organs.

One major change that occurs as the body ages is a process termed, 'thymic involution'. The thymus is the organ where T cells mature. T cells constitute an extremely important, highly specialized population of lymphocytes that have many functions, ranging from killing bacteria to assisting other cell types of the immune system.

This review covers a summary of the immune system, links between the neuroendocrine system, sex hormones and the immune system, autoimmune diseases related to alterations in sex hormones, mainly with reference to estrogen deficiency in the menopause, and hormone replacement therapy (HRT) and immune functions.

OVERVIEW OF THE IMMUNE SYSTEM

The immune system is an interactive network of lymphoid organs, cells, humoral factors and cytokines. The essential function of the immune system in host defense is best illustrated when it goes wrong: underactivity resulting in the severe infections and tumors of immunodeficiency, overactivity in allergic and autoimmune disease[2].

Immunity is divided into two parts determined by the speed and specificity of reactions. The immune system eliminates foreign material in two ways: natural/innate immunity and adaptive/specific immunity.

Natural immunity produces a relatively unsophisticated response that prevents access of pathogens to the body and provides immediate host defense. This is a primitive evolutionary response that occurs without the need of prior exposure to similar pathogens. For example, macrophages and granulocytes engulf invading micro-organisms at the site of entry. These macrophages are estrogen-sensitive.

Adaptive immunity is the hallmark of the immune system of higher animals. This response consists of antigen-specific reactions through T lymphocytes and B lymphocytes. Specific immunity comprises two types of immune response: humoral immunity, in which antibodies are produced, and cellular immunity, which involves cell lysis by specialized lymphocytes (cytolytic T cells). Adaptive immunity is characterized by an anamnestic response that enables immune cells to, 'remember' the foreign antigenic encounter, and by the use of cytokines for communication and regulation of the innate immune response[3].

Immune cells mediate their effects by releasing cytokines and thus establishing particular microenvironments. T-helper (Th) lymphocytes originating from the thymus play a major role in creating a specific microenvironment for a particular organ or tissue. T-helper cells are subdivided functionally by the pattern of cytokines they produce[4]. On stimulation, precursor Th0 lymphocytes become either T-helper 1 or T-helper 2 cells. The difference between these cells is only in the cytokines secreted; they are morphologically indistinguishable. However the responses they generate are very different. Th1 cytokines induce mainly a cell-mediated inflammatory response and inhibit Th2 differentiation. Th1 cells secrete interleukin-2 (IL-2) and interferon-γ (IFN-γ), setting the basis for a proinflammatory environment. A Th1 response, is essential to the host to control the replication of intracellular pathogens, but possibly contributes to the pathogenesis of autoimmune diseases such as rheumatoid arthritis and multiple sclerosis. Conversely, Th2 cells produce IL-4, -5, -6 and -10, which are predominantly involved in antibody production. Thus, the Th2 response is associated with allergic disease. The actions of the two types of lymphocyte are closely intertwined, both acting in concert and responding to counterregulatory effects of their cytokines.

Thus, T lymphocytes play a major role in the immune response. They have been found to be susceptible to dysregulated function with aging, and these alterations affect both antibody- and cell-mediated responses[5].

In addition, the concept of the immune system has advanced from merely response to infectious agents to include a variety of complex situations and interactions with most, if not all, of the body's systems. For the purpose of understanding, Mor[3] assumes a division of these interactions into classical immune regulation and non-immune regulation by leukocytes. Each of the components of non-immune regulation is sensitive to the reproductive milieu and therefore to gonadal function. The elements of non-immune regulation include stimuli, effector cells, signals and target cells. Chiefly among these are the circulating monocytes that arise in the bone marrow and are the precursors to the tissue macrophages. In many organs, estrogen regulates the number of tissue macrophages. Thus, gonadal steroids represent primary signals for non-immune regulation. Acting via steroid receptors they can regulate monocyte number, cytokine production by monocytes and differentiation of monocytes into macrophages in the tissues. Monocytes contain estrogen receptors, but macrophages contain both aromatase and estrogen receptors. They respond to estradiol by secretion of cytokines, which can act in an autocrine or paracrine manner to regulate cell number and cell function.

Also, considerable evidence has accumulated suggesting that the interaction between estrogens and cells of the immune system can have non-immune regulatory effects. Thus, the role of estrogens in the prevention of bone loss is mediated by mechanisms involving the inhibition of proinflammatory cytokines by bone marrow cells. Moreover, disorders frequently affecting women after the menopause, such as cardiovascular disease, osteoporosis and neurodegenerative disorders, can be ascribed to the loss of sex hormone-dependent regulation of physiological functions, as well as to a modification of the non-immune regulatory functions of resident immune cells[3].

NEUROENDOCRINE AND IMMUNE SYSTEMS

Until recently, the immune system was considered to constitute a largely autonomous self-regulating system. However, it is now clear that the immune system interacts with the neuroendocrine system and with virtually all tissues and organs, and that the central nervous system is the highest immunoregulatory organ, controlling immune and inflammatory reactions with the aid of classical hormones, neuroptides and neurotransmitters. A failure of this central neuroimmunoregulatory network invariably leads to disease, which may be a consequence of hyperactivity (for example, autoimmune diseases, allergy, chronic inflammatory conditions) or hypoactivity (immunodeficiency, susceptibility to infectious disease, cancer, etc.) of the immune system[6]. The evidence that suggests interactions between the immune system and the neuroendocrine system comes from several observations. First, immune and neuroendocrine cells share common signal molecules and receptors; second, hormones and neuropeptides can alter the functional activities of immune cells; and third, the immune system is innervated by noradrenergic sympathetic and peptidergic nerve fibers. These nerve fibers are in direct contact with lymphocytes and macrophages, performing neuroeffector functions and releasing neurotransmitters that exert direct effects on the immune function. Finally, the immune system and its products, such as cytokines, can modulate the function of neural and endocrine systems[7]. Communications between the immune and neuroendocrine systems utilize both hormonal and neural mechanisms. The hypothalamic–pituitary–adrenal (HPA) axis and hypothalamic–pituitary–gonadal (HPG) axis function as a neuroendocrine circuit, incorporating complex feedback mechanisms that preserve homeostasis. Cytokine effects on neural and endocrine systems include activation of the HPA and HPG axes. The cytokines IL-1 and IL-6, in particular, are crucial factors in the activation of the neuroendocrine system[8–10].

SEX HORMONES AND THE IMMUNE SYSTEM

It has long been suspected that there is a strong interaction between sex hormones and the immune system. Numerous *in vitro* and *in vivo* experiments have demonstrated that sex hormones affect and modify the action of cells of the immune system.

Sex hormones have been shown to modulate a great variety of mechanisms involved in the immune response, including thymocyte maturation and selection, cell trafficking, and cytokine and monokine production; lymphocyte proliferation; and expression of adhesion molecules and human leukocyte antigen (HLA)-class receptors.

Estrogens have stimulating effects on B-cell function, which seem dependent on inhibition of suppressor T cells; estrogens increase B-cell response and antibody production. On the other hand, progesterone and androgens depress antibody production. The above observations suggest that estrogens enhance B cell-mediated diseases but suppress T cell-dependent conditions. Androgens appear to

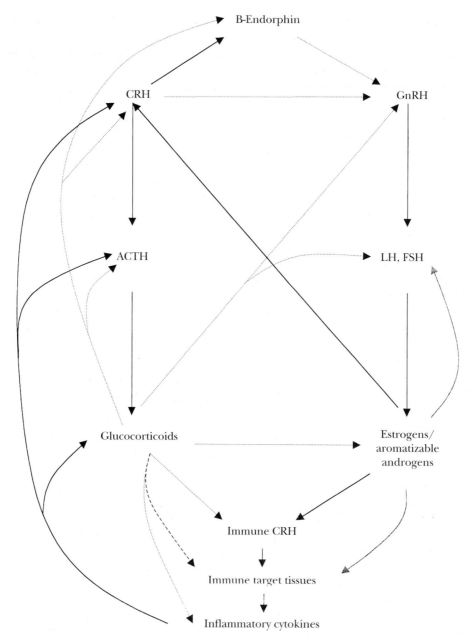

Figure 1 A model of the interaction between the hypothalamic–pituitary–adrenal (HPA) and hypothalamic–pituitary–gonadal (HPG) axes and the immune/inflammatory response. Solid black lines indicate stimulation, broken lines inhibition and dashed lines conditional inhibition or stimulation. Interactions between the axes are bidirectional. The HPA axis inhibits the HPG axis at multiple levels. Estrogens may stimulate the corticotropin-releasing hormone (CRH) neuron, and therefore the HPA axis; and the peripheral production of immune CRH, and hence the immune/inflammatory response. Immune CRH exerts proinflammatory effects; consequent cytokine production activates the HPA axis and glucocorticoids dampen the inflammatory response. ACTH, adrenocorticotropic hormone; GnRH, gonadotropin-releasing hormone; LH, luteinizing hormone; FSH, follicle stimulating hormone. Reproduced with permission from Vamvakopoulos NC, Chrousos GP. Hormonal regulation of human corticotropin-releasing hormone gene expression: implications for the stress response and immune/inflammatory reaction. *Endocr Rev* 1994;15:409–20[12]. ©The Endocrine Society

suppress both B-cell and T-cell immune responses, and virtually always suppress disease expression[11].

In addition, sex hormones may affect the immune system not only by direct effects on immune-competent cells but indirectly through changes in the HPA axis.

The HPA axis inhibits the reproductive axis at many levels (Figure 1); thus, corticotropin-releasing hormone (CRH) inhibits the gonadotropin-releasing hormone (GnRH) neuron of the hypothalamic arcuate nucleus directly, and via β-endorphins. As the GnRH neuron has no estradiol receptors, estradiol may act through hypothalamic CRH to inhibit GnRH secretion, and hence exert negative feedback through this mechanism. Glucocorticoids inhibit GnRH secretion as well as gonadotropin and gonadal steroid hormone production. Conversely, estradiol appears to exert positive effects on CRH production both in the hypothalamus and peripheral tissues[13].

Estradiol stimulates the expression of adhesion molecules by immune cells[14] while inhibiting the production of IL-6, an inflammatory cytokine, which plays a major role in the control and termination of inflammation directly via inhibition of tumor necrosis factor-α (TNF-α) and IL-1 production, and indirectly via stimulation of glucocorticoid secretion and activation of the acute phase of reaction. Hence, we can conclude that gonadal axis hormones, directly and indirectly through the HPA axis, alter the tone of the immune system and the quantity and quality of the inflammatory responses. These complex interactions between the HPA axis and immune and gonadal systems may prove to be fundamental in the genesis and perpetuation of autoimmune disease[15].

SEX DIFFERENCES IN THE IMMUNE RESPONSE

The immune system is clearly sexually dimorphic. Physiological, experimental and clinical data confirm differences in immune responses between the sexes. Therefore, gender emerges

as one of the most important epidemiological risk factors for the development of autoimmune diseases. For instance, data on the incidence of a great variety of autoimmune diseases show that females represent the majority of patients affected in most of the conditions: 85% in Hashimoto's thyroiditis and Grave's disease, over 90% in systemic lupus erythematosus and Sjögren's syndrome, and 65–75% in Addison's disease, myasthenia gravis and rheumatoid arthritis[16]. Females have higher immunoglobulin levels and stronger humoral and cell-mediated immune responses[17].

During the reproductive years, females tend to have more a vigorous immune response, stronger antibody response to immunization and infection, increased production of autoreactive autoimmune antibodies, increased resistance to the induction of immunological tolerance and a greater ability to reject tumors and homografts[3], compared with males.

CHANGES IN IMMUNE SYSTEM DURING THE MENOPAUSE

The menopause represents a low-estrogen state, and possibly a Th1 (type 1) immune environment. During the menopause, deficiency of estrogen results in a failure of estrogen's regulation of the immune system. It is now generally agreed that the immune responses may polarize into cytokine environments characteristic of Th1 and Th2 cells. In general, the normal reproductive woman has a strong tendency to respond to foreign antigens by developing a Th1 (type 1) immune response (cell-mediated) and by expressing high levels of proinflammatory cytokines[3].

In menopausal women, the number of peripheral blood monocytes is increased and the percentage of estrogen receptor-positive monocytes is relatively decreased. Furthermore, estrogen replacement therapy for a period of 3 months led to a decline in the numbers of monocytes to the values observed in young women and an increase in percentage of estrogen receptor-positive monocytes. Declining estrogen levels may facilitate the development of cell-mediated autoimmune diseases such as rheumatoid arthritis, whereas high estrogen levels may promote autoimmune diseases associated with humoral immunity such as systemic lupus erythematosus[3].

AUTOIMMUNE DISEASES AND THE MENOPAUSE

For years scientists and physicians have suspected that estrogens and other steroid hormones play a role in autoimmune diseases. A shifting balance between cellular (Th1) and humoral (Th2) immunity is theorized to underlie the etiology of many autoimmune conditions. Rheumatoid arthritis (RA) strikes women chiefly during the peri- and post-menopausal periods. Mounting evidence suggests that RA may develop in response to the sudden drop in adrenal and gonadal steroid hormones induced by the menopause, which creates a shift towards the Th1 immune response. Thus, the predominance of this disease among women suggests that sex hormones may modulate immune susceptibility[18]. The reasons for the sex bias in autoimmune diseases are unclear, but may include factors such as sex-related differences in immune responsiveness and response to infection, sex steroid effects and other sex-linked parameters. Women may have greater susceptibility to autoimmune diseases, in part because of more robust immune responses, yet have a better prognosis, perhaps as a result of heightened recovery mechanisms. Estrogen has a biphasic effect on the normal immune response, and in autoimmune diseases estrogens suppress T cell-dependent immune function but stimulate T cell-independent, B cell-dependent humoral immunity.

Notably, RA in postmenopausal women is associated with accelerated bone reabsorption, compared with RA in premenopausal women. However, RA is uncommon in men under the age of 45, but the risk increases markedly in older age groups[19]. These observations suggest that factors regulating the gender differences are linked to aging and reproductive functions.

Although an understanding of the mechanisms is clearly incomplete, sufficient data are available to suggest that one of the mechanisms through which adrenal and gonadal hormones act is via their regulatory effects on TNF-α, IL-12 and IL-10 production by activated macrophages[20].

Research into neuroendocrine–immune interactions over the past few years indicates that hormones are important contributory factors in RA, and may be involved in both the altered responses to inflammatory insults with the development of chronic inflammatory disease and the microvascular dynamics.

There is evidence that deficient levels of gonadal androgens (testosterone and dihydro-testosterone) and adrenal androgens (dehydro-epiandrosterone sulfate, DHEAS) are present and even pre-exist in both male and female subjects affected with RA. Females have significantly reduced levels of DHEAS, while in males the consistent finding is low testosterone levels. DHEAS can counteract the immuno-suppressive effects of corticosteroids by enhancing IL-2 and IFN production, and thus enhance Th1 cellular responses. On the other hand, gonadal androgens inhibit macrophage activation by abolishing IL-6, TNF-α and IL-1 production[21]. Thus, from currently available data reviewed above, it can be concluded that patients with RA have a predominantly pro-inflammatory hormonal milieu which promotes the development of chronic inflammatory disease.

In vivo and *in vitro* studies have demonstrated that sex hormones interfere with a number of putative processes involved in the pathogenesis of RA, including immunoregulation, interaction with inflammatory mediators and the cytokine system, and a direct effect on the cartilage itself[22]. All these observations point towards the importance of gonadal hormones. However, trials on the potential therapeutic use of sex hormones in RA are limitred. Further work is necessary to determine whether the role of sex hormones is as central protagonist or supporting cast in the complex arena of rheumatoid arthritis[15].

HORMONE REPLACEMENT THERAPY AND THE IMMUNE SYSTEM

Hormone replacement therapy (HRT) confers many health benefits to postmenopausal women. Despite links between estrogens and immune function prior to the menopause, the immune status of women receiving HRT has not been rigorously investigated[23].

Mor[3] has found that, during the climacteric, the function of the immune system becomes more similar to that in men. This alteration is in both function and cellular composition. The number of circulating macrophage precursors (monocytes) increases during the menopause. This estrogen-regulated function could be due to an increase of bone marrow precursors or a decrease of cell migration into tissues. HRT decreases the monocyte number to levels found in premenopausal women. Moreover, in animal studies, ovariectomy up-regulates myeloid cell differentiation into the monocyte–macrophage lineage and increases thymic weight, while estrogen replacement therapy decreases the number of thymocytes and the size of the thymus.

Futhermore, in a prospective study Kamada and colleagues[24] have shown the effect of HRT on postmenopausal changes of lymphocytes and T cell subsets. Since endocrinosenescence occurs simultaneously with immunosenescence, they aimed to determine whether or not lymphocytes and T cell subsets were altered in postmenopausal women. HRT induced a significant increase in the percentage of lymphocytes, but showed no effect on aberrations of naive cells and memory/activated cells. Therefore, HRT prevents the decline in lymphocytes observed in postmenopausal women, but appears not to influence the observed alteration in T cell subsets.

Porter and colleagues[23] studied the immune effects of HRT in postmenopausal women, and their findings showed a reversal of immune alterations associated with normal aging, suggesting that preservation or improvement of immune function may be associated with the use of HRT.

Fahlman and associates[25] examined the effects of long-term HRT on selected indices of resting immune function in postmenopausal women. From this study, they concluded that women taking HRT had increased lymphocyte blastogenesis and decreased natural cell-mediated cytotoxicity, compared with controls.

Research focused on immunology and the menopause is yet scarce; more investigations will be necessary to further our understanding of the aging process of the ovaries in general.

SUMMARY

The immune system is a function of the body profoundly affected by aging.

The essential function of the immune system in host defense is best illustrated when it goes wrong; underactivity resulting in the severe infections and tumors of immunodeficiency, overactivity in autoimmune and allergic diseases.

During the menopause, a deficiency of estrogen results in a failure of estrogen's regulation of the immune system. Estrogen can modify immune cell function and, consequently, immune activities. For instance, the role of estrogen in the prevention of bone loss is mediated by immune mechanisms involving the inhibition of proinflammatory cytokines by bone marrow cells. Moreover, disorders frequently affecting women after the menopause, such as cardiovascular disease, osteoporosis and neurodegenerative disorders, can be ascribed to the loss of sex hormone-dependent regulation of physiological functions, as well as to a modification of the non-immune functions of resident immune cells.

In addition, gender and sex hormones exert powerful effects on the susceptibility to, and progression of, numerous human and experimental autoimmune diseases. This has been attributed to direct immunological effects of sex hormones that exert a clear gender dimorphism on the immune system. Globally, estrogens depress T cell-dependent immune function and diseases. The menopause represents a low-estrogen state and possibly a type 1 immune environment. Androgens suppress both T cell and B cell immune responses, and virtually always result in the suppression of disease expression. Declining estrogen levels may facilitate the development of T-cell mediated diseases such as rheumatoid arthritis. As well defects in the hypothalamic–pituitary–adrenal axis have been proposed to play an important role in the pathogenesis of autoimmune diseases. Adrenal and gonadal deficiency facilitates excessive macrophage production of TNF and IL-12 that characterizes rheumatoid arthritis.

Current evidence indicates that the neuroendocrine system is the highest regulator of immune inflammatory reactions. The hypothalamus–pituitary–adrenal axis constitutes the most powerful circuit regulating the immune system. Abnormalities of neuroimmunoregulation contribute to the etiology of autoimmune disease, chronic inflammatory disease, immunodeficiency and allergic disorders.

Hormone replacement therapy confers many health benefits to postmenopausal women. Despite links between estrogen and immune function prior to the menopause, the immune status has not been rigorously investigated. The number of circulating macrophage precursors (monocytes) increases during the menopause. HRT decreases the monocyte number to levels found in premenopausal women, and some of the impairment observed in the menopause can be restored after HRT. Although much is currently known about the menopausal process, much is yet to be explained. Currently, there are more questions than answers related to links between sex hormones, the menopause and the immune system. However, with the current advances in molecular biology, answers to most of these questions may be found in the near future.

References

1. Kamel HK, Mooradian AD, Mir T. Biological theories of aging. In Morley JE, van den Berg L, eds. *Endocrinology of Aging.* Totowa: Humana Press, 1999;1–6
2. Parkin J. An overview of the immune system. *Lancet* 2001;357:1177–89
3. Mor G. Sex hormones and the immune system. http://info.med.yale.edu/obgyn (2002)
4. Swain SL, Bradley LM, Croft M. Helper T-cell subsets: phenotype, function, and the role of lymphokines in their development. *Immunol Rev* 1991;123:115–44
5. Bartolomi C, Guidi L, Tricerri A, *et al.* Aging of the immune system. In *Immunology and Aging in Europe.* EUCAMBIS. IOS Press, 2000
6. Berczi I, *et al.* The immune effects of neuropeptides. *Ballière's Clin Rheumatol* 1996;4:228–49
7. Chikanza IC, Grossman AB. Neuroendocrine immune responses to inflammation: the concept of the neuroendocrine immune loop. *Balliere's Clin Rheumatol* 1996;10:200–17
8. Navarra P, Tsasgarahis S, Fria MS, *et al.* Interleukin 1 and 6 stimulate the release of corticotropin-releasing hormone from rat hypothalamus *in vitro*, via the eicosanoid cyclooxygenase pathway. *J Endocrinol* 1991;128:37–34
9. Matta S, Weatherbee J, Sharp BM, *et al.* A central mechanism is involved in the secretion of ACTH in response to IL6 in rats. Comparaison to an interaction with IL1. *Neuroendocrinology* 1992; 56:516–25
10. Dinarello CA, Wolf SM. The role of interleukin-1 in disease. *N Engl J Med* 1993;328:106–13
11. Da Silva JPA. Sex hormones and glucocorticoids: interaction with the immune system. *Ann NY Acad Sci* 1998;840:103–15
12. Vamvakopoulos NS, Chrousos GP. Hormonal regulation of human corticotropin-releasing hormone gene expression: implications for the stress response and immune/inflammatory reaction. *Endocr Rev* 1994; 15:409–20
13. Torpy DJ, Chrousos GP. The three way interactions between the hypothalamic–

pituitary–adrenal and gonadal axes and the immune system. *Ballière's Clin Rheumatol* 1996; 10:182–93

14. Cid MC, Klinman HK, Grant DS, *et al.* Estradol enhances leukocyte binding to tumor necrosis factor stimulated endothelial cells via an increase in TNF induced adhesion molecules E-selectin, intercellular adhesion molecule type 1. *J Clin Invest* 1994; 93:17–25

15. Wilder RL. Neuroendocrine–immune system interactions and autoimmunity. *Ann Rev Immunol* 1995;13:307–38

16. Da Silva JPA, Mall G. The effects of gender and sex hormones on outcome in rheumatoid arthritis. *Ballière's Clin Rheumatol* 1992;6:193–219

17. Ahmed S. Gender and risk of autoimmune diseases; possible role of estrogenic compounds. *Environ Health Perspect* 1900;107(Suppl 5): 681–4

18. Masi AT, Da Silva JPA, Cutolo M. Perturbations of hypothalamic–pituitary–gonadal axis and adrenal androgens (AA) functions in rheumatoid arthritis. *Ballière's Clin Rheumatol* 1996; 10:295–332

19. Chikanza IA. The neuroendocrine immunology of rheumatoid arthritis. *Balliere's Clin Rheumatol* 1996;10:274–8

20. Cutolo M, Seriolo B, Villagio B, *et al.* Androgens and estrogens modulate the immune and inflammatory responses in rheumathoid arthritis. *Ann NY Acad Sci* 2002;966:131–42

21. Giltay ER, van Schaadenburg D, Gooren L, *et al.* Dehydroepiandrosterone sulfate in patients with rheumatoid arthritis. *Ann NY Acad Sci* 1998;00:152–3

22. Da Silva JPA, Pers SH, Perreti M, *et al.* Sex steroids affect glucocorticoid response to chronic inflammation and to interleukin 1. *J Endocrinol* 1993; 136:389–97

23. Porter VR, Greendale GA, Schockem M, *et al.* Immune effects of hormone replacement therapy in postmenopausal women. *Exp Gerontol* 2001;36:311–26

24. Kamada M, Ihara M, Maegawa M, *et al.* Effect of hormone replacement therapy on post-menopausal changes of lymphocytes and T-cell subsets. *J Endocrinol Invest* 2000; 23:376–82

25. Fahlman MM, Boardley D, Flynn MG, *et al.* Effects of hormone replacement therapy on selected indices of immune function in post-menopausal women. *Gynecol Obstet Invest* 2000; 50:189–93

19

Contribution of assisted reproduction technology to the understanding of early ovarian aging

D. Nikolaou and G. Trew

INTRODUCTION

In 1998, te Velde and colleagues proposed a very important theory regarding ovarian aging[1]. According to this theory, all major reproductive milestones preceding the menopause show a similar age variation to that of the menopause itself, and the time intervals between them and the menopause are more or less fixed. The reproductive milestones are the age of onset of reduced fertility (30 years on average), age of rapid decline of fertility (37 years on average), age of total loss of fertility (41 years on average) and age of loss of menstrual regularity (45 years on average). Furthermore, the same, mainly genetic, factors[2] that affect the time of the menopause also determine the time of all reproductive milestones that precede the menopause (Figure 1).

The average age at menopause is 51 years, although there is wide variation[3]. Te Velde and colleagues suggested that age at menopause is likely to be a 'perfect, albeit retrospective' marker of the reproductive life span of an individual woman (Figure 2). In support of this hypothesis, it has been shown that the time interval between the loss of menstrual regularity and the menopause is 6–7 years, regardless of age at menopause[4]. With regard to the total loss of fertility, te Velde and colleagues[1] quoted data showing that the age of last delivery for Canadian women in the 19th century showed

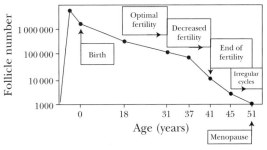

Figure 1 Normal ovarian aging: the menopause and the preceding major reproductive milestones, in relation to age and number of remaining follicles in the ovaries. Reproduced with permission from te Velde ER, *et al.* Age at menopause as a marker of reproductive aging. *Maturitas* 1998;30:119–25[1]

the same variation as the age of menopause, but 10 years earlier. The time of onset of reduced fertility is difficult to ascertain. An important contribution of assisted conception has been to provide indirect evidence that the time interval between onset of accelerated decline of fertility and menopause must also be fixed.

BASIS OF THE FIXED-INTERVALS HYPOTHESIS

The basis of the fixed-intervals hypothesis is the mathematics of follicular depletion in the ovaries. Faddy and co-workers[5], based on pathological data sets[6–8], proposed a mathematical model to describe the age-related decline in

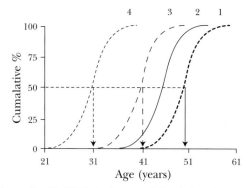

Figure 2 Te Velde's theory of fixed time intervals between major reproductive milestones preceding the menopause: the cumulative age at menopause (1), the age of transition from cycle regularity to irregularity (2), the end of female fertility (3) and the beginning of subfertility (4). Reproduced with permission from te Velde ER, *et al.* Age at menopause as a marker of reproductive aging. *Maturitas* 1998;30:119–25[1]

population of small follicles in the human ovary. Their study confirmed earlier suspicions that the rate of follicle disappearance increased with age[6,7], and demonstrated that the rate more than doubled when numbers fell to the critical figure of 25 000 at around 37 years of age (Figure 3).

Based on their bi-exponential model, they estimated the impact of step reductions of follicle numbers on age at menopause. For example, a unilateral oophorectomy before the age of 30 years would not lower follicle numbers below 25 000, and so the rate of disappearance would continue at the lower rate for some years before a more rapid depletion began. The threshold number of 1000 remaining follicles (menopause) would then be reached at around the age of 44 (Figure 4).

All these projections about the age at menopause after step reductions in follicle number

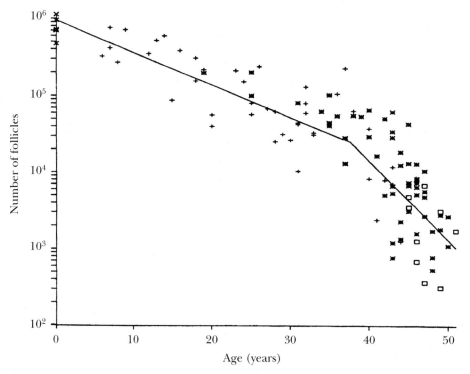

Figure 3 Bi-exponential model of declining follicle numbers in pairs of human ovaries from neonatal age to 51 years old. Data were obtained from studies of Block[6], Richardson and colleagues[7] and Gougeon and Chainy[8]. Reproduced with permission from Faddy MJ, *et al.* Accelerated disappearance of ovarian follicles in mid-life: implications for forecasting menopause. *Hum Reprod* 1992;7:1342–6[5]

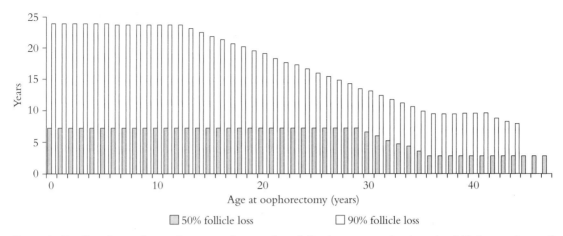

Figure 4 Predicted numbers of menstrual years lost following step reductions in follicle numbers of 50 or 90% at the ages indicated. The predictions are truncated before the age of 50 years because few women reach the menopause later than the mid-sixth decade of life. Reproduced with permission from Faddy MJ, *et al.* Accelerated disappearance of ovarian follicles in mid-life: implications for forecasting menopause. *Hum Reprod* 1992;7:1342–6[5]

were based on the assumption that the change in exponential rate was determined by a critical number rather than a critical age *per se*, as if the ovary measured biological time according to numbers of follicles remaining rather than chronologically. Menopause occurs when the remaining number of resting follicles in the ovaries falls below a critical number, which has been estimated at 1000 follicles. For the average healthy woman who becomes menopausal at the age of 51, an accelerated loss and accelerated qualitative decline of follicles has started at around the age of 37, when only 25 000 resting follicles remain in the ovaries. This is about 13 years before the menopause. It is reasonable to assume, therefore, that for women who become menopausal by the age of 45, the critical point of 25 000 remaining follicles in the ovaries has been reached by the age of 32.

In understanding ovarian aging, a crucial point is that quantity and quality of remaining oocytes are closely correlated. Brook and colleagues[9] found that an earlier cessation of reproductive life in the mouse, brought on by unilateral oophorectomy, resulted in the earlier onset of irregular cyclicity and an earlier rise in aneuploidy. In their discussion, the authors favored the view that there was a continuum of age-related aneuploidy in women, governed not by chronological, but by biological age. Similar findings have been reported more recently following oophorectomies in humans[10,11]. The original cause of age-related deterioration of oocyte quality has been an issue of scientific debate for some time[12–15], although it is generally accepted that the main mechanism is meiotic non-disjunction. One theory, which would explain the findings of Brook and colleagues, is that differentiation of oocyte quality is already established, to some degree, in fetal life, and the best oocytes are simply recruited and selected first, so that oocytes of inferior quality remain at a more advanced age. Another approach has been that the deterioration of oocyte quality is due to accumulation of damage in the DNA of the oocyte as a woman grows older. More recently, the 'two-hit' model of non-disjunction appears to combine all the previous theories on oocyte aging[15,16].

EXPERIENCE GAINED FROM ASSISTED REPRODUCTION

The term used in assisted conception to describe a woman's reproductive potential, in terms of both number and quality of remaining oocytes, is ovarian reserve[17]. The *in vitro* fertilization (IVF) procedure itself can be viewed as an extended dynamic assessment of ovarian reserve. Success rates with IVF depend mainly on the age of the female partner, and decline significantly in the late 30s[18] (Figure 5).

An important contribution of assisted reproduction has been to clarify the relevant contributions of the factors 'sperm', 'oocyte' and 'endometrium' to the decline of fertility observed with age. Studies with donated sperm have shown that the age-related decline in fertility is not caused primarily by the sperm[19]. The advantage of these studies is that the age of the sperm donor is more or less fixed, and therefore the age-related variation is essentially attributable to the woman. For couples where the female partner is 35 years of age or older, the conception rates are half the rates of women up to the age of 25 (Figure 6).

Studies using donated oocytes[20] have shown that the age-related decline in fertility is not primarily caused by the endometrium, either. Women over the age of 40 or postmenopausal, who are treated with hormone replacement therapy and are given oocytes or embryos from younger women, achieve good endometrial development and clinical pregnancy rates. *In vitro* studies, in IVF programs, have shown that the follicles of women in their late 30s have fewer granulosa cells, with decreased mitosis, increased apoptosis and a poorer steroid and glucoprotein production compared with younger women[21]. At the same time, the oocytes within these follicles exhibit abnormal nuclear and cytoplasmic maturation[22–28]. Exactly the same pattern that is seen in the success rates of assisted conception is observed in the way natural fertility declines in various populations around the world (Figure 7).

Mathematical models, developed in these natural fertility populations, have also suggested that the observed sharp decline of

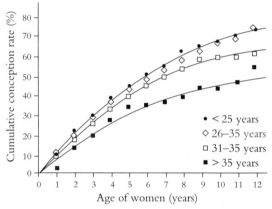

Figure 6 Results of donor insemination in 2193 nulliparous women with azoospermic husbands. Reproduced with permission from Schwarz D, Mayaux MJ. Female fecundity as a function of age: results of artificial insemination in 2193 nulliparous women with azoospermic husbands. *N Engl J Med* 1982;306:404–6[19]

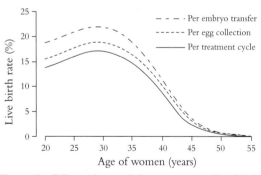

Figure 5 Effect of age of the woman on live birth rate per cycle started, per egg collection and per embryo transfer. Data are from the Human Fertilisation and Embryology Authority, including all *in vitro* fertilization treatment cycles and outcomes registered between August 1991 and April 1994. Reproduced with permission from Templeton A, *et al.* Factors that affect outcome of *in-vitro* fertilization treatment. *Lancet* 1996;348:1402–6[18]

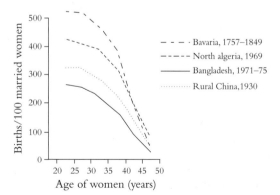

Figure 7 Age-specific marital fertility rates for natural fertility populations. Reproduced with permission from O'Connor KA, *et al.* Declining fecundity and ovarian aging in natural fertility populations. *Maturitas* 1998;30:127–36[29]

fertility in the late 30s is not caused by non-fertilization, but rather by increased early pregnancy loss, and is attributed to a deterioration of oocyte quality[29,30]. This sharp decline of reproductive potential in the late 30s, observed in epidemiological studies, is accompanied by a sharp increase of clinically observed aneuploidy and early pregnancy loss[31,32].

The next important contribution of IVF was to show that the rate of decline of ovarian reserve varies between individuals. In every IVF program there is a proportion of relatively young women who respond poorly to ovarian stimulation and have very low success rates, despite their age. It has been universally observed that increasing the amount of ovarian stimulation beyond a certain limit does not usually improve the outcome[33], and neither do various stimulation protocols or adjuvant treatments that have been tried[34,35]. Once a woman has responded poorly to a reasonable amount of ovarian stimulation, her chances of success in future IVF cycles are low[36–38]. Although relatively young, these women behave reproductively as women in their late 30s or early 40s.

BASIS OF THE LINK BETWEEN RESPONSE TO IVF AND RESTING FOLLICULAR POOL

The basis of the link between response to IVF and number of resting follicles in the ovary, which makes IVF suitable for assessing the ovarian reserve of an individual, lies in the physiology of follicular development. It has been suggested that the size of the cohort of follicles more than 2 mm, which is the cohort of follicles likely to respond to exogenous gonadotropin stimulation during IVF, may be a reflection of the actual resting follicle pool. According to the model of follicular development proposed by Gougeon[39], from a size of 2 mm the follicles enter the 'rapid' growth phase and and become more dependent on follicle stimulating hormone (FSH)[39–41] (Figure 8). During the late luteal phase, the 2–5-mm follicles, which have entered the preantral stage 70 days earlier, become 'selectable' follicles (class 5) and constitute the pool of follicles from

which the one destined to ovulate in the subsequent cycle is selected[42]. Their number in the late luteal phase strongly decreases with advancing age, with an abrupt drop in women over the age of 40[43].

Several studies, both in patients undergoing assisted conception and in healthy volunteers, have shown the potential of antral follicular count by ultrasound to predict ovarian responsiveness and ovarian biological age[44–52] (Figure 9). In a review of ovarian reserve screening tests by Broekmans and colleagues[53], the antral follicular count had a positive likelihood ratio of 3 and was abnormal in 11% of patients. A prospective study was published in 2002[54] assessing various predictors of poor ovarian response in IVF. As a single predictor, the antral follicle count appeared to have the best discriminative potential for poor response, expressed by the largest area under the curve (AUC) of 0.87. It also appeared to be the best predictor in the subsequent multivariate analysis, as it was selected first.

DATA FROM IVF SUGGEST A COVARIATION BETWEEN AGE OF RAPID DECLINE OF REPRODUCTIVE POTENTIAL AND AGE OF MENOPAUSE

A further extremely important contribution of IVF was to show that 'poor responders' enter the menopause earlier. In other words, the variability of age of poor response is not just similar, but parallel to the age of loss of menstrual cyclicity and age of menopause. This observation supports the theory of fixed intervals between reproductive landmarks and validates the IVF cycle as a model for the development of suitable screening tools for early ovarian aging. Total non-response to ovarian stimulation, which is an extreme situation, is likely to represent total loss of fertility. Poor response does not have a standard definition, although it probably should be defined as fewer than four follicles developing following stimulation[52] with at least 300 IU of exogenous FSH/day in a long protocol[36]. There are differences in the way that 'poor response' is defined in various studies[36]. Furthermore, it is difficult

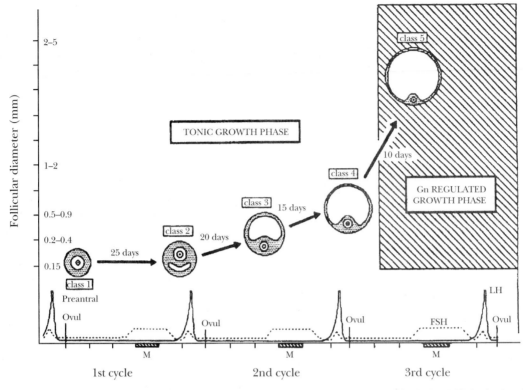

Figure 8 Dynamics of the development of follicles belonging to the cohort from which the follicle destined to ovulate will be selected. From size 2 mm (class 5, selectable follicles), the follicles become more responsive to follicle stimulating hormone (FSH) and enter a rapid growth phase. Ovul, ovulation; M, menstruation; LH, luteinizing hormone; Gn, gonadotropin. Reproduced with permission from Gougeon A. Regulation of ovarian follicular development in primates: facts and hypotheses. *Endocrine Rev* 1996;17:121–55[39]. ©The Endocrine Society

to ascertain the exact age of onset of poor response for each patient. However, it is likely that 'poor response', in most cases, represents a stage somewhere between the onset of accelerated decline of ovarian reserve (25 000 remaining follicles) and total loss of fertility.

An important case series was published in 1997[55]. Twelve infertile women, initially diagnosed as having unexplained or anovulatory infertility, who had a normal baseline hormonal profile and did not respond to repeated ovarian stimulation with gonadotropins, developed ovarian failure within a few months. The mean age of the patients in that group was 39.8 years (range 34–43), and the mean early follicular serum FSH at first evaluation was 5.4 IU/l and, following the diagnosis of non-response to ovarian stimulation, 53.5 IU/l. The mean time

elapsed between the two tests was 8.8 months. The authors concluded that non-response to gonadotropin stimulation might be the first detectable sign of impending menopause.

Based on this interesting observation, we carried out a controlled retrospective cohort study in the IVF unit of Hammersmith Hospital, to see whether an extremely poor response to ovarian stimulation would be associated with an earlier menopause[56]. All patients aged 35–40 who had cancelled IVF cycles for non-response between 1991 and 1993 were asked to report on the subsequent development of menopausal symptoms, menopause or commencement of hormone replacement therapy. A control group consisted of patients of the same age and with similar medical history, who had IVF the same year and responded well. We accepted as

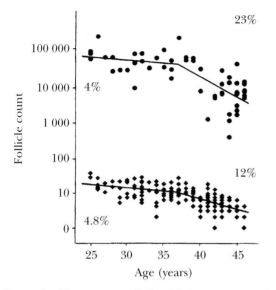

Figure 9 Upper curve: relationship between natural log-transformed primordial follicle count obtained from histological studies and chronological age in a group of 58 women. The yearly relative decline in follicle number is given for both regression lines. Lower curve: relationship between log-transformed number of antral follicles obtained by ultrasound scanning in the early follicular phase of the cycle and chronological age in a group of 162 regularly cycling, fertile women. Reproduced with permission from Scheffer GJ, *et al.* Antral follicle counts by transvaginal ultrasonography are related to age in women with proven natural fertility. *Fertil Steril* 1999;72:845–51[50]

extremely poor response ('non-response') the absence of follicles more than 10 mm diameter on vaginal ultrasound scan or a peak estrogen level of less than 300 pmol/l, despite receiving at least 150 IU of human menopausal gonadotropin (hMG) for at least 9 days, i.e. 1350 IU of hMG. Eleven of the 12 patients of the non-response group developed menopausal symptoms within 7 years, compared with only four of 24 in the control group ($p < 0.0001$). Similarly, eight of 12 non-responders either entered the menopause or started using hormone replacement therapy, compared with only four of 24 in the control group ($p < 0.0001$). The median age at development of menopausal symptoms in the study group was 40 years (38–45), and the median time difference between non-response and menopausal symptoms was 4 years (1–7).

These data were first presented at a meeting of the British Fertility Society in October 1999 and published in 2002[56]. The observation that the time interval between non-response and loss of menstrual cyclicity was 4 years would agree with the predictions of the fixed-intervals hypothesis[1]. In the following 2 years, two similar studies were presented at the American Society for Reproductive Medicine[57,58]. The first was carried out in Milan, Italy[57]. It was a controlled study to evaluate the menstrual status and reproductive outcome of patients who underwent an IVF treatment between 1993 and 1997 showing poor response, and to compare these findings with those of a population of normal responders who underwent IVF at the same age and in the same period. Poor response was defined as fewer than three follicles > 10 mm at stimulation day 6. One hundred and nine eumenorrheic poor responders to IVF treatment were matched to 101 controls of the same age. The mean age at the IVF attempt was not different between patients and controls (35.8 versus 35.7 years). Patients and controls were interviewed by phone regarding their actual menstrual status and their reproductive outcome during the years following the IVF cycle. At the time of interview, seven patients and no controls had a premature menopause with a mean onset period after IVF of 3.3 years ($p = 0.016$). The mean age of menopause of these seven patients was 40.8 years. Forty pregnancies were achieved in 33 of 101 controls in the period between the IVF attempt and the interview (20 spontaneous and 20 induced), and 23 pregnancies in 20 of 109 poor responders (12 spontaneous and 11 induced) ($p < 0.02$)

The other study took place in London, UK[58]. It was a retrospective cohort study of 110 women and 170 controls who underwent assisted reproductive techniques (ART) between 1987 and 1998. Ovarian function and reproductive outcome were assessed by postal questionnaire sent in 2000/2001. All women were < 40 years at the time of treatment, and had regular menstrual cycles. The study group ($n = 110$) were women who underwent ovarian stimulation with 450 IU gonadotropins daily for a minimum of 8 days and had either: a cycle cancelled due to poor follicular development (≤ 3 follicles), or ≤ 3 eggs obtained at egg collection. The control group ($n = 170$) were women for whom ≥ 6 eggs were obtained at egg collection following gonadotropin ovarian stimulation at a dose appropriate for their age (150 IU if < 30, 225 IU if 30–35 or 300 IU if > 35 years). Poor responders to ovarian stimulation were significantly more likely to be amenorrheic (6 versus 0.3%) and to suffer menstrual irregularities (19 versus 5%) and/or vasomotor symptoms (27 versus 10%) 5 years after the treatment cycle. The total pregnancy rate of poor responders (spontaneous and as a result of ART) was significantly less than that of the control group.

New evidence for a link between the number of retrieved oocytes at IVF and age at menopause came in 2002 from a nested case–control study involving 12 IVF clinics in The Netherlands[59]. Participants were part of a nationwide Dutch cohort study (the OMEGA Project) of 26 428 women diagnosed with subfertility problems in all 12 IVF clinics in The Netherlands between 1 January 1980 and 1 January 1995. The main purpose of the OMEGA study is to examine the risk of hormone-related cancers in women who received hormone stimulation for IVF. Women who were alive on 1 January 1997 were mailed a questionnaire to obtain information on gynecological disorders before and after subfertility treatment. Trained research assistants obtained data from the medical files on gynecological history, subfertility diagnosis and fertility hormones used before IVF treatment, and detailed information about each subsequent IVF treatment. Each patient who experienced a natural menopause at or before 46 years ($n = 38$) was individually matched to five controls ($n = 190$) who had not yet entered the menopause at the time the patient became postmenopausal. Women with a poor response (0–3 oocytes) had a relative risk of 11.6 (95% confidence interval 3.9–34.7) of having an early menopause, compared with women who had a normal response (> 3 oocytes).

EARLY OVARIAN AGING AS A SEPARATE CLINICAL ENTITY: DEFINITION, EPIDEMIOLOGY, SYMPTOMS, SEQUELAE, SCREENING AND PREVENTION

Assuming a fixed interval of 13 years between the age of accelerated decline of fertility (25 000 follicles) and the menopause, it can be speculated that women who become menopausal by the age of 45 will have experienced an accelerated decline of fertility before the age of 32 (25 000 remaining follicles) and a total loss of fertility by the age of 36 (Figure 10). Nevertheless, they may continue to be otherwise asymptomatic, with regular menstrual cycles, for a few more years. These women should perhaps be classified under a new clinical entity, 'early ovarian aging'[60]. This is a condition potentially suitable for screening in the general population, starting in the early 30s[56]. Epidemiological studies have shown that 10% of women in the general population become menopausal by the age of 45 years[61,62], and therefore it is estimated that 10% of women in the general population might be at risk of early ovarian aging (Figure 10).

In the years following diagnosis at the age of 32 or less, these women will have similar reproductive potential to that of a 37-year-old woman, and could experience increased incidence of dizygotic twinning[63–67], increased incidence of aneuploidy and miscarriage[11,68–71], unexplained subfertility[72–74] and relatively poor response to ovarian stimulation[55–59]. Assuming a fixed time-difference between reproductive milestones[1,15,75], fertility will not be lost completely for 4 years on average following diagnosis. Menstrual cycles will continue to be regular, although relatively short, for 6–8 more years on average[4]. Furthermore, these women might exhibit other physical and possibly mental and psychological signs compatible with accelerated general aging[76–86].

An important contribution of assisted reproduction has been the development of tests for the assessment of ovarian reserve. Starting in 1987[87], there has been increasing interest in this area. Among the tests already in use are basal

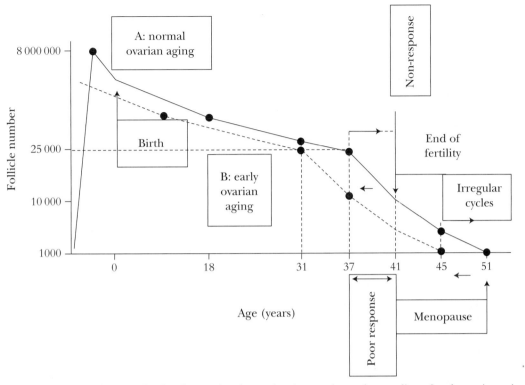

Figure 10 The contribution of assisted reproduction technology to the understanding of early ovarian aging. Data from *in vitro* fertilization suggest that there is a parallel variation between the accelerated decline of reproductive potential and the menopause. This supports te Velde's hypothesis of fixed intervals between reproductive milestones. On the basis of a fixed interval of 13 years between the onset of accelerated decline of fertility (25 000 remaining follicles) and the menopause, it can be speculated that women who become menopausal by age 45 have experienced an accelerated decline of fertility before the age of 32. These women are classified under a separate clinical entity, 'early ovarian aging'. It is estimated that 10% of asymptomatic women aged 32 or less fall into this category and the condition is suitable for screening. Adapted with permission from te Velde ER, *et al.* Age at menopause as a marker of reproductive aging. *Maturitas* 1998;30:119–25[1]

biochemical markers, such as day-2 FSH and inhibin B, dynamic assays, such as the clomiphene stimulation test, the exogenous FSH stimulation test and the gonadotropin-releasing hormone analog (GnRHa) stimulation test, biophysical markers, such as antral follicular counts, ovarian volumes and Doppler studies, and ovarian biopsies[44–54,72,73,87–95]. The driving force for the initial development of these tests was the desire to predict IVF outcome. However, some of them might be suitable as screening tools for early ovarian aging in the general population. As discussed above, small antral follicular counts have been shown to be very promising, although there are clearly many issues to be resolved. A crucial issue is whether the cohort of antral follicles in the late 30s represents the size of the pool of resting follicles reliably enough. Serum levels of anti-Müllerian hormone have more recently been shown to have a strong correlation with the number of antral follicles and they decrease over time[96]. This and other similar new markers warrant further evaluation. Ultimately, it is hoped that, with developments in molecular genetics, it will become possible to construct 'DNA fingerprints' that will identify women with a genetic predisposition to 'early ovarian aging'[15].

Screening for early ovarian aging would be much more effective in high-risk groups.

Assuming that the same, mainly genetic, factors that affect the time of menopause will also determine all preceding reproductive milestones that depend on the number of remaining resting follicles in the ovaries, a high-risk group for early ovarian aging would include women with a family history of early menopause[2,62,97-101]. Other possible acquired factors may include: chemotherapy, radiotherapy, pelvic surgery[102-104], pelvic infections or tubal disease[104,105], severe endometriosis[106] and heavy smoking[62,107,108].

With regard to primary prevention, smoking, pelvic infection and surgical interventions may be avoidable. In recent years, the tendency to postpone child-bearing[109-111] has led to more attempts to start a family at a more advanced age, and this has contributed considerably to the increase in incidence of infertility[111-113]. Screening for 'early ovarian aging' in the early 30s could provide information to women on which to base rational decisions about their fertility, without risking involuntary childlessness. In the longer term, advances in molecular reproductive biology and pharmacology may enable us to develop drugs or interventions that will delay the accelerated decline of ovarian reserve in some women.

CONCLUSION

In vitro fertilization, a major scientific breakthrough of the 20th century, opened new horizons in medicine, such as preimplantation genetic diagnosis and embryonic stem-cell therapy. A further important contribution of IVF has been the better understanding of reproductive aging. Among other things, data from IVF cycles suggest that the age of onset of rapid decline of fertility has a variability that is parallel to the variability of age at menopause. This supports te Velde's general hypothesis of fixed intervals between reproductive milestones. On the basis of a fixed interval of 13 years between the onset of accelerated decline of fertility (25 000 remaining follicles) and the menopause, it can be speculated that women who become menopausal by age 45 have experienced an accelerated decline of fertility before the age of 32. These women can be classified under a separate clinical entity, 'early ovarian aging', which possibly affects 10% of the general population, and is suitable for screening (Figure 10). Moreover, IVF provides a model for the development of ovarian reserve tests, some of which could enable us to detect early ovarian aging in asymptomatic young women in the general population.

References

1. te Velde ER, Dorland M, Broekmans FJ. Age at menopause as a marker of reproductive ageing. *Maturitas* 1998;30:119–25
2. De Bruin JP, Bovenhuis H, Van Noord PAH, *et al.* The role of genetic factors in age at natural menopause. *Hum Reprod* 2001;16: 2014–18
3. Khaw KT. Epidemiology of the menopause. *Br Med Bull* 1992;48:249–61
4. den Tonkelaar I, te Velde ER, Looman CW. Menstrual cycle length preceding menopause in relation to age at menopause. *Maturitas* 1998;29:115–23
5. Faddy MJ, Gosden RG, Gougeon A, Richardson SJ, Nelson JF. Accelerated disappearance of ovarian follicles in mid-life: implications for forecasting menopause. *Hum Reprod* 1992;7: 1342–6
6. Block EA. Quantitative morphological investigations of the follicular system in women; variations at different ages. *Acta Anat* 1952; 14:108–23
7. Richardson SJ, Senikas V, Nelson JF. Follicular depletion during the menopausal transition: evidence for accelerated loss and ultimate

exhaustion. *J Clin Endocrinol Metab* 1987;65: 1231–7

8. Gougeon A, Chainy GB. Morphometric studies of small follicles in ovaries of women at different ages. *J Reprod Fertil* 1987;81:433–42

9. Brook JD, Gosden RG, Chandley AC. Maternal ageing and aneuploid embryos: evidence from the mouse that biological and not chronological age is the important influence. *Hum Genet* 1984;66:41–5

10. Hardy R, Kuh D. Reproductive characteristics and the age at inception of the perimenopause in a British national cohort. *Am J Epidemiol* 1999;149:612–20

11. Freeman S, Yang Q, Allran K, Taft L, Sherman S. Women with a reduced ovarian complement may have an increased risk for a child with Down syndrome. *Am J Hum Genet* 2000;66: 1680–3

12. Henderson SA, Edwards RG. Chiasma frequency and maternal age in mammals. *Nature (London)* 1968;218:22–8

13. Gaulden ME. Maternal age effect: the enigma of Down syndrome and other trisomic conditions. *Mutat Res* 1992;296:69–88

14. Eichenlaub-Ritter U. Parental age-related aneuploidy in human germ cells and offspring: a story of past and present. *Environ Mol Mutagen* 1996;28:211–36

15. te Velde ER, Pearson PL. The variability of female reproductive ageing. *Hum Reprod* 2002;8:141–54

16. Lamb NE, Feingold E, Savage A, *et al.* Characterisation of susceptible chiasma configurations that increase the risk for maternal non-disjunction of chromosome 21. *Hum Mol Genet* 1997;6:1391–9

17. Wallach EE. Pitfalls in evaluating ovarian reserve. *Fertil Steril* 1995;63:12–14

18. Templeton A, Morris J, Parslow W. Factors that affect outcome of *in-vitro* fertilization treatment. *Lancet* 1996;348:1402–6

19. Schwartz D, Mayaux MJ. Female fecundity as a function of age: results of artificial insemination in 2193 nulliparous women with azoospermic husbands. Federation CECOS. *N Engl J Med* 1982;306:404–6

20. Sauer MV. The impact of age on reproductive potential: lessons learned from oocyte donation. *Maturitas* 1998;30:221–5

21. Seifer DB, Naftolin F. Moving toward an earlier and better understanding of perimenopause. *Fertil Steril* 1998;69:387–8

22. Munne S, Lee A, Rosenwaks Z, Grifo J, Cohen J. Diagnosis of major chromosome aneuploidies in human preimplantation embryos. *Hum Reprod* 1993;8:2185–91

23. Munne S, Alikani M, Giles T, Grifo J, Cohen J. Embryo morphology developmental rates and maternal age are correlated with chromosomal abnormalities. *Fertil Steril* 1995;64:382–91

24. Benadiva CA, Kligman I, Munne S. Aneuploidy in human embryos increases significantly with maternal age. *Fertil Steril* 1996;66:248–55

25. Battaglia DE, Goodwin P, Klein NA, Soules MR. Influence of maternal age on meiotic spindle assembly in oocytes from naturally cycling women. *Hum Reprod* 1996;11:2217–22

26. Lim AS, Tsasok MFH. Age-related decline in fertility: a link to degenerative oocytes? *Fertil Steril* 1997;68:265–71

27. Volarcik K, Sheean L, Golfarb J, Abdul-Karim FW, Hunt P. The meiotic competence of *in-vitro* matured human oocytes is influenced by donor age: evidence that folliculogenesis is compromised in the reproductively aged ovary. *Hum Reprod* 1998;13:154–60

28. Zucotti M, Garagna S, Redi CA, Forabosco A. Folliculogenesis: effects of ageing on the meiotic and developmental competence of oocytes. *Gonadotrophins and Fertility in the Woman.* Serono Fertility Series Volume 3. Rome: Serono, 1999;21–32

29. O'Connor KA, Holman DJ, Wood JW. Declining fecundity and ovarian ageing in natural fertility populations. *Maturitas* 1998;30:127–36

30. Holman DJ, Wood JW, Campbell KL. Age-dependent decline of female fecundity is caused by early fetal loss. In te Velde ER, Pearson PL, Broekmans FJ, eds. *Female Reproductive Ageing.* Lancaster, UK: Parthenon Publishing 2000: 123–36

31. Hecht CA, Hook EB. Rates of Down's syndrome at livebirth by one-year maternal age intervals in studies with apparent close to complete ascertainment in populations of European origin: a proposed revised rate schedule for use in genetic and prenatal screening. *Am J Med Genet* 1996;62:376–85

32. Andersen NAM, Wohlfahrt J, Christens P, Olsen J, Melbye M. Maternal age and fetal loss: population based register linkage study. *Br Med J* 2000;24:1708–12

33. Out HJ, Braat DD, Lintsen RM, *et al.* Increasing the daily dose of recombinant follicle stimulating hormone (Puregon) does not compensate for the age-related decline in retrievable oocytes after ovarian stimulation. *Hum Reprod* 2000;15:29–35

34. Karande V, Gleicher R. A rational approach to the management of low responders in *in-vitro* fertilization: opinion. *Hum Reprod* 1999;14: 1744–8

35. Keay SD. Poor ovarian response to gonadotrophin stimulation – the role of adjuvant treatments. *Hum Fertil* 2002;5(Supp):S46–52

36. Keay SD, Liversedge NH, Marthur RS, Jenkins JM. Assisted conception following poor

response to gonadotrophin stimulation. *Br J Obstet Gynaecol* 1997;104:521–7

37. van Rysselberge M, Puissant F, Barlow P, *et al.* Fertility prognosis in IVF treatment of patients with cancelled cycles. *Hum Reprod* 1989; 4:663–6

38. Jenkins JM, Davies DW, Devonport H, *et al.* Comparison of 'poor' responders with 'good' responders using a standard buserelin/human menopausal gonadotrophin regime for *in vitro* fertilization. *Hum Reprod* 1991;6:918–21

39. Gougeon A. Regulation of ovarian follicular development in primates: facts and hypotheses. *Endocr Rev* 1996;17:121–55

40. Adashi EY. *The Ovarian Follicular Apparatus. Reproductive Endocrinology, Surgery and Technology.* Philadelphia: Lippincott-Raven, 1996: Ch 2, 17–40

41. Macklon NS, Fauser BCJM. Follicle development during the normal menstrual cycle. *Maturitas* 1998;30:181–8

42. Gougeon A, Lefevre B. Evolution of the diameters of the largest healthy and atretic follicles during the human menstrual cycle. *J Reprod Fertil* 1983;69:497–502

43. Gougeon A. Ovarian follicular growth in humans: ovarian aging and population of growing follicles. *Maturitas* 1998;30:137–42

44. Pache TD, Wladimiroff JW, de Jong FH, Hop WC, Fauser BCJM. Growth patterns of nondominant ovarian follicles during the normal menstrual cycle. *Fertil Steril* 1990;54: 638–42

45. Reuss ML, Kline J, Santos R, Levin B, Timor-Tritsch I. Age and the ovarian follicle pool assessed with transvaginal ultrasonography. *Am J Obstet Gynecol* 1996;174:624–7

46. Thomas C, Nuojua-Huttunen S, Martikainen H. Pretreatment transvaginal ultrasound examination predicts ovarian responsiveness to gonadotrophins in *in vitro* fertilization. *Hum Reprod* 1997;12:220–3

47. Pellicer A, Ardiles G, Neuspiller F, *et al.* Evaluation of the ovarian reserve in young low responders with normal basal levels of follicle-stimulating hormone using three-dimensional ultrasonography. *Fertil Steril* 1998; 70:671–5

48. Chang MY, Chiang CH, Hsieh TT, Soong YK, Hsu KH. Use of the antral folicle count to predict the outcome of assisted reproductive technologies. *Fertil Steril* 1998;69:505–10

49. Sharara FI, Lim J, McClamrock HD. The effect of pituitary desensitization on ovarian volume measurements prior to *in vitro* fertilization. *Hum Reprod* 1999;14:183–5

50. Scheffer GJ, Broekmans FJM, Dorland M, *et al.* Antral follicle counts by transvaginal ultrasonography are related to age in women with proven natural fertility. *Fertil Steril* 1999;72: 845–51

51. Tan SL, Child TJ, Gulekli B. *In vitro* maturation and fertilization of oocytes from unstimulated ovaries: predicting the number of immature oocytes retrieved by early follicular phase ultrasonography. *Am J Obstet Gynecol* 2002; 86:684–9

52. Beckers NG, Macklon NS, Eijkemans MJC, Fauser BCJM. Women with regular menstrual cycles and a poor response to ovarian hyperstimulation for *in vitro* fertilization exhibit follicular phase characteristics suggestive of ovarian ageing. *Fertil Steril* 2002;78:291–7

53. Broekmans FJ, Scheffer GJ, Bancsi LF, *et al.* Ovarian reserve tests in infertility practice and normal fertile women. *Maturitas* 1998;30: 205–14

54. Bancsi LF, Broekmans FJ, Eijkemans MJ, *et al.* Predictors of poor ovarian response in *in vitro* fertilization: a prospective study comparing basal markers of ovarian reserve. *Fertil Steril* 2002; 77:328–36

55. Farhi J, Homburg R, Ferber A, Orvieto R, Ben Rafael Z. Non-response to ovarian stimulation in normogonadotrophic, normogonadal women: a clinical sign of impending onset of ovarian failure pre-empting the rise of basal follicle stimulating hormone levels. *Hum Reprod* 1997;12:241–3

56. Nikolaou D, Lavery S, Turner C, Margara R, Trew G. Is there a link between an extremely poor response to ovarian hyperstimulation and early ovarian failure? *Hum Reprod* 2002; 17:1106–11

57. Crosignani PG, Ragni G, Guermandi E, *et al.* Menopause and pregnancy outcome in the follow-up of IVF poor responders: a case–control study [Abstract]. *Fertil Steril* 2000;74 (Suppl 1):S169

58. Lawson R, Touchy TE, Taylor A, *et al.* 'Poor response' to ovarian stimulation: a sign of incipient ovarian failure [Abstract]. *Fertil Steril* 2001;76(Suppl 1):S160

59. De Boer EJ, Den Tonkelaar I, te Velde ER, *et al.* A low number of retrieved oocytes at *in vitro* fertilization treatment is predictive of early menopause. *Fertil Steril* 2002;77:978–85

60. Nikolaou D, Templeton A. Early ovarian ageing: a hypothesis. *Hum Reprod* 2003; in press

61. Treloar AE. Menstrual cyclicity and the perimenopause. *Maturitas* 1981;3:49–64

62. van Noord PA, Dubas JS, Dorland M, Boersma H, te Velde E. Age at natural menopause in a population-based screening cohort: the role of menarche, fecundity and lifestyle factors. *Fertil Steril* 1997;68:95–102

63. Wyshak G. Twinning rates among women at the end of their reproductive span and their

relation to age at menopause. *Am J Epidemiol* 1975;102:170–8

64. Turner G, Robinson H, Wake S, Martin N. Dizygous twinning and premature menopause in fragile X syndrome. *Lancet* 1994;344:1500

65. Martin NG, Heath AC, Turner G. Do mothers of dizygotic twins have earlier menopause? *Am J Med Genet* 1997;69:114–6

66. Milhan S. Pituitary gonadotrophin and dizygotic twinning. *Lancet* 1964;2:566

67. Lambalk CB, Koning CH, Braat DD. The endocrinology of dizygotic twinning in the human. *Mol Cell Endocrinol* 1998;145:97–102

68. Nasseri A, Murkherjee T, Grifo JA, *et al.* Elevated day 3 serum follicle stimulating hormone and/or estradiol may predict fetal aneuploidy. *Fertil Steril* 1999; 71:715–18

69. van Montfrans JM, Dorland M, Oosterhuis G, *et al.* Increased concentrations of follicle-stimulating hormone in mothers with Down's syndrome. *Lancet* 1999;353:1853–54

70. van Montfrans JM, van Hooff MH, Martens F, Lambalk CB. Basal FSH, estradiol and inhibin B concentrations in women with a previous Down's syndrome affected pregnancy. *Hum Reprod* 2002;17:44–7

71. Trout S, Seifer D. Do women with unexplained recurrent pregnancy loss have higher day 3 serum FSH and estradiol values? *Fertil Steril* 2000;74:335–7

72. Scott RT, Leonardi MR, Hofman GE, *et al.* A prospective evaluation of clomiphene citrate challenge test screening of the general infertility population. *Obstet Gynecol* 1993;82: 539–44

73. Hofmann GE, Sosnowski J, Scott RT, Thie J. Efficacy of selection criteria of ovarian reserve screening using the clomiphene citrate challenge test in a tertiary fertility centre population. *Fertil Steril* 1996;66:49–53

74. Leach RE, Moghissi KS, Randolph JF, *et al.* Intensive hormone monitoring in women with unexplained infertility: evidence for subtle abnormalities suggestive of diminished ovarian reserve. *Fertil Steril* 1997;68: 413–20

75. te Velde ER, Scheffer GJ, Dorland M, Broekmans FJ, Fauser BCJM. Developmental and endocrine aspects of normal ovarian ageing. *Mol Cell Endocrinol* 1998;145:67–73

76. Dorland M, van Kooij RJ, te Velde ER. General ageing and ovarian ageing. *Maturitas* 1998; 30:113–18

77. Epstein CJ, Martin GM, Schultz AL, Motulski AG. Werner's syndrome: a review of its symptomatology, natural history, pathologic features, genetics and relationship to the natural ageing process. *Medicine* 1966;45: 177–221

78. Bundey S. Clinical and genetic features of ataxia–telangiectasia. *Int J Radiat Biol* 1994; 66:s23–9

79. Carr J, Hollins S. Menopause in women with learning disabilities. *J Intellect Disabil Res* 1995;39:137–9

80. Martin GM, Oshima J. Lessons from human progeroid syndromes. *Nature (London)* 2000; 408:263–6

81. Snowdon DA, Kane RL, Beeson WL, *et al.* Is early natural menopause a biologic marker of health and ageing? *Am J Public Health* 1989; 79:70

82. Snowdon DA. Early natural menopause and the duration of postmenopausal life. Findings from a mathematical model of life expectancy. *J Am Geriatr Soc* 1990;38:402–8

83. Cooper GS, Sandler DP. Age at natural menopause and mortality. *Ann Epidemiol* 1998; 8:229–35

84. Cooper GS, Baird DD, Weinberg CR, Ephross SA, Sandler DP. Age at menopause and childbearing patterns in relation to mortality. *Am J Epidemiol* 2000;151:620–3

85. Perls TT, Alpert R, Fretts RC. Middle aged mothers live longer. *Nature (London)* 1997; 389:133

86. Schupf N, Kapell D, Lee JH, Ottman R, Mayeux R. Increased risk of Alzheimer's disease in mothers of adults with Down's syndrome. *Lancet* 1994;344:353–6

87. Navot D, Rosenwaks Z, Margalioth EJ. Prognostic assessment of female fecundity. *Lancet* 1987;2:645–7

88. Sharara F, Scott R, Seifer D. The detection of diminished ovarian reserve in infertile women. *Am J Obstet Gynecol* 1998;179:804–12

89. Barnhart K, Osheroff J. Follicle stimulating hormone as a predictor of fertility. *Curr Opin Obstet Gynaecol* 1998;19:227–32

90. Bharnhart K, Osheroff J. We are over-interpreting the predictive value of serum follicle-stimulating hormone levels. *Fertil Steril* 1999;72:8–9

91. Gulekli B, Bulbul Y, Onvural A, *et al.* Acuracy of ovarian reserve tests. *Hum Reprod* 1999; 14:2822–6

92. Lass A, Brindsen P. The role of ovarian volume in reproductive medicine. *Hum Reprod Update* 1999;5:256–66

93. Engmann L, Sladkevecios P, Agrawal R, *et al.* Value of ovarian stromal blood flow velocity measurement after pituitary supresion in the prediction of ovarian responsiveness and outcome of *in-vitro* fertilization treatment. *Fertil Steril* 1999;71:22–9

94. Lass A. Assessment of ovarian reserve – is there a role for ovarian biopsy? *Hum Reprod* 2001;16:1055–7

95. Buckman A, Heineman M. Ovarian reserve testing and the use of prognostic models in patients with subfertility. *Hum Reprod* 2001;7: 581–90

96. de Vet A, Laven JSE, de jong FH, Themmen APN, Fauser BCM. Antimullerian hormone serum levels: a putative marker for ovarian ageing. *Fertil Steril* 2002;77:357–62

97. Cramer DW, Huijuan XMPH, Harlow BL. Family history as a predictor of early menopause. *Fertil Steril* 1995;64:740–5

98. Torgerson DJ, Thomas RE, Campbell MK, Reid DM. Alcohol consumption and age of maternal menopause are associated with menopause onset. *Maturitas* 1997;26:21–5

99. Torgerson DJ, Thomas RE, Reid DM. Mothers' and daughters' menopausal ages: is there a link? *Eur J Obstet Gynaecol* 1997;74:63–6

100. Snieder H, MacGregor A, Spector T. Genes control the cessation of a woman's reproductive life: a twin study of hysterectomy and age at menopause. *J Clin Endocrinol Metab* 1998; 83:1875–80

101. Treloar SA, Do K, Martin NG. Genetic influences on the age at menopause. *Lancet* 1998;352:1084–5

102. Lass A, Ellenbogen A, Croucher C, *et al.* Effect of salpingectomy on ovarian response to super-ovulation in an *in vitro* fertilization–embryo transfer program. *Fertil Steril* 1998;70:1035–8

103. Tulandi T, Sammour A, Valenti D, *et al.* Ovarian reserve after uterine artery embolization for leiomyomata. *Fertil Steril* 2002;78:197–8

104. Keay SD, Liversedge NH, Jenkins JM. Could ovarian infection impair ovarian response to gonadotrophin stimulation? *Br J Obstet Gynaecol* 1998;105:252–4

105. Sharara F. 'Poor responders' to gonadotropins and levels of antibodies to *Chlamydia trachomatis*? *Fertil Steril* 1998;1:388–9

106. Barnhart K, Dunsmoor R, Coutifaris C. Effect of endometriosis on *in vitro* fertilization. *Fertil Steril* 2002;77:1148–55

107. Feichtinger W, Papalambrou K, Poehl M, Kridchker U, Neumann K. Smoking in *in-vitro* fertilization: a meta-analysis. *Clin Assist Reprod Genet* 1997;14:596–9

108. Augood C, Duckitt K, Templeton A. Smoking and female infertility: a systematic review and meta-analysis. *Hum Reprod* 1998;13:1532–9

109. Gosden R, Rutherford A. Delayed childbearing. *Br Med J* 1995;311:1585–6

110. Breart G. Delayed childbearing. *Eur J Obstet Gynaecol Reprod Biol* 1997;75:71–3

111. Astolfi P, Ulizzi L, Zonta LA. Selective cost of delayed childbearing. *Hum Reprod* 1999; 14:572–3

112. Council of Europe. *Recent Demographic Developments in Europe 2000.* Strasbourg: Council of Europe, 2000

113. van Zonneveld, Scheffer GJ, Broekmans FJM, te Velde ER. Hormones and reproductive ageing. *Maturitas* 2001;38:83–94

20

Efficacy of and tolerance towards different kinds of hormone replacement therapy

J. Donát

INTRODUCTION

Essential for good compliance with hormone replacement therapy (HRT) is the appropriate choice of estrogen and progestin, their dosage and the form of administration. An individual approach to the choice of drug is the first condition of successful long-term therapy. Treatment has to be efficacious, with a minimum of adverse side-effects. Ineffectual treatment with adverse side-effects often results in withdrawal within the first month of therapy. This may engender distrust or fear, and, as a consequence, permanent refusal of such treatment. Not only is the appropriate choice of drug, dose and form of administration necessary, but also full information on possible adverse side-effects, which for the most part disappear within the first 3 months of treatment.

TYPES OF ESTROGENS, DOSAGE AND ADMINISTRATION

The main circulating estrogen in the premenopause is 17β-estradiol, produced in the ovarian granulosa cells by conversion from testosterone. Another circulating estrogen is estrone, produced during the conversion of estradiol and by peripheral conversion from androstenedione in fatty tissue. In the postmenopause, estrone produced by peripheral conversion from androstendione is the main circulating estrogen. Estradiol and estrone are the most frequent components of HRT preparations.

Natural and synthetic estrogens may be used in HRT. Natural estrogens include 17β-estradiol, estradiol valerate and estriol, which are human hormones, and conjugated vegetal and equine estrogens (CEE). The basic component of CEE is estrone sulfate, and preparations also contain non-human estrogens, for example equilin and equilinin. These bind to estrogen receptors and have a long half-life. Synthetic estrogens are still used in some oral HRT preparations, primarily ethinylestradiol. They are more efficacious than natural estrogens, as may be seen in their effects on liver function and fibrinolytic and coagulation factors, as well as an increased risk of hypertension and thromboembolism especially in users of hormonal contraceptives. Estrogen is most frequently administered orally. Alternative formulations are transdermal (patch), percutaneous (gel), subcutaneous (implants), intranasal (spray) and vaginal (tablets, cream and rings). Oral administration has a two-fold specific effect not seen with any of the other methods. First, conversion to estrone occurs in the intestinal mucosa. This results in a change of the premenopausal condition where the estradiol/estrone ratio is in favor of estradiol. Conversion of estradiol to estrone does not depend on the type of oral estrogen. The other specific effect of oral estrogens is the so-called 'first-pass' effect in the liver. Absorbed estrogen enters the liver via the portal vein, and is then metabolized 35–95% into the inactive estrone-3-glucuronide. This means that oral estrogen doses must be substantially higher than non-oral doses to obtain similar therapeutic plasma levels.

Estrogens vary in their dose equivalence and their effect on target tissues. Oral micronized estradiol 1 mg is equivalent to CEE 0.625 mg, piperazine estrone sulfate 0.625 mg, esterified estrogens 0.75 mg and ethinylestradiol 0.005–0.015 mg. Today, the trend is to minimize estrogen doses. Findings on the efficacy and safety of and tolerance towards lower estrogen doses in HRT are key to the compliance problem. Recent studies suggest that lower estrogen doses may provide benefits similar to those with the currently used standard doses[1], while at the same time reducing the incidence of side-effects. For example, doses of 1 mg estradiol and 0.3 mg CEE relieve acute symptoms of the climacteric syndrome, have a bone-sparing effect, relieve vaginal atrophy and result in minimal side-effects[2–4].

SPECIAL FEATURES OF TRANSDERMAL AND PERCUTANEOUS ADMINISTRATION

Transdermal patches have been used in Europe since 1985. The results of the first four Estraderm® studies by Whitehead and co-workers[5,6] and Place and colleagues[7,8] were presented at the 4th International Congress on the Menopause in Orlando, Florida. Findings from both single-center and multicenter studies soon revealed that the transdermal system was more efficacious and better tolerated than conjugated estrogens, and did not affect liver proteins[9].

Transdermal administration has improved during the past decade, and is being used more and more. A satellite symposium of the XIV FIGO Congress[10] discussed HRT methods and alternatives to oral administration. Nachtigall[11] had evaluated both the advantages and the disadvantages of oral and transdermal HRT delivery, and suggested that the benefit of transdermal systems was that they secure the

therapeutic effect with lower doses and uniform estradiol release. Owing to 'direct estrogen infusion' with no effect on liver protein production, transdermal delivery is suitable for women presenting with certain health conditions.

It was reported at the 8th International Congress on the Menopause in Sydney in 1996 that, of all types of HRT application, transdermal systems are used most frequently with oral administration coming next, while vaginal methods (rings delivering estradiol) are used less often and implants are rare[12]. However, the situation in the Czech Republic is different. Oral administration is used most often and transdermal patches represent a third of the total amount of prescribed HRT, although their application is increasing. Vaginal HRT administration is quite unsatisfactory; so far, vaginal rings delivering estradiol have not been approved for clinical use in the above country.

Basically, all kinds of administration, with the exception of oral and vaginal estriol, have a very similar effect; there are, of course, some differences owing to the individuality of patients and the symptoms for which HRT is indicated.

Some particular traits may be seen in transdermal and percutaneous administration not seen with oral drugs, and they may be beneficial under specific conditions. Such advantages result from the following properties[10,13,14]:

(1) Hormones bypass the gastrointestinal tract;

(2) Hormones are absorbed directly from the skin into the blood circulation and diffused to target organs before passing through the liver, i.e. there is no 'first-pass' effect;

(3) In the case of oral estradiol administration as much as 70% of the hormone is converted into estrone and thus the efficacy is lower. The estradiol/estrone ratio in transdermal application is approximately 1, i.e. the natural premenopausal balance. Transdermal therapy therefore has an optimum pharmacokinetic profile, and estradiol blood levels reach their peak faster and are more stable;

(4) Triacylglycerol levels in the lipid profile do not rise;

(5) The positive effect on bone density may be quicker with transdermal delivery than after oral administration;

(6) There are fewer adverse side-effects.

The indication area is basically the same for transdermal and percutaneous HRT as for HRT generally. However, transdermal HRT can be prescribed in the presence of some pathological conditions that do not allow oral therapy, or when such therapy is less effective than transdermal patches. These conditions include:

(1) After thrombophlebitis or deep vein thrombosis;

(2) Liver disease with abnormal liver function;

(3) More serious osteoporosis with a higher risk of fractures;

(4) Dyslipidemia with higher triacylglycerols;

(5) Gastrointestinal and gall-bladder problems;

(6) Other side-effects of oral HRT.

In clinical practice, transdermal patches and percutaneous gel (Oestrogel® and Estreva®) reduce the incidence of hot flushes and eliminate all signs of estrogen deficiency, and thus improve the quality of life of women. They raise neither blood pressure nor blood sedimentation rate factors (fibrinogen and antithrombin III). They reduce plasma levels of total cholesterol and of low-density lipoprotein (LDL) cholesterol. This effect seems to be associated with a rise of serum estradiol concentration and increased activity of LDL receptors. A cross-study involving gel, transdermal patches and oral estradiol carried out to compare the pharmacokinetic indicators of various kinds of estradiol (E_2) administration revealed that Oestrogel, Estreva and Estraderm resulted in stable E_2 and estrone (E_1) concentrations, while the E_2/E_1 ratio was similar to that in women with an active menstrual cycle. Percutaneous Oestrogel (1.5 mg dosage) resulted in least individual variability. Oral Estrace® exhibited better biological availability, but conspicuous changes of level with time and a non-physiological E_1 level[15]. As far as E_2 biological availability in transdermal preparations using a matrix patch is concerned, a statistically significant increase in E_2 serum levels after a week of application was found with both Dermestril 50® and Climara® at a 1% significance level for both drugs[16]. E_2 levels remained stable with both preparations over a period of 4 weeks, and the nature of changes was very similar. Both medicaments had a very good clinical effect. The Kupperman index improved with Dermestril from an average of 20 points to 4.6 after 4 weeks' administration, and the result was similar with Climara. In a study of 186 women, von Holst and Salbach[17] evaluated the efficacy of and tolerance towards a 7-day transdermal E_2 patch versus placebo in women after hysterectomy with postmenopausal complaints. They assessed the Kupperman index, a score of urogenital complaints and adverse dermal side-effects of the patch in three treatment cycles. Compared with placebo, the patch was well tolerated, and genuinely attenuated mild and severe vasomotor symptoms in women after hysterectomy; the onset of this effect was rapid and it persisted for 7 days. Although our group[15] used a different 7-day E_2 patch (in the above-mentioned study[17] the patch used was Fem7®), our results are similar. The effects of transdermal and percutaneous forms of estradiol and the nature of changes in hormone levels are known from the literature; the situation is somewhat different with vaginal and intranasal estradiol.

When E_2 biological availability was assessed after daily Oestrogel or Estreva application, a statistically significant increase in serum E_2 levels was found already after 1 week, and the nature of the rise was very similar to that found with Climara transdermal application[18]. Thus, Oestrogel represents a valuable first-choice drug in HRT indications. It provides fast biological availability and stable E_2 levels.

Estreva is a new gel preparation containing an estradiol dose of 0.1% (the daily dose of gel, 1.5 g, provides the recommended daily dose of E_2, 1.5 mg), administered with three squeezes of the pump dispenser. It contains glycol derivatives that completely dissolve E_2 in a hydro-alcohol medium and allow a lower ethanol content in the gel base. The nature of E_2 levels seen in our patients is indicative of a persisting statistically significant rise in E_2 serum levels already within the first week of administration. Pharmacokinetic data[15], followed during the first 24 h after administration of the same daily dose of 1.5 mg of E_2 in the gel, presented a smooth rise of E_2 and E_1 to a maximum within 12 h after administration; the authors found no statistically significant differences in E_2 and E_1 values with the reference gel. The values of serum E_2 seen in our study[19] with the administration of an identical dose were significantly higher, and corresponded to the values Scott and colleagues[15] found after the administration of a daily dose of 3 mg. The biological availability of E_2 with a daily dose of 3 mg of E_2 was greater than with the reference gel. With this dose, the maximum serum levels are reached very quickly, within 2–4 h after administration. Our results[19] obtained 12 h after administration of the gel presented significantly higher E_2 levels, yet essentially their nature corresponds to the maximum found 12 h after administration by other authors[15]. In these cases we found significantly higher serum E_2 values after a daily dose of 1.5 mg of E_2, but the relatively small set of patients does not allow a reliable comment. Oral estrogen therapy is the priority for patients presenting problems with skin tolerance of the patch adhesive and/or adverse side-effects.

CHARACTERISTICS OF INTRANASAL ADMINISTRATION

The intranasal form of estradiol, Octodiol® (Aerodiol®), is a new delivery form that works on the principle of the pulsed nature of changes in E_2 levels. Our results[19] confirm a significant reduction of the Kupperman index with a daily E_2 dose of 300 mg. Studd and colleagues[20] found this to be the optimum dose for 80% of women. A significant decrease in the Kupperman index sets in after 4 weeks, with a maximum decrease reached after 12 weeks of treatment. The intensity and number of hot flushes decreases similarly to those found with oral E_2 in a daily dose of 2 mg[20]. Also, the effect is similar to that of transdermal E_2 in a daily dose of 50 μg[21,22]. Compared with placebo, the Kupperman index decreases after 1 week of intranasal therapy, and after 3 weeks this decrease is statistically significant[20]. The effect is long-lasting, as shown by the study of Gompel and associates[23]. After 12 weeks there was a statistically significant decrease of the Kupperman index at a level of $p < 0.001$. In accordance with data from the literature, our results show that the treatment has a minimum of adverse side-effects. Mattsson and colleagues[22] and Lopes and co-workers[21] found that use of Octodiol results in a smaller occurrence of mastalgia than that with oral or transdermal HRT. In women with a preserved uterus Octodiol presents fewer cases of irregular bleeding than with oral or transdermal E_2[21,22]. Octodiol gives stable absorption and high biological availability[19], i.e even small doses may be administered. Our results confirm a persisting biological ratio of E_1/E_2. Studd and colleagues[20] found that Octodiol does not produce changes in mucociliary clearance or mucus viscosity of the nasal mucosa. Local symptoms are responsible for less than 3.5% of withdrawals from treatment, as against 5–8% with transdermal therapy[20]. The compliance with Octodiol in long-term treatment is very good. After 1 year it is still taken by 85% of women[21,23]. In our study, we found a relatively high fluctuation of E_2 levels with a statistically significant rise only after 1 week of treatment, which could, theoretically, indicate a lower absorption of the drug than with other parenteral forms. However, it must be taken into consideration that our values were measured 12 h after nasal administration of the drug. None the less, the mean E_2 values throughout the period of the study were within the range of premenopausal values or transdermal HRT values. They indicated a possible effect after 24 h.

PLASMA LIPOPROTEINS AND SELECTIVE HRT IN CLINICAL PRACTICE

Dyslipidemia participates in the onset of cardio-vascular disease, or, expressed more clearly, in the development of coronary ischemia, in one-third of patients. It is important, therefore, to examine lipids as a certain risk indicator both before hormone replacement and during HRT. Long-term monitoring of lipid metabolism indicators is required; this is sometimes rather difficult owing to the great variability of input parameters and individual differences in HRT effect. Lipid evaluation must be carried out in every study in a way that would eliminate as much as possible any distortion, both positive and negative.

In a continuous study[16] we investigated lipid profiles with various HRT methods. This was a short-term study; we studied a few sets of patients treated with conjugated estrogens (Presomen® 0.625 mg and Oestrofeminal® 0.6 mg) with and without medroxypro-gesterone acetate (MPA) (daily dose 5 mg) and with 17β-estradiol using a transdermal system (Estraderm® 50 and 25) with and without MPA for a period of 1–2 years. The goal of the study was to evaluate the effect of different HRT methods on plasma lipoprotein levels in postmenopausal women, and to determine the best possible form of HRT delivery to dys-lipidemic patients. The following values were determined before HRT and at specific intervals in a total of 98 women treated with HRT: plasma lipid levels including total cholesterol, high-density lipoprotein (HDL) cholesterol, LDL cholesterol, triacylglycerol and LDL/HDL ratio, and hormone levels including luteinizing hormone (LH), follicle stimulating hormone (FSH) E_2, E_1, prolactin and, in some cases, thyroid stimulating hormone, tri-iodothyronine, thyroxine and parathormone. Statistical analysis of differences in all monitored values was carried out using both paired and unpaired t-tests. Attention was paid to determination of differences in the following values before and during treatment between groups on estrogen monotherapy and in combination with MPA; and between groups on oral therapy with conjugated estrogens (Presomen®, Oestrofeminal®) at a daily dose of 0.625 mg and transdermal administration (Estraderm® TTS 50 and/or TTS 25).

Patients were divided into nine groups in the following way:

(1) Patients treated with transdermal estradiol:

    (a) Estraderm® 50 and normolipidemia;

    (b) Estraderm® 50 and dyslipidemia;

    (c) Estraderm® 50 + MPA and normo-lipidemia;

    (d) Estraderm® 50 + MPA and dyslipidemia;

    (e) Estraderm® 25 + MPA and dyslipidemia;

(2) Patients treated with conjugated estrogens:

    (a) Presomen® 0.625 mg in monotherapy;

    (b) Presomen® 0.625 mg + MPA;

    (c) Oestrofeminal® 0.625 mg in mono-therapy;

    (d) Oestrofeminal® 0.625 mg + MPA.

Average age and time elapsed since natural or artificial menopause were comparable in all groups. Patients on estrogen monotherapy had undergone a hysterectomy; those with the MPA combination had an intact uterus. The groups were identical; all followed patients were examined before starting HRT and then after 6, 12, 18 and sometimes even 24 months. This suggests that the results obtained may be considered relatively accurate. An interesting finding is that with Estraderm® there was deterioration of the studied parameters of lipid metabolism in cases of normolipidemia, but we should be careful in evaluating such results as the values remained within physiological limits. Patients after hysterectomy and with dyslipid-emia treated with Estraderm® 50 presented significantly increased E_2 levels only after 18 months and a favorable effect on all lipid meta-bolism indicators, but these were not statistically significant. Statistically significant lower HDL cholesterol levels at a 1% level of significance were found in the group on combined therapy with Estraderm® 50 + MPA and dyslipidemia after 1 year of treatment. Estraderm® TTS 25 + MPA (daily dose 2.5 mg) was prescribed to perimenopausal women without any conspicuous estrogen deficiency. No statistically significant results were found in women with normolipidemia. With regard to oral conjugated estrogens, women after hysterectomy were on therapy with Presomen® alone (daily dose of 0.625 mg). Lower LDL cholesterol levels and LDL/HDL ratio were found in women with dyslipidemia after 1 year of treatment, but this was not statistically significant. Results were even better after 18 months' therapy. The total picture of lipid metabolism was favorable.

After 24 months of therapy, the E_2 level increased, which was significant at a 5% level. After therapy with Oestrofeminal® alone (daily dosage of 0.625 mg) in dyslipidemia, no significant differences in levels were found after 12 months of treatment and no differences were found in women with dyslipidemia treated with Presomen® 0.625 mg + MPA 5 mg. Of course, we were interested in the relationship between lipid levels in patients treated with transdermal estradiol and in those on oral conjugated estrogens. Statistical comparison in both groups was performed of both initial values and those measured during therapy. After 12 months of HRT, statistically significantly lower values were found in the Oestrofeminal® group (1% significance) as well as significantly lower LDL cholesterol concentration and LDL/HDL ratio (1% significance). On the basis of the above, we believe that the effect of conjugated estrogens is more favorable.

Interpretation of the relationship between HRT and plasma lipoproteins is not easy, as we noted at the end of our study; it requires the assessment of identical groups comparable in the following basic parameters: menopause both natural and induced, duration of menopause, initial E_2 and FSH levels, strict differentiation between normolipidemia and dyslipidemia, and stable type of HRT with or without progestogens. It is sometimes difficult to secure stability of an HRT method as a number of patients change HRT depending on their compliance, or in the case of side-effects. To determine the effect of HRT on lipoproteins in the case of normolipidemia may be questionable: 'adverse changes' remain within the standard range. HRT has a positive effect on plasma lipoproteins in cases of dyslipidemia. Conjugated estrogens have a greater effect on plasma lipoproteins. Oestrofeminal® reduces cholesterol and LDL cholesterol more significantly than Estraderm®. MPA does not significantly affect the favorable influence of conjugated estrogens, but it can reduce the favorable effect of Estraderm® on HDL cholesterol. The results have revealed that it is always necessary to adopt a selective approach to hormone replacement, depending on whether the woman has undergone a hysterectomy and whether the woman is normolipidemic or dyslipidemic.

VAGINAL ESTROGEN THERAPY

Vaginal estrogens may be used as tablets, globules, suppositories, cream, rings or pessaries. The following estrogens are used for vaginal administration in the Czech Republic: estradiol (Vagifem® tablets) and estriol (Ortho-Gynest® suppositories and cream, Ovestin® suppositories and cream). Vaginal absorption depends on several factors, i.e. thickness of the vaginal wall, its vascular supply and blood return, occurrence of inflammatory changes and pathological microbes. A little greater absorption may be seen in an atrophic vaginal wall. With a thicker wall and the reappearance of glandula, estrogen systemic absorption reduces markedly. Vaginal administration is thus less suitable for treatment of vasomotor problems and for the prevention of osteoporosis and cardiovascular disease, but it is good for treating urogenital problems.

Estrogens have a specific effect of stimulation on urogenital tissues, i.e. the vagina, cervix, urethra and trigone of the bladder. The result is regeneration of the vaginal epithelium and proliferation of the urethral epithelium with rapid improvement of urogenital problems caused by atrophy, such as vaginal dryness, soreness, itching and burning, dyspareunia and problems with urination defined as the urethral syndrome. There is neither endometrium proliferation nor vaginal bleeding with vaginal HRT, especially when estriol is used, so there is no need for progesterone administration to women with an intact uterus. In the case of vulvar skin atrophy, a possible factor predisposing to dystrophic changes, vaginal estrogen cream may be indicated. Pruritus, tingle, paresthesia and tendency to inflammatory changes of the skin are first signs, which should indicate HRT.

Postmenopausal vulvovaginitis therapy should be performed in three areas:

(1) Alleviation of complaints and cure of acute inflammation: non-specific anti-inflammatory and antimicrobial therapy;

(2) Targeted antimicrobial therapy based on results of tissue cultures and microbial sensitivity: both local and general therapy using chemotherapy and antibiotics;

(3) Long-term estrogen therapy to eliminate or relieve symptoms of atrophy of the vulvar skin and epithelium: local, general therapy or their combination depending on the patient's condition.

After local estrogen therapy, symptoms of vaginal atrophy improve in a few days; with vulvar atrophy improvement is seen usually after 2–3 weeks.

Strategies for treatment of the urethral syndrome depend on the severity of symptoms. Local and vaginal estriol (cream, suppositories, globules) is recommended for treating mild initial complaints. At the beginning of therapy it is administered daily, and then every other day after alleviation. Moderate symptoms of mucosal atrophy should be treated using a combination of general and local estrogen therapy (vaginal estradiol or total estradiol with local estriol). In severe complaints caused by mucosal atrophy, any infection should be cured first and then long-term administration of combined HRT, total oral treatment or trans-dermal therapy with vaginal estrogens is indicated.

Although vaginal E_2 has proved efficacious in the urogenital area, its possible systemic effect has not been taken into consideration in some studies. Obviously, this is affected by the condition of the vaginal mucosa, its absorption capacity, secondary infection and so on. As early as 1984, Martin and colleagues[24] published a study in which they established, already within 1 h after administration of a vaginal tablet containing 0.5 mg of micronized estradiol, a 5.3-fold rise in E_2 serum levels and a 1.5-fold rise of E_1 levels. They also determined a corresponding significant decrease in LH and FSH levels. According to their results, vaginal absorption of micronized E_2 into the systemic circulation was rapid and efficacious. Moreover, patients readily accepted and tolerated well the vaginal path of administration. In this respect, our results[18] tally with this earlier study. According to the literature[25], in women with a preserved uterus, vaginal administration twice weekly did not result in endometrial hyperstimulation. After 1 year of treatment endometrial proliferation was found in only 6% of cases, and after 2 years atrophy of the endometrium was found in 100% of cases.

BIOLOGICAL AVAILABILITY OF ESTRADIOL WITH DIFFERENT HRT METHODS

The basic precondition of biological availability of E_2 in the various methods of HRT administration is to achieve premenopausal and well-balanced E_2 blood levels in both short- and long-term profiles and a favorable ratio of E_2 and E_1 levels. This problem was investigated in our case studies. We found that with vaginal E_2 application a statistically significant rise in E_2 blood levels appeared as early as 2 weeks after the beginning of therapy and persisted, with a marked improvement of the Kupperman index, for 4 weeks (short-term profile)[18]. On the basis of this observation, we prepared a study comparing the effects of different methods of HRT application on the biological availability of E_2 in a group of 80 postmenopausal women[18,19]. The goals of our study were the following:

(1) To assess the effect of E_2 administration on gonadotropin serum levels of LH, FSH, E_1 and E_2;

(2) To evaluate the biological availability of E_2 with transdermal, percutaneous, intranasal and vaginal HRT as related to the nature of changes in serum levels;

(3) To assess possible advantages and disadvantages of different HRT methods and their potential mutual substitutability.

The group was divided according to HRT methods into the following subgroups:

(1) Transdermal E_2 (Climara®);

(2) Percutaneous E_2 (Oestrogel® and Estreva®);

(3) Intranasal E_2 (Octodiol®);

(4) Vaginal E_2 (Vagifem®).

The studied parameters, i.e. serum LH, FSH, E_1 and E_2, were analyzed statistically using the non-parametric Wilcoxon method for the paired t-test and the Mann–Whitney method for the unpaired t-test. Simultaneously the Kupperman index was also studied.

The following results were obtained in a short-term 4-week HRT profile:

(1) A statistically significant rise in E_2 levels with all therapeutic methods (transdermal, percutaneous, intranasal and vaginal): with transdermal, percutaneous and intranasal administration after 1 week and with vaginal therapy after 2 weeks (Figure 1);

(2) A statistically significant rise in E_1 levels with percutaneous (Oestrogel®) and intranasal administration after 1 week (Figure 1), and a statistically significant drop in LH and FSH levels with both transdermal and percutaneous applications after 1 week (Figure 2);

(3) A conspicuous drop in the Kupperman index with all four methods of administration (Figure 3).

We drew the following conclusions from the above results

(1) All four HRT methods induced a rapid rise in E_2 levels up to almost double values (to the premenopausal level), after 1 week with transdermal, percutaneous and intranasal administration, and in 2 weeks with vaginal therapy;

(2) E_2 levels were well-balanced in all four therapeutical methods without any risk of hyperstimulation of the target organs;

(3) E_1 levels did not change with transdermal and vaginal administration but they rose nearly three-fold with percutaneous therapy; the final E_2/E_1 ratio was, however, normal in a 12-month profile (Figure 4);

(4) All four HRT methods had a good clinical effect on climacteric symptoms;

(5) Theoretically, depending on E_2 availability, all four methods can be equally efficient and mutually substitutable.

Our experience suggests that examination of E_1 and E_2 blood levels is useful. It is especially important in the postmenopausal period, as it provides information on the current E_2 level, which is the basic precondition of biological availability, and on the efficacy of the selected therapeutical method. Hormone level determination may be decisive for the choice of an HRT method from the viewpoint of individual selective HRT.

CONCLUSIONS

Parenteral forms of administration ensure a rapid onset of action and attenuation of complaints within 1–2 weeks of treatment. Their advantage is that they achieve steady serum levels of E_2, similar to premenopausal levels. They bypass the gastrointestinal tract and the liver and thus present fewer adverse side-effects, especially gastrointestinal; they are a smaller burden for the liver and for the venous system; and in the lipid spectrum they do not raise triglycerides. We prefer them in patients pre-

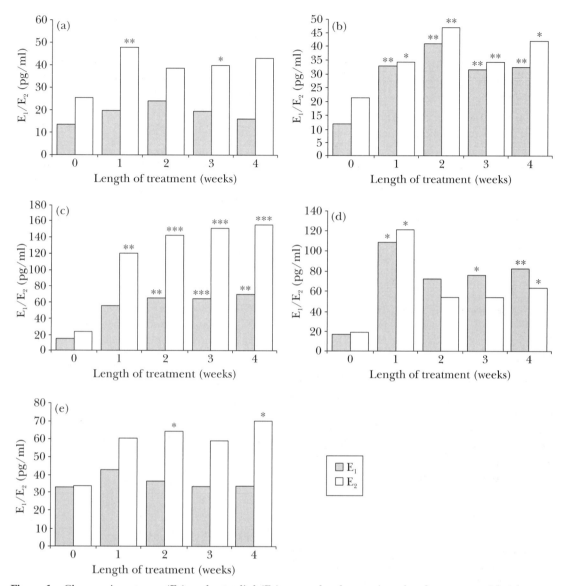

Figure 1 Changes in estrone (E_1) and estradiol (E_2) serum levels over 4 weeks of treatment with (a) transdermal (Climara®), (b) and (c) percutaneous (Oestrogel®, Estreva®), (d) intranasal (Octodiol®) and (e) vaginal (Vagifem®) estradiol replacement therapy. ***p < 0.001, **p < 0.01, *p < 0.05, versus baseline

senting with hepatic disorders, after thrombo-embolic events and in hypertriglyceridemia. The investigated parenteral HRT forms presented, over a 4-week study period, a rapid and significant reduction of acute symptoms of the climacteric. It was most pronounced with transdermal estrogen administration. Equally interesting is the vaginal administration of E_2 in relation to its systemic effect. In addition to the treatment of urovaginal symptoms of an organic estrogen deficiency syndrome, we are justified in expecting with this therapy also a favorable impact on vasomotor symptoms of the climacteric. This is, in a way, indicated by the profile of peripheral E_2 levels with this treatment. A rise of E_2 levels was statistically

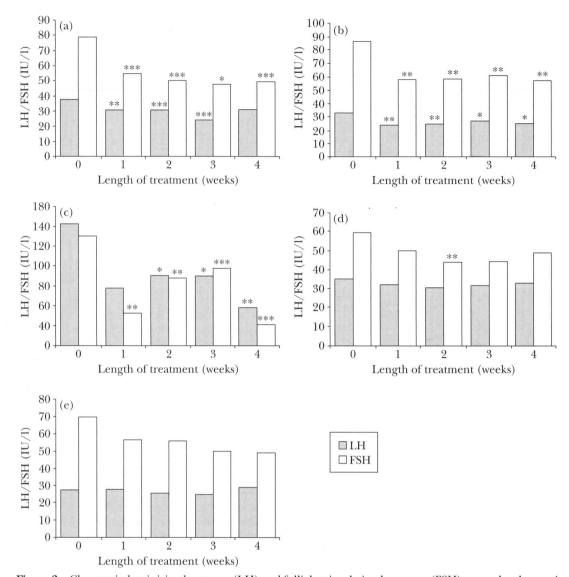

Figure 2 Changes in luteinizing hormone (LH) and follicle stimulating hormone (FSH) serum levels over 4 weeks of (a) transdermal (Climara®), (b) and (c) percutaneous (Oestrogel®, Estreva®), (d) intranasal (Octodiol®) and (e) vaginal (Vagifem®) estradiol replacement therapy. ***$p < 0.001$, **$p < 0.01$, *$p < 0.05$, versus baseline

significant, although less pronounced and slower than with other forms. All other HRT forms presented a similar statistically significant rise of E_2 levels and a drop of FSH levels. Lower E_2 levels with Octodiol®, compared with transdermal and percutaneous HRT, correspond to the pulsed nature of the drug, with E_2 levels reaching their maximum soon after admin-

istration; we found such values, however, 12 h after administration, i.e. long after the pulse peak. A statistically significant rise of E_1 could be seen with percutaneous gels and an unfavorable E_1/E_2 ratio, especially with Oestrogel®. A similar rise of E_1 with intranasal administration was, however, accompanied by an adequate rise of E_2, so that the E_1/E_2 ratio remained within

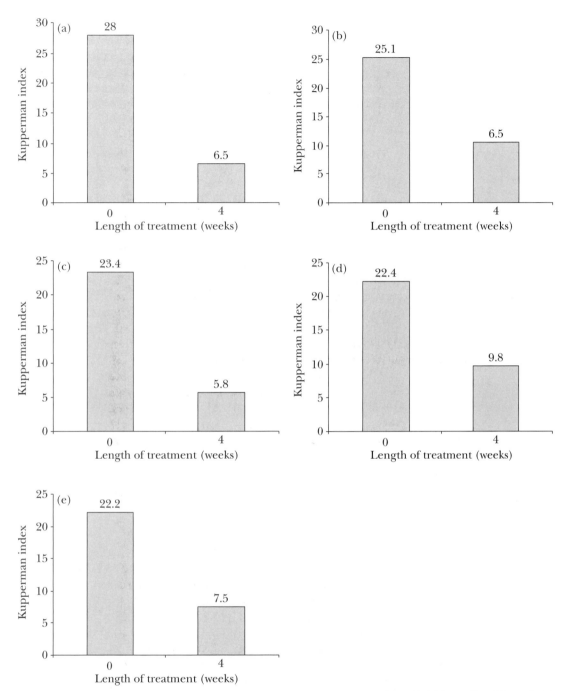

Figure 3 Changes in Kupperman index over 4 weeks of (a) transdermal (Climara®), (b) and (c) percutaneous (Oestrogel®, Estreva®), (d) intranasal (Octodiol®) and (e) vaginal (Vagifem®) estradiol replacement therapy

normal limits. With all the evaluated HRT types we saw good efficacy, tolerance and no adverse side-effects.

With Octodiol®, patients appreciate the speed and ease of administration, discrete form and rapid onset of effect. With regard

209

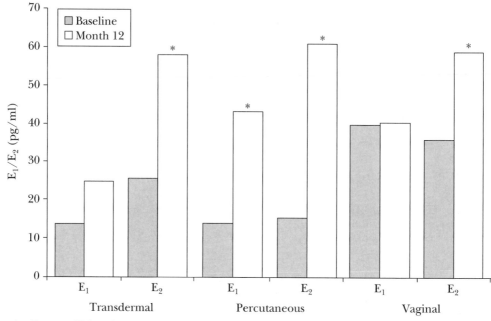

Figure 4 Estrone (E_1) and estradiol (E_2) serum levels before and after 12 months of treatment with transdermal (Climara®), percutaneous (Oestrogel®) and vaginal (Vagifem®) estradiol replacement therapy. *$p < 0.05$, versus baseline

to compliance at the beginning of treatment, all the investigated types of HRT seem appropriate, and it will be solely up to the patient which form she prefers for comfort. Parenteral forms of estrogen therapy applied percutaneously, intranasally or vaginally seem to be effective in relieving acute vasomotor and subacute urogenital symptoms of estrogen deficiency, and are mutually interchangeable when side-effects appear. In addition, percutaneous and intranasal estrogen application forms allow individual low-dose treatment with the use of minimal efficacious doses.

References

1. Notelovitz M, Leniham JP, McDermott M, *et al.* Initial 17β-estradiol dose for treating vasomotor symptoms. *Obstet Gynecol* 2000;95:726–31
2. Archer DF, Arce JC. Differences in bleeding profile between women receiving three different continuous-combined regimens: a randomized, double-blind trial. Presented at the *North American Menopause Society 11th Annual Meeting*, Orlando, Florida, September 2000
3. Archer DF. Safety and side effects of low-dose ERT/HRT. Justifying the trend to low-dose ERT/HRT. Presented at the *North American Menopause Society 12th Annual Meeting*, New Orleans, Louisiana, October 2001
4. Utian WH, Shoupe D, Bachmann G, *et al.* Relief of vasomotor symptoms and vaginal atrophy with lower doses of conjugated equine estrogens and medroxyprogesterone acetate. *Fertil Steril* 2001;75:1065–79
5. Whitehead MI, Padwick ML, Endacott J, Pryse-Davies J. Endometrial responses to transdermal estradiol administration. *Am J Obstet Gynecol* 1985;152:1079–84

6. Padwick ML, Endacott J, Whitehead MI. Efficacy, acceptability and metabolic effects of transdermal estradiol in the management of postmenopausal women. *Am J Obstet Gynecol* 1985; 152:1085–91

7. Place VA, Powers M, Darley PE, *et al.* A double-blind comparative study of Estraderm and Premarin in the amelioration of postmenopausal symptoms. *Am J Obstet Gynecol* 1985;152:1092–9

8. Powers MS, Schenkel L, Darley PE, *et al.* Pharmacokinetics and pharmacodynamics of transdermal dosage forms of 17β-estradiol: comparison with conventional oral estrogens used for hormone replacement. *Am J Obstet Gynecol* 1985;152:1099–106

9. Utian WH. Transdermal estradiol overall safety profile. *Am J Obstet Gynecol* 1987;156:1335–8

10. Lobo RA. Estrogen replacement: the evolving role of alternative delivery systems. *Am J Obstet Gynecol* 1995;173:981

11. Nachtigall LE. Emerging delivery systems for estrogen replacement: aspects of transdermal and oral delivery. *Am J Obstet Gynecol* 1995; 173:993–7

12. Fraser IS, Wang Y. New delivery systems for hormone replacement therapy. In Wren B, ed. *Progress in the Management of the Menopause. Proceedings of the 8th International Congress on the Menopause.* Carnforth, UK: Parthenon Publishing, 1997:58–67

13. Christiansen C, Alexandersen P. Future management of HRT for the prevention and treatment of osteoporosis, state of the art. Presented at the *IV European Congress on Menopause*, Vienna, October 1997

14. Stevenson JC, Cust MP, Gangar KF, *et al.* Effects of transdermal versus oral hormone replacement therapy on bone density in spine and proximal femur in postmenopausal women. *Lancet* 1990;335:265–9

15. Scott RT Jr, Ross B, Anderson C, Archer DF. Pharmacokinetics of percutaneous estradiol: a crossover study using a gel and a transdermal system in comparison with oral micronised estradiol. *Obstet Gynecol* 1991;77:758–64

16. Donát J. *Hormonální Substitucní Terapie [Hormone Replacement Therapy].* Hradec Králové, Czech Republic: *Domena* 1999:133–45

17. von Holst T, Salbach B. Efficacy and tolerability of a new 7-day transdermal estradiol patch versus placebo in hysterectomized women with postmenopausal complaints. *Maturitas* 2000;34: 143–53

18. Donát J. Efficacy and tolerance of different kinds of ERT. In Aso T, Yanaihara T, Fujimoto S, eds. *The Menopause at the Millenium. Proceedings of the 9th International Menopause Society World Congress on the Menopause.* Carnforth, UK: Parthenon Publishing 2000:381–90

19. Donát J, Kvasnicka J, Šormová I. Efficacy and tolerance of different kinds of ERT. *J Menopause* 2002;9:10

20. Studd J, Pornel B, Marton I, *et al.* Efficacy and acceptability of intranasal 17β-oestradiol for menopausal symptoms: randomised dose–response study. *Lancet* 1999;353:1574–6

21. Lopes P, Merkus HMWM, Nauman J, *et al.* Randomized comparison of intranasal and transdermal estradiol. *Obstet Gynecol* 2000;94:906–12

22. Mattsson LA, Christiansen C, Colau JC, *et al.* Clinical equivalence of intranasal and oral 17β-estradiol for postmenopausal symptoms. *Am J Obstet Gynecol* 2000;182:545–52

23. Gompel A, Bergeron C, Jondet M, *et al.* Endometrial safety and tolerability of Aerodiol (intranasal estradiol) for 1 year. *Maturitas* 2000; 36:209–15

24. Martin PL, Greaney MO, Burnier AM, *et al.* Estradiol, estrone and gonadotropin levels after use of vaginal estradiol. *Obstet Gynecol* 1984;63: 441–4

25. Mettler L, Olsen PG. Long-term treatment of atrophic vaginitis with low-dose estradiol vaginal tablets. *Maturitas* 1991;14:23–31

21

Vaginal estrogens: is there a role for their use?

W. H. Cronje and J. Studd

INTRODUCTION

It is well known that estrogen alleviates symptoms of the menopause such as vasomotor disturbances and urogenital atrophy. Various articles have also attributed a protective effect on osteoporosis[1], cardiovascular disease[2] and stroke[3] as well as possibly Alzheimer's disease[4]. This view, with regard to protection against cardiovascular disease and stroke, has now been challenged by the Women's Health Initiative study[5]. It should be stressed that the combination of conjugated equine estrogens and medroxyprogesterone was perhaps not ideal, and additionally the women in this study were too old to allow assessment of primary protection. Various routes of delivering estrogen have been explored over the years: oral tablets, transdermal patches and gel, subcutaneous implants and the vaginal route via creams, tablets, pessaries and rings. The former three are more widely used by physicians. The reason for these different forms of hormone replacement therapy (HRT) is that none of them are totally without problems. Table 1 gives the advantages and disadvantages of the various methods. There are many reasons for discontinuation of HRT[6] (Table 2), and rates of discontinuation within 1 year vary between 20 and 60%. Up to 30% of patients do not even pick up their prescription from the pharmacy[7]. It has also been recognized by many that some women require relief from, for example, urogenital symptoms without wanting to suffer the common side-effects of HRT such as the return of monthly bleeds and fear of cancer. A further

10–25% of women receiving systemic HRT with adequate control of symptoms such as hot flushes still suffer from the symptoms of urogenital aging[8].

UROGENITAL AGING

It is estimated that 10–40% of all postmenopausal women suffer from urogenital aging[9]. Whereas vasomotor symptoms resolve over time, the climacteric symptoms of hypoestrogenic urogenital atrophy persist and often worsen. These are vaginal dryness, dyspareunia and symptoms from the lower urinary tract, including incontinence, urethritis and recurrent urinary tract infections[10]. Women often do not associate these symptoms with the climacteric, as they can appear long after the menopause. More emphasis has been put on the prevention of osteoporosis and cardiovascular disease than on the alleviation of these local symptoms. The problem is compounded by the fact that women are often too embarrassed to discuss their symptoms openly, and it is of no help that sexual difficulties often complicate matters.

Clinicians experience difficulties in trying to treat older women, as they are less likely to tolerate side-effects of estrogen such as uterine withdrawal bleeding, breakthrough bleeding and breast tenderness. These occur especially at the doses of estrogen required to alleviate vasomotor symptoms. Furthermore, some women have contraindications to the use of

Table 1 Advantages and disadvantages of different forms of hormone replacement therapy

Advantages	Disadvantages
Oral therapy	
Easy to administer	easy to forget
Easy to stop	gastrointestinal side-effects
No accumulation	variable absorption
Beneficial effect on cholesterol	oral conversion to estrone
Wide choice of preparations	more minor side-effects
Patches and gel	
Easy to administer	can be forgotten
Easy to stop	occasional skin reactions
Avoids first-pass metabolism	may come off accidentally
Beneficial effect on cholesterol	more expensive than tablets
Released directly into bloodstream	cosmetic effects poor
Physiological estradiol/estrone ratio	
Low-dose pure estradiol	
Implants	
Guaranteed compliance	minor surgery
Pure estradiol	accumulation
Avoids first-pass metabolism	pellet may need to be removed
Physiological estradiol/estrone ratio	progestogen to be given orally
Testosterone can also be given	possible tachyphylaxis

Table 2 Factors associated with non-use of hormone replacement therapy

Safety concerns about effects on the breast, endometrium and thrombosis
Not medically recommended
Lack of information
Fear of weight gain
Fear of cancer
Bleeding and progestogenic side-effects
'Unnatural'

systemic estrogens, yet should not have to suffer the debilitating symptoms of urogenital aging.

Older women are more likely to suffer from urinary tract infections owing to changes in the vaginal flora associated with the menopause. Estrogen in premenopausal women leads to colonization of the vagina by lactobacilli. This in turn leads to the production of lactic acid from glycogen, which maintains low vaginal pH with concomitant inhibition of organisms associated with urogenital infections. Estrogen also enhances pelvic blood flow, and thus the vaginal epithelium is kept healthy by the moisturization from an adequate transudate[11].

Bearing all of this in mind, the issue of a possible role for locally administered vaginal estrogens has become a focus point.

METABOLISM OF ESTROGENS

Cholesterol and its esters act as a substrate for steroid hormones, and the basic skeletons of these hormones are therefore similar[12]. Cholesterol, through mediation by the cytochrome P-450, is converted into pregnenolone. This molecule is the precursor for ovarian steroidogenesis via a series of complex interactions of positive and negative feedback systems in the ovary, anterior pituitary and hypothalamus. The most important estrogen produced by the premenopausal ovary is 17β-estradiol. It is unique because almost all of it is synthesized in the granulosa cells from androgenic precursors derived from theca cells. The range of estradiol levels varies widely throughout the menstrual cycle[13]. With age, ovulation becomes less frequent, with lower plasma levels of 17β-estradiol.

Estrone is the second major estrogen found in humans, and it is the principal estrogen of the menopause. It is formed mainly from the metabolism of 17β-estradiol and aromatization of androstenedione in adipose tissue. The estradiol/estrone ratio usually remains greater than 1 during the menstrual cycle. After the menopause, this ratio changes, as 17β-estradiol levels fall significantly whereas aromatization of androstenedione continues in adipose tissue. The estradiol/estrone ratio therefore reverses, and there is no deficiency of estrone.

The third estrogen found in women is estriol. It is not secreted by the ovary but thought to be a peripheral metabolite of estradiol and estrone[14].

During this metabolism of estradiol to estrone and estriol there is a reduction in estrogenic potency.

All these estrogens, estrone, estradiol and estriol, as well as synthetic estrogens are currently used as vaginal preparations.

VAGINAL ESTROGENS

Estrogen is readily absorbed through the vaginal epithelium[15]. However, it is true that although a daily dose of 50 µg of estradiol is necessary to relieve vasomotor symptoms, daily doses as low as 7–10 µg can produce relief of urogenital symptoms[16].

The reason for this absorption is the lipophilic nature of estrogens[17]. Rapid absorption follows vaginal administration of estradiol, with minimal changes in estrone levels due to avoidance of the first-pass effect in the liver. This suggests very little metabolism of estradiol during absorption by the vaginal epithelium. Various studies have confirmed this. Martin and colleagues[18] showed that 0.5 mg of micronized estradiol is absorbed rapidly and efficiently into the systemic circulation, without major conversion of estradiol to estrone as seen with oral estrogens. At this dose, the estradiol was absorbed systemically with suppression of gonadotropin levels. This confirmed the earlier findings of Schiff and associates[19]. The question is, how much estrogen is needed to avoid systemic effects if this is indeed what is desired?

It is therefore necessary to take care when selecting the dose to be administered, as systemic absorption does occur except if the

dose is very low. Nilsson and Heimer[20] used vaginal tablets containing 10 and 25 µg of 17 β-estradiol in a double-blind cross-over study. They found that maturation of the vaginal epithelium occurred with both doses, confirmed by cytology and use of the maturation index. There was no effect on plasma gonadotropin or estrone levels, but an initial rise in estradiol levels occurred in the first 6–8 h with decreased absorption as the vaginal epithelium became more mature. This confirmed the findings of Pschera and co-workers[21], who found that absorption was significantly higher in an atrophic vaginal epithelium. Handa and colleagues[22] used low-dose vaginal estrogens (0.3 mg of conjugated estrogens, administered three nights a week for 6 months) and found satisfactory relief in 95% of cases. Vaginal cellular maturation improved significantly, and there were no significant changes in endometrial thickness or serum estrogen levels. Endometrial proliferation occurred in one case. Follow-up was 6 months, longer than in the Nilsson study. Weiderpass and co-workers[23] found only a very weak association between vaginal application of low-potency estrogen formulations and relative risk of endometrial neoplasia in a population-based case–control study in Sweden.

Heimer and Samsioe[16] argue that there is a therapeutic window where estrogens can relieve the symptoms of urogenital atrophy without stimulating the endometrium. Various possibilities for this unique response are discussed, but no definite answer has yet been found. The density of estrogen receptors in the vagina and paravaginal tissues is not high enough to explain this phenomenon, and it is not known whether functional status or a longer half-life of these receptors would explain it. Another possibility is that there is less attenuation of estrogenic potency through retarded metabolism in urogenital tissues, but even this possibility would not fully explain the differences in estradiol metabolism.

There are also problems with vaginal estrogens[24]. Under-treatment leads to inadequate relief of symptoms, while over-treatment could lead to endometrial stimulation, despite the findings of Horwitz and Feinstein[25] that there was no causal association between vaginal estrogens and endometrial cancer in two case-controlled studies. It is now widely accepted that Rigg and colleagues[15] were correct in cautioning against the possible effects of vaginal estrogens on the endometrium. Other authors[26,27] have demonstrated the systemic absorption of doses such as 1.25 mg of conjugated estrogens and 0.2 mg of micronized estradiol. In addition to the effects on the endometrium, creams, tablets and pessaries are also found to be messy, absorption is variable and administration intervals are irregular[28].

ESTRIOL

Another option to avoid endometrial stimulation is usage of the weak estrogen estriol, which is believed not to be systemically absorbed or have endometrial effects because of its short half-life, probably due to shorter nuclear permanence. Its potency is also many times less than that of estradiol[29]. Because of this short-acting effect, it does not appear to lead to cellular multiplication and differentiation or the synthesis of progesterone receptors. For this reason, estriol was studied to evaluate its effect on the vaginal epithelium. Bottiglione and co-workers[30] showed that there was no significant difference between 0.5 and 1.0 mg estriol in their effect on genital symptoms, but that there was a dose-related difference related to other symptoms of the menopause. Kikovic and associates[31] showed that there was no endometrial stimulation after 16 weeks of treatment with estriol, but their number of patients was very small. Mattson and Cullberg[32] confirmed these findings, although their follow-up period was only 8 weeks (and there was no control group in either of the above studies). They did, however, find subjective relief of urogenital symptoms in all the women in their study. They also showed estriol cream to be superior to suppositories as far as cervical mucus and vaginal cytology assessment was concerned. These studies and others[33,34] showed very little effect of vaginal estriol on various hormones including luteinizing hormone, follicle stimulating hormone, prolactin, sex hormone-binding globulin and estradiol and estrone. Estriol levels initially rose sharply followed by a steady decline.

In a meta-analysis of estrogen therapy, Cardozo and colleagues[35] found low-dose vaginal estrogens to be as effective as systemic therapy for the treatment of urogenital atrophy, with least absorption of estriol compared with estradiol and estrone.

In addition to symptoms associated with vaginal dryness, approximately one in every eight women over the age of 60 suffers from recurrent urinary symptoms[36]. Raz and Stamm[37] showed that 0.5 mg estriol cream intravaginally was superior to placebo in reducing this incidence of urinary tract infections.

VAGINAL RINGS

Another vehicle for delivering estrogen is the estradiol-releasing silicone vaginal ring. The reasons for trying to find an alternative method of vaginal administration have already been mentioned. A pilot study showed that two-thirds of hysterectomized women found a placebo intravaginal ring acceptable[38]. All these women were taking alternative forms of HRT, and it could therefore be expected that a vaginal ring that actually contains hormones would be tolerated even better. Until recently the main use of vaginal rings was the delivery of low-dose estradiol (Estring®). This ring was designed for a constant low release of 7.5 μg estradiol in 24 h. This intravaginal delivery system uses a soft, flexible silicone ring with a core section containing a 2-mg reservoir of 17β-estradiol[24]. The surrounding silicone sheath acts as a diffusion barrier, which allows a uniform, sustained release of minute amounts of estradiol over 90 days. This leads to controlled local delivery with stable but low systemic levels of estradiol. Levels of estradiol remain comfortably within the normal postmenopausal range after an initial rise in the first 8 h. Henriksson and co-workers[39] compared the use of a low-dose estradiol vaginal ring with 0.5 mg estriol vaginal pessaries. They found that both methods were equally effective in restoring the vaginal pH.

Histopathological assessment of vaginal maturation showed the ring to be superior to the pessaries. Pessaries were also found to be significantly less comfortable than the ring, and patients previously using pessaries strongly preferred the ring. The same authors[40] also showed Estring to be a highly effective and well-accepted mode of delivery in the long term for urogenital atrophy, over a period of 1 year. Other studies[24,41-43] comparing use of the ring with various other forms of vaginal estrogens have also found results comparable, with satisfaction rates as high as 84% as reviewed by Bachmann[44]. The same author[45] reviewed 11 reports of clinical trials with the estradiol vaginal ring. The conclusion was that in 946 women treated with the ring for up to 96 weeks there was a good response regarding patient comfort and physical and cytological examination. No serious adverse events occurred and the ring was well tolerated. The greatest advantage, however, was that the ring was almost always significantly preferred to other forms of vaginal estrogens.

Furthermore, Eriksen[46] compared users of Estring to an untreated control group in a randomized, open, parallel-group study to examine the effect of treatment on recurrent urinary tract infections. The vaginal ring was found to have a significant effect on prevention of recurrent infection. The mechanism by which this is explained is that estrogen restores the atrophic mucosa and increases the number of lactobacilli, thus leading to the cascade described previously.

The logical next step in development of the vaginal ring is investigating whether it will be suitable for the delivery of sufficient levels of estrogen to be used as systemic HRT. Nash and colleagues[47,48] have addressed this issue recently after the concept was introduced in 1981[49]. In the first study, three different doses of estradiol were used to determine whether sufficient levels in the effective estrogen replacement range could be reached *in vivo*. Relief of menopausal symptoms was reported in all women. Estradiol levels achieved were compatible with the control of menopausal symptoms as well as bone loss. There was also a significant reduction in total and low-density lipoprotein cholesterol. This study, however, was not placebo-controlled, numbers were small and the duration of treatment was very short.

The later study was conducted over a period of 6 months and showed a significant improvement in vasomotor symptoms and vaginal conditions. Again, there was no placebo arm.

Menoring® (Galen), a ring delivering adequate levels of circulating estradiol[50] for periods of 3 months to relieve a wide range of systemic symptoms[51], has recently been released.

CONCLUSIONS

Seen in the light of high discontinuation rates and patient reluctance to use systemic HRT, it would seem that vaginal estrogens have a role to play for postmenopausal women. That the use of HRT is certainly beneficial is a matter of education of the public, to remove often unnecessary biases against estrogen replacement therapy. Until such a time that clinicians and women are prepared to be more positive towards HRT, it would seem wrong not to treat the debilitating symptoms of urogenital aging. Certainly, the older woman with urogenital atrophy who does not wish to be subjected to the side-effects of systemic treatment would benefit from low-dose estrogens to alleviate very disturbing symptoms. This also applies to women in whom systemic treatment is contraindicated who wish to live a life without constant vaginal symptoms or urinary tract infections. The role is further extended to those women who need topping up of their systemic treatment. It is very important to remember that low-dose regimens are not an alternative to systemic HRT. If studies show that higher doses of estrogens with continuous combined progestogens offer the same advantages as other forms of HRT, this may well become an alternative form of replacement therapy with its own benefits. A vaginal ring capable of attaining adequate levels of systemic estradiol to offer all the advantages of such a treatment seems an entertaining idea, especially if concomitant progestogens can be administered via the same route. One particular factor that makes this form of administration appealing is that women can forget about HRT for periods of 3 months, yet still have enough control to remove the ring at certain times should they so wish. It should not be forgotten that HRT is an excellent form of preventive medicine with far more advantages than disadvantages. Any new idea that may therefore help to combat the high discontinuation rates or offer an alternative to women who cannot or do not want to tolerate current forms of administration should at least be considered.

References

1. Lufkin EG, Wahner HW, O'Fallon WM, *et al.* Treatment of postmenopausal osteoporosis with transdermal estrogen. *Ann Intern Med* 1992;117: 1–9

2. Stampfer MJ, Willet WC, Colditz GA, *et al.* A prospective study of postmenopausal estrogen therapy and coronary heart disease. *N Engl J Med* 1985;313:1044–9

3. Paganini-Hill A, Ross RK, Henderson BE. Postmenopausal estrogen treatment and stroke – a prospective study. *Br Med J* 1988;297:519–22

4. Henderson VW, Paganini-Hill A, Emanuel CK, *et al.* Estrogen replacement therapy in older women: comparisons between Alzheimer's disease cases and non-demented control subjects. *Arch Neurol* 1994;51:896–900

5. Rossouw JE, Anderson GL, Prentice RL, *et al.* Risks and benefits of estrogen plus progestin in healthy postmenopausal women: results from the Women's Health Initiative randomised controlled trial. *J Am Med Assoc* 2002;288:321–33

6. Domoney C, Studd J. Continuation with hormone replacement therapy. In Studd J, ed. *The Management of the Menopause 2000.* Carnforth, UK: Parthenon Publishing, 2000;35–48

7. Ravnikar VA. Compliance with HRT. *Am J Obstet Gynecol* 1987;156:1332–4

8. Smith RJN, Studd JWW. Recent advances in hormone replacement therapy. *Br J Hosp Med* 1993;49:799–809

9. Greendale GA, Judd JL. The menopause: health implications and clinical management. *J Am Geriatr Soc* 1993;41:426–36

10. Samsioe G. Urogenital aging – a hidden problem. *Am J Obstet Gynecol* 1998;178(Suppl): 245S–9S

11. Notelovitz M. Urogenital atrophy and low-dose vaginal estrogen therapy. *Menopause* 2000;7: 140–2

12. Al-Azzawi F. Endocrinological aspects of the menopause. *Br Med Bull* 1992;48:262–75

13. Gabrielsson J, Wallenbeck I, Birgerson L. Pharmacokinetic data on estradiol in light of the Estring concept. *Acta Obstet Gynecol Scand* 1996;75(Suppl 163):26–31

14. Speroff L, Glass RH, Kase NG. *Clinical Gynecologic Endocrinology and Infertility,* 4th edn. Baltimore. MD: Williams and Wilkins, 1989;16

15. Rigg LA, Hermann H, Yen SSC. Absorption of estrogens from vaginal creams. *N Engl J Med* 1978;298:195–7

16. Heimer G, Samsioe G. Effects of vaginally delivered estrogens. *Acta Obstet Gynecol Scand* 1996;75(Suppl 163):1–2

17. Stumpf PG. Pharmacokinetics of estrogen. *Obstet Gynecol* 1990;75(Suppl):9S–17S

18. Martin PL, Greaney MO, Burnier AM, *et al.* Estradiol, estrone and gonadotrophin levels after use of vaginal estradiol. *Obstet Gynecol* 1984;63:441–4

19. Schiff I, Tulchinsky D, Ryan KJ. Vaginal absorption of estrone and 17β-estradiol. *Fertil Steril* 1977;28:1063–5

20. Nilsson K, Heimer G. Low-dose oestradiol in the treatment of urogenital estrogen deficiency – a pharmacokinetic and pharmacodynamic study. *Maturitas* 1992;15:121–7

21. Pschera H, Hjerpe A, Carlstrom K. Influence of the maturity of the vaginal epithelium upon the absorption of vaginally administered estradiol-17β and progesterone in postmenopausal women. *Gynecol Obstet Invest* 1989;27: 204–7

22. Handa VL, Bachus KE, Johnston WW, *et al.* Vaginal administration of low-dose conjugated estrogens: systemic absorption and effects on the endometrium. *Obstet Gynecol* 1994; 84:215–14

23. Weiderpass E, Baron JA, Adami H, *et al.* Low-potency estrogen and risk of endometrial cancer: a case–control study. *Lancet* 1999;353: 1824–8

24. Ayton RA, Darling GM, Murkies AL, *et al.* A comparative study of safety and efficacy of continuous low dose oestradiol released from a vaginal ring compared with conjugated equine estrogen vaginal cream in the treatment of postmenopausal urogenital atrophy. *Br J Obstet Gynaecol* 1996;103:351–8

25. Horwitz RI, Feinstein AR. Intravaginal estrogen creams and endometrial cancer. *J Am Med Assoc* 1979;241:1266–7

26. Martin PL, Yen SSC, Burnier AM, *et al.* Systemic absorption and sustained effects of vaginal estrogen creams. *J Am Med Assoc* 1979;242:2699–700

27. Deutsch S, Ossowski R, Benjamin I. Comparison between degree of systemic absorption of vaginally and orally administered estrogens at different dose levels in postmenopausal women. *Am J Obstet Gynecol* 1981;139:967–8

28. Vartiainen J, Wahlström T, Nilsson C-G. Effects and acceptability of a new 17β-oestradiol-releasing vaginal ring in the treatment of post-menopausal complaints. *Maturitas* 1993;17:129–37

29. Esposito G. Estriol: a weak estrogen or a different hormone? *Gynecol Endocrinol* 1991;5:131–53

30. Bottiglione F, Volpe A, Esposito G, *et al.* Transvaginal estriol administration in postmenopausal women: a double blind comparative study of two different doses. *Maturitas* 1995;22:227–32

31. Kikovic PM, Cortes-Prieto J, Milojevic S, *et al.* The treatment of postmenopausal vaginal atrophy with Ovestin vaginal cream or suppositories: clinical, endocrinological and safety aspects. *Maturitas* 1980;2:275–82

32. Mattson L, Cullberg G. A clinical evaluation of treatment with estriol vaginal cream versus suppository in postmenopausal women. *Acta Obstet Gynecol Scand* 1983;62:397–401

33. Haspels AA, Luisi M, Kikovic PM. Endocrinological and clinical investigations in postmenopausal women following administration of vaginal cream containing oestriol. *Maturitas* 1981;3:321–7

34. Punnonen R, Vilska S, Gronroos M, *et al.* The vaginal absorption of estrogens in postmenopausal women. *Maturitas* 1980;2:321–6

35. Cardozo L, Bachmann G, McClish D, *et al.* Meta-analysis of estrogen therapy in the management of urogenital atrophy in postmenopausal women: second report of the Hormones and Urogenital Therapy Committee. *Obstet Gynecol* 1998;92:722–7

36. Romano JM, Kaye D. UTI in the elderly: common yet atypical. *Geriatrics* 1981;36:113–15

37. Raz R, Stamm WE. A controlled trial of intravaginal estriol in postmenopausal women with recurrent urinary tract infections. *N Engl J Med* 1993;329:753–6

38. Spencer CP, Cooper AJ, Ross D, *et al.* Patient acceptability of and tolerance to a placebo intravaginal ring in hysterectomized women: a pilot study. *Climacteric* 1999;2:110–14

39. Henriksson L, Stjernquist M, Boquist L, *et al.* A comparative multicenter study of the effects of continuous low-dose estradiol released from a new vaginal ring versus estriol pessaries in postmenopausal women with symptoms and signs of urogenital atrophy. *Am J Obstet Gynecol* 1994;171:624–32

40. Henriksson L, Stjernquist M, Boquist L, *et al.* A one-year multicenter study of efficacy and safety of a continuous, low-dose, estradiol-releasing vaginal ring (Estring) in postmenopausal women with symptoms and signs of of urogenital aging. *Am J Obstet Gynecol* 1996;174:85–92

41. Barentsen R, Van de Weijer PHM, Schram JHN. Continuous low dose estradiol released from a vaginal ring versus estriol vaginal cream for urogenital atrophy. *Eur J Obstet Gynecol Reprod Biol* 1997;71:73–80

42. Bachmann G, Notelovitz M, Nachtigall L, *et al.* A multicentre comparative study of the safety and efficacy of a low dose estradiol vaginal ring and conjugated estrogen cream for postmenopausal urogenital atrophy. *Prim Care Update Obstet Gynecol* 1997;4:109–15

43. Fraser AS, Ayton R, Farrell E, *et al.* A multicentre Australian trial of low-dose estradiol therapy for symptoms of vaginal atrophy using a vaginal ring as a delivery system. *Maturitas* 1995;22(Suppl):S41

44. Bachmann G. Estradiol-releasing vaginal ring delivery system for urogenital atrophy. *J Reprod Med* 1998;43:991–8

45. Bachmann G. The estradiol vaginal ring – a study of existing clinical data. *Maturitas* 1995;22 (Suppl):S21–9

46. Eriksen BC. A randomised, open, parallel-group study on the preventive effect of an estradiol-releasing vaginal ring (Estring) on recurrent urinary tract infections in postmenopausal women. *Am J Obstet Gynecol* 1999;180:1072–9

47. Nash HA, Brache V, Alvarez-Sanchez F, *et al.* Estradiol delivery by vaginal rings: potential for hormone replacement therapy. *Maturitas* 1997;26:27–33

48. Nash HA, Alvarez-Sanchez F, Mishell DR, *et al.* Estradiol-delivering vaginal rings for hormone replacement therapy. *Am J Obstet Gynecol* 1999;181:1400–6

49. Englund DE, Victor A, Johansson EDB. Pharmacokinetics and pharmacodynamic effects of vaginal oestradiol administration from silastic rings in postmenopausal women. *Maturitas* 1981;3:125–33

50. McNamee B, De Vries T. Pharmacokinetic characterisation of an estradiol acetate intravaginal ring delivering 0.05 mg/day estradiol to healthy postmenopausal women. Presented at the *North American Menopause Society Meeting*, New Orleans, Louisiana, October 2001

51. Buckler H, Perry W. The effect on climacteric symptoms of estrogen replacement therapy with a novel estradiol acetate intravaginal ring in postmenopausal women. Presented at the *British Menopause Society Meeting*, Birmingham, UK, June 2001

22

Pulsed estrogen therapy: a new concept in hormone replacement therapy

N. Panay and J. Studd

INTRODUCTION

The efficacy of estrogen replacement therapy (ERT) in relieving vasomotor and urogenital symptoms associated with the menopause is well established[1–3]. Estrogen supplementation also provides additional long-term clinical benefits by reducing postmenopausal bone loss and bone fractures[4–6], and may have beneficial effects on cardiovascular[7] and neuro-cognitive functions[8,9].

The two most widely used forms of estrogens are conjugated equine extracts and 17β-estradiol. Currently, the oral and transdermal routes are the most commonly used in the administration of ERT. Both routes are effective in relieving menopausal symptoms but are associated with a number of clinical disadvantages[10,11]. Orally administered estrogen is subject to first-pass hepatic and intestinal effects and consequently this route requires high doses to be effective (1–2 mg/day), with significant intra- and interpatient variability[12]. Although transdermal patches have circumvented some of the drawbacks of oral therapy, they present additional problems, such as wide inter-individual variations in absorption rate (including the presence of poor absorbers)[13], the loss of 4–8% of patches due to poor adhesion[14], and local skin reactions[15,16]. Furthermore, this route provides a relatively constant delivery of hormone but at least 2–10 mg must be applied to the skin to obtain the passage of 50 μg of estradiol per day.

Despite the benefits of ERT, its use is currently limited to a minority of postmenopausal women and among those treated, the average duration of treatment is no greater than 18–24 months. This problem of compliance is mainly due to undesirable and uncomfortable side-effects such as mastalgia and bleeding.

A better understanding of the mechanism of estrogen action has allowed the development of compounds with specific action according to the tissue, such as specific estrogen receptor modulators (SERMs) or tibolone, but these compounds are less effective than estrogen in alleviating climacteric symptoms or preventing postmenopausal bone loss. Progress in endocrinology has also shown that due to the complex cellular machinery, differences in the kinetics of stimulation of estrogen receptors may also result in different reactions at the tissue level. The nasal mucosa offers a large surface for absorption, which avoids first-pass intestinal and hepatic metabolism and allows a rapid increase of drug concentration in plasma, resulting in a rapid diffusion at the tissue level. Several hormones such as calcitonin and luteinizing hormone-releasing hormone (LHRH) analogs are already administered successfully using this route[17].

S21400 (Aerodiol®, 17β-estradiol) with its original pharmacokinetic profile leading to transient hormonal exposure and brief stimulation of estrogen receptors, introduces a new concept in HRT: the 'pulsed estrogen therapy' (PET).

PHARMACOKINETICS

Aerodiol® is an aqueous formulation of 17β-estradiol for nasal administration, which uses randomly methylated β-cyclodextrin, a novel polysaccharide excipient, which increases steroid aqueous solubility about 1000 fold[18]. The estradiol–cyclodextrin complex easily dissociates when in contact with the nasal mucosa. Estradiol is readily absorbed whereas the cyclodextrin component is swallowed and eliminated in the faeces.

The pharmacokinetic profile of Aerodiol® was characterized in a study including 36 postmenopausal women[19]. It differs from that of oral or transdermally administered estradiol. The intranasal route provides a 'pulsed' plasma concentration profile, characterized by high, rapidly-achieved maximal plasma concentrations of estradiol, 10–30 min after administration, followed by a relatively quick return to levels of untreated postmenopausal women within 8–12 hours. For example, Cmax of estradiol after 300 μg of Aerodiol®, administered as a single daily dose, is more than 10-fold than after transdermal and oral dosing (Figure 1).

Systemic exposure following Aerodiol® treatment is dose-dependent and does not differ whether given as a single dose or as two doses split over a day. Compared with oral (2 mg/day) and transdermal (50 μg/day) estradiol, which give sustained plasma levels over the day, a similar estimated 24-hour exposure to estradiol (measured as area under curve) was provided by all three formulations.

The bioavailability of Aerodiol® is 25%, seven times greater than that following oral administration as a consequence of the first-pass effect. This enables the administration of lower doses, and above all ensures particularly small variations in absorption.

Avoiding this first-pass metabolism, intranasally administered 17β-estradiol is particularly well-tolerated, and the estrone/estradiol (E1/E2) ratio is close to 1, the physiologic ratio[19,20], compared with the oral route, which has an E1/E2 ratio of 4 (Figure 2).

MODE OF ACTION

Although a plateau of estradiol plasma level has been claimed to be necessary for ERT efficacy, no clear link between estradiol concentration and symptoms has ever been demonstrated. There is no clear threshold value above which estradiol concentrations should be maintained and total systemic exposure to estradiol may be a more reliable index of estrogenic impregnation and activity. Indeed, the pharmacokinetic profile of Aerodiol®, with a pulsed exposure, is consistent with the current understanding of the mechanism of action of estradiol[21]. After estradiol enters the cell, the binding to specific

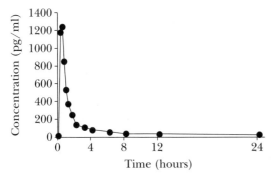

Figure 1 Mean plasma concentrations of estradiol after intranasal administration of 300 μg 17β-estradiol. Reproduced with permission from Devissaguet J-P, *et al. Eur J Drug Metab Pharmacokinet* 1999[19]

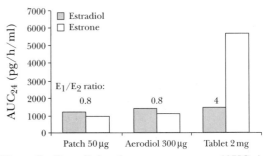

Figure 2 Estradiol and estrone exposures (AUC$_{24}$). Reproduced with permission from Devissaguet J-P, *et al. Eur J Drug Metab Pharmacokinet* 1999[19]

nuclear receptors triggers a cascade of events leading to a delay in protein synthesis and to physiologic effects occurring 12–48 hours after tissue exposure. The PET provided by Aerodiol® may take advantage of this inertia in biologic response. In fact, the better tolerance observed with PET could be explained by the influence of a short duration of exposure to estradiol on biologic response. Thanks to its unique pharmacokinetic profile, producing a brief stimulation of estrogens receptors[22,23], Aerodiol® acts in a distinctive way on cofactors and alters the response of breast and uterine tissue. The beneficial clinical consequences of this different mode of action have been observed in two well-designed trials comparing Aerodiol® 300 µg/day with oral estradiol 2 mg/day or transdermal estradiol 50 µg/day[24,25].

Because of the pulsed pharmacokinetic profile of plasma estradiol, the efficacy of Aerodiol® on climacteric symptoms is thought to be related to total daily hormonal exposure rather than to estradiol serum concentration. The sustained efficacy of the estradiol pulse seen with Aerodiol® over a 24-hour dosing inter-val is supported by the finding that PET is effective against night sweats, despite being administered in the morning. When the treatment could be administered either in the morning or in the evening, vasomotor symptoms were similarly alleviated, regardless of time of intake[26,27].

EFFICACY

Efficacy on climacteric symptoms

The efficacy of PET on climacteric symptoms has been established versus placebo[23,27] and compared to that of transdermal and oral estradiol[24,25].

Two large studies including 418 and 659 postmenopausal women compared Aerodiol® with oral estradiol and placebo[23,24], and showed that Aerodiol® reduced postmenopausal symp-toms in a dose-dependent manner as shown by the significant reduction in the Kupperman Index (KI) (Figure 3).

The change in KI was chosen as the primary efficacy criterion because this index quantifies

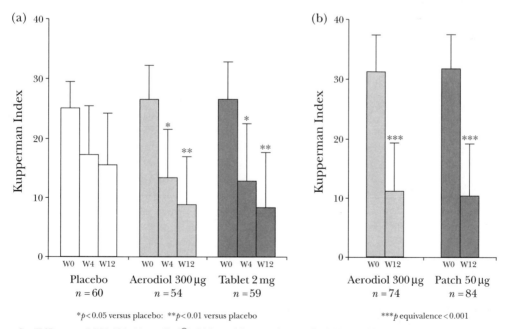

*p < 0.05 versus placebo: **p < 0.01 versus placebo   ***p equivalence < 0.001

Figure 3 Efficacy of S21400 (Aerodiol®) 300 µg/day, oral estradiol (2 mg/day) and patch (50 µg/day) on Kupperman Index; w, week. (a) Reproduced with permission from Studd J, *et al. Lancet* 1999[23]; (b) reproduced with permission from Lopes P, *et al. Obstet Gynecol* 2000[25]

both the incidence and severity of postmeno-pausal symptoms in a weighted manner and has been extensively validated[28].

The 300 µg/day dosage, one spray in each nostril once daily, appeared to be at least as effective as oral estradiol 2 mg/day[29].

A further double-blind study including 165 patients confirmed the efficacy and safety of the PET on climacteric symptoms in highly symp-tomatic postmenopausal women[27]. Aerodiol® 300 µg/day had a faster onset of therapeutic activity than the lower dose (150 µg/day), significantly decreasing the number of moderate-to-severe vasomotor symptoms com-pared with placebo from the second week of treatment; Aerodiol® 150 µg/day significantly decreased symptoms from week 8 compared with placebo. No change in the efficacy of Aerodiol® was found during episodes of infectious rhinitis[27].

A randomized crossover study involving 358 women compared Aerodiol® 300 µg/day with transdermal 17β-estradiol (delivering 50 µg/day)[26]. Efficacy was compared between groups using the KI and vasomotor symptoms at week 12. The two dosage systems produced significant reductions in KI and in the occur-rence of hot flushes and night sweats at week 12. Alleviation of climacteric symptoms was statistically equivalent in the two groups ($p < 0.001$).

Efficacy on bone turnover and bone mineral density

Osteoporosis affects women after menopause and results from an accelerated rate of bone loss mainly due to the effects of estrogen deficiency on the bone remodeling system.

Estrogen supplementation, using either oral or transdermal routes, has been shown to decrease bone turnover, prevent postmeno-pausal bone loss, and significantly reduce fracture risk in both early and late postmeno-pausal women.

The effect of Aerodiol® in normalizing bone turnover was demonstrated in randomized studies versus placebo and oral or transdermal estradiol treatment[30–32].

After 1 year of treatment with intranasal estradiol (300 µg/day), both resorption (uri-nary type I collagen C telopeptides) and forma-tion (osteocalcin, serum bone alkaline phos-phatase (BAP) and serum type I collagen N-terminal extension propeptide (PINP)) markers decreased, reaching the levels in premenopausal women[30].

The effect of Aerodiol® in preventing post-menopausal bone loss was shown in a study versus patch[31], on bone mineral density (BMD) measured after 1 year at the lumbar spine and hip. Dual energy X-ray absorptiometry (DEXA) values increased on average by 2.1% at the lumbar spine and by 1.2% at the hip without any difference between the two treatments – E2 patch 50 µg and Aerodiol® 300 µg[31].

Very recent data from a 2-year randomized placebo controlled study has demonstrated the efficacy of Aerodiol® 150 or 300 µg/day in the prevention of bone loss in early postmeno-pausal women at the spine, hip and forearm[32]. At the lumbar spine, the increase in BMD was 2.2 and 4% respectively with Aerodiol® 150 µg and 300 µg/day, respectively, compared with a decrease of 3.4% in the placebo group for the patients who received the treatment over 2 years.

SAFETY AND TOLERANCE

Breast tolerance and safety

In the intranasal/oral estradiol comparison trial, the incidence of mastalgia was significantly lower with Aerodiol® 300 µg/day than with oral estradiol 2 mg/day (by a mean of 13%; 90% confidence interval (CI): –19.5 to –6.5)[24].

Futhermore, women treated with Aerodiol® suffered significantly less severe mastalgia than women treated with oral estrogen (1 versus 5.2%, $p < 0.01$).

Similarly, in the intranasal/transdermal comparative trial, moderate and severe mastalgia was less frequent in the intranasal group (7.2 versus 15.5%, $p = 0.02$)[26].

The mammary safety of PET has been assessed in both *in vitro* and *in vivo* studies. Results of the comparison of the *in vitro* effects of PET and continuous estradiol treatments on gene expression and cell proliferation indicated that the total exposure to estradiol was more important than the total concentration in accounting for the effect of estrogen on gene expression and cell proliferation. Compared with untreated controls, there were no substantial differences between pulsed and continuous estradiol treatment for the same 24-hour period of exposure in: the extent and time-course of genomic responses studied up to 24 hours; the extent of the dose-dependent proliferation of human estrogen-receptor-positive cancer cells and in the proliferation of normal human breast cells[33].

Mammary safety of PET was studied *in vivo* in a well-recognized experimental model using mammary tumors chemically induced by 7,12-dimethylbenz[a]anthracene (DMBA) in the rat. Potency of both continuous and pulsed estrogen therapy was assessed by the measurements of uterus weight. Results demonstrated that PET led to a significantly lower tumor incidence ($p = 0.05$) and to lower mammary tumor development rates than continuous estrogen therapy[34].

Endometrial safety

Endometrial safety was also assessed during the development of S21400 (Aerodiol®). There were no cases of atypia, hyperplasia or cancer in 311 women treated for 12 months with Aerodiol® with various progestogens administered at recommended doses (medroxyprogesterone acetate, dydrogesterone, chlormadinone acetate, promegestone and natural progesterone). The endometrium was mostly atrophic (34%) or secretory (39%) leading to an adequate progestational response rate of 97%[35].

Nasal tolerance and safety

Results from studies comparing the acceptability of Aerodiol® with that of placebo and oral estradiol control groups confirm that Aerodiol® was well-tolerated locally. The most common effects are minor local symptoms, such as prickling or sneezing lasting only a few minutes after administration and persisting for only a few weeks. Their frequency decreases during treatment, falling to 9% after 1 year. Ear, nose and throat examinations, including rhinoscopy and mucociliary clearance, systematically performed on 304 women after 3 and 6 months of treatment and in cases of premature withdrawal of treatment due to local symptoms (rhinoscopy only) did not show any major alterations of the nasal mucosa[24,25].

OVERALL TOLERABILITY

No clinically relevant changes were observed in laboratory parameters, body weight, or diastolic or systolic blood pressure[36] with S21400 (Aerodiol®).

DOSAGE AND ADMINISTRATION

The recommended initial dosage of Aerodiol® is one spray in each nostril per day (300 μg/day) and can be given cyclically 25–28 days/month or continuously every day. Oral progestogen at recommended doses has to be added for non-hysterectomized women for at least 12 days of each cycle. If there are signs of hyper- or hypo-estrogenization, the usual dosage of 300 μg/day can be decreased to 150 μg/day (one spray per day) or increased to up to 600 μg/day (four sprays per day). In that case a delay of 30 minutes should be observed between each administration in the same nostril.

Combined sequential regimens of estrogen and progestin are associated with cyclic withdrawal bleeding, often poorly tolerated by women over 50 years old[37]. This can be avoided by the use of continuous combined hormone replacement therapy (ccHRT), which may result in greater compliance with therapy. Women on sequential Aerodiol® and progestogen could be switched to a continuous combined regimen after 1 year. They should be informed that initial breakthrough bleeding usually settles after 3–6 months of usage.

Intranasal estradiol retains its efficacy in patients with blocked or streaming noses. If the nasal passages are severely blocked, intranasal estradiol can be administered temporarily buccally (at twice the intranasal dosage), by spraying and rubbing the intranasal estradiol onto the gums.

CONCLUSIONS

S21400 (Aerodiol®) introduces a brand new concept in HRT: pulsed estrogen therapy. PET, a brief once-daily exposure of target tissues to a small dose of natural 17β-estradiol, produces high therapeutic efficacy over 24 hours, thus avoiding continuously elevated plasma estrogen levels. Data collected during the clinical development have shown that Aerodiol® provides excellent clinical efficacy in relieving climacteric symptoms and in the prevention of postmenopausal bone loss. It is at least as effective as continuous estrogen therapies, but is better tolerated than oral and transdermal treatments with significantly less frequent mastalgia and a lower incidence of uterine bleeding. Initial breast safety data are encouraging.

Aerodiol®, the first PET, increases acceptability and compliance, offering a new approach to HRT to physicians and women.

References

1. Kupperman HS, Blatt MGH, Wiesbader H, Filler W. Comparative clinical evaluation of estrogenic preparations by the menopausal and amenorrheal indices. *J Clin Endocrinol* 1953;13:688–703

2. Belchetz PE. Hormonal treatment of postmenopausal women. *N Engl J Med* 1994;330:1062–71

3. Greendale GA, Lee NP, Arriola ER. The menopause. *Lancet* 1999;353:571–80

4. Christiansen C, Christensen MS, McNair P, *et al.* Prevention of early postmenopausal bone loss: controlled 2-year study in 315 normal females. *Eur J Clin Invest* 1980;10:273–9

5. Michaelsson K, Baron JA, Farahmand BH, *et al.* Hormone replacement therapy and risk of hip fracture: population-based case–control study. *Br Med J* 1998;316:1858–63

6. The Writing Group for the Women's Health Initiative Investigators. Risk and benefits of estrogen plus progestin in healthy postmenopausal women. *J Am Med Assoc* 2002;288:321–33

7. Ettinger B, Friedman GD, Bush T, *et al.* Reduced mortality associated with long-term postmenopausal estrogen therapy. *Obstet Gynecol* 1996;87:6–12

8. LeBlanc ES, Janowsky J, Chan BKS, *et al.* Hormone replacement therapy and cognition. Systematic review and meta-analysis. *J Am Med Assoc* 2001;285:1489–99

9. Kyomen HH, Hennen J, Gottlieb GL, *et al.* Estrogen therapy and noncognitive psychiatric signs and symptoms in elderly patients with dementia. *Am J Psychiatry* 2002;159:1225–7

10. O'Connell MB. Pharmacokinetic and pharmacologic variation between different estrogen products. *J Clin Pharmacol* 1995;35:18S–24S

11. de Lignieres B, Basdevant A, Thomas G, *et al.* Biological effects of estradiol-17-beta in postmenopausal women: oral versus percutaneous administration. *J Clin Endocrinol Metab* 1986;62:536–41

12. Longcope C, Gorbach S, Goldin B, *et al.* The metabolism of estradiol: oral compared with intravenous administration. *J Steroid Biochem* 1985;23:1065–75

13. Stanczyk FZ, Shoupe D, Nunez V, *et al.* A randomized comparison of nonoral estradiol delivery in postmenopausal women. *Am J Obstet Gynecol* 1988;159:1540–6

14. Amy JJ, Balmer JA, Baumarten K, *et al.* A randomized study to compare the effectiveness, tolerability and acceptability of two different transdermal estradiol replacement therapies: the transdermal HRT Investigators Group. *Int J Fertil Menopausal Stud* 1993;38:5–11

15. Frenkel Y, Kopernik G, Lazer S, *et al.* Acceptability and skin reactions to transdermal estrogen replacement therapy in reaction to climate. *Maturitas* 1994;20:31–6

16. Grebe SK, Adams JD, Feek CM. Systemic sensitization to ethanol by transdermal estrogen patches. *Arch Dermatol* 1993;129:379–80

17. Jones NS, Quraishi S, Mason JD. The nasal delivery of systemic drugs. *Int J Clin Pract* 1997;51: 308–11

18. Nogradi M. Dimethyl-ß-cyclodextrin. *Drugs Future* 1984;9:577–8

19. Devissaguet J-P, Brion N, Lhote O, *et al.* Pulsed estrogen therapy: pharmacokinetics of intranasal 17-beta-estradiol (S21400) in postmenopausal women and comparison with oral and transdermal formulations. *Eur J Drug Metab Pharmacokinet* 1999;24:265–71

20. Hermens WA, Belder CW, Merkus JM, *et al.* S21400 (Aerodiol®) administration to oophorectomised women. *Eur J Obstet Gynecol Reprod Biol* 1991;40:35–41

21. Lindsay R, Dempster DW, Jordan VC, eds. *Estrogens and Antiestrogens: Basic and Clinical Aspects.* Philadelphia: Lipincott-Raven 1997: 43–62

22. Robinson JA, Spelsberg T. Mode of action at the cellular level with specific reference to bone cells. *Estrogens Antiestrogens* 1997;5:43–62

23. Studd J, Pornel B, Marton I, *et al.*, for the S21400 (Aerodiol®) Study Group. Efficacy and acceptability of intranasal 17β-estradiol for menopausal symptoms: randomised dose-response study. *Lancet* 1999;353:1574–8

24. Mattsson LA, Christiansen C, Colau JC, *et al.* Clinical equivalence of intranasal and oral 17β-estradiol for postmenopausal symptoms. *Am J Obstet Gynecol* 2000;182:545–52

25. Lopes P, Merkus HMWM, Nauman J, *et al.* Randomized comparison of intranasal and transdermal estradiol. *Obstet Gynecol* 2000;96: 906–12

26. Lopes P, Rozenberg S, de Graaf J, *et al.* S21400 (Aerodiol®) versus the transdermal route: perspectives for patient preference. *Maturitas* 2001;38(Suppl.1):S1–S58

27. Rozenbaum H, Chevallier O, Moyal M, *et al.* Efficacy and tolerability of pulsed estrogen therapy: a 12-week double-blind placebo-controlled study in highly symptomatic postmenopausal women. *Climacteric,* 2002;5:249–58

28. Wiklund I, Karlberg J, Mattson LA. Quality of life of postmenopausal women on a regimen of transdermal estradiol therapy: a double blind placebo-controlled study. *Am J Obstet Gynecol* 1993;168:824–30

29. Panay N, Toth K, Pelisser C, Studd J. Dose-ranging studies of a novel intranasal estrogen replacement therapy. *Maturitas* 2001;38 Suppl 1:S15–22

30. Garnero P, Tsouderos Y, Marton I, *et al.* Effects of intranasal 17β-oestradiol for menopausal symptoms: randomized dose-response study. *J Clin Endocrinol Metab* 1999;84:2390–7

31. Ribot C, Trémollières F, Pornel B, *et al.* Postmenopausal bone loss is prevented by pulsed estrogen therapy: a comparison with the transdermal patch. *Gynecol Endocrinol* 2000;14 (Suppl 2):230, abstract S25

32. Christiansen C, Bagger Y, Chetaille E, *et al.* Prevention of postmenopausal bone loss with pulsed estrogen therapy by nasal route: a randomized double-blind, placebo-controlled study. *Osteoporosis Int* 2002;13:O41

33. Cavaillès V, Gompel A, Portois MC, *et al.* Comparative activity of pulsed or continuous estradiol exposure on gene expression and proliferation of normal and tumoral human breast cells. *J Mol Endocrinol* 2002;28:165–75

34. Kerdelhué B, Jolette J. The influence of the route of administration of 17β-estradiol, intravenous (pulsed) versus oral, upon DMBA-induced mammary tumour development in ovariectomised rats. *Breast Cancer Res Treat* 2002; 73:13–22

35. Gompel A, Bergeron C, Jondet M, *et al.* Endometrial safety and tolerability of S21400 (Aerodiol®) for 1 year. *Maturitas* 2000; s36:209–15

36. Dooley M, Spencer CM, Ormrod D. Estradiol-Intranasal: a review of its use in the management of menopause. *Drugs* 2001;61:2243–62

37. Panay N, Studd J. Progestogen intolerance and compliance with HRT in menopausal women. *Hum Reprod Update* 1997;3:159–71

23

Dyspareunia: clinical approach in the perimenopause

A. Graziottin

INTRODUCTION

The gynecologist is increasingly asked to address his/her patients' sexual complaints. This is mandatory when the woman complains of pain during intercourse, clinically known as 'dyspareunia', from ancient Greek, meaning 'difficult mating'. No other physician has the same competence in evaluating all the potential biological causes of dyspareunia, particularly during and after the menopause, when endocrine, dystrophic and age correlated etiologies become prominent as the woman ages[1].

In the Diagnostic and Statistical Manual of Mental Disorders, fourth edition (DSM IV)[2], dyspareunia is defined as follows: ' recurrent or persistent genital pain associated with intercourse; the disturbance causes considerable distress and interpersonal difficulties; the disturbance is not exclusively due to vaginismus or lack of lubrication, nor is it due to any other disturbance on the Axis I, or the direct physiological effects of a substance or of a general medical condition.'

Unfortunately, the DSM-IV classification arbitrarily eliminates the major biological factors of coital pain[3–7], which must be addressed if the symptoms are to be etiologically cured. The exclusion of 'a general medical condition' keeps the following, among others, out of the diagnostic field: the menopause, which is the most frequent condition leading to vaginal dryness and coital pain in middle age, due to the loss of sexual hormones[3–5]; diabetes,

with reduced lubrication due to microangiopathy, and vascular diseases (atherosclerosis, hypercholesterolemia, smoking, age)[6]; and urological conditions increasingly associated with sexual disorders as the woman ages[7]. Vascular diseases in women (as in men) are still under-diagnosed causes of arousal disorders, one of the major physio-pathologic contributors to vaginal dryness and sexual pain. The new International Consensus Development Conference on female sexual disorders (FSD)[8] has changed the classification to a general category of 'sexual pain disorders' that includes dyspareunia and vaginismus and a new entry, 'non-coital sexual pain disorders', conceptualized as 'recurrent or persistent genital pain induced by non-coital sexual stimulation' (Table 1). As in the previous DSM-IV classification, sub-types of 'lifelong' versus 'acquired and generalized' versus 'situational' are maintained, but again, a new entry helps to describe a comprehensive diagnosis. The third sub-type, 'etiologic origin', includes four possibilities: 'organic', 'psychogenic', 'mixed' and 'unknown', finally stressing the importance of biologic factors and therefore encouraging a more balanced, integrated diagnostic approach between biologic and psychogenic causes.

Sexual comorbidity is frequently reported in women, addressing well both the physiologic interdependence of different aspects of the sexual response (desire, arousal, orgasm,

Table 1 Classification of sexual pain disorders. Adapted with permission from Basson R, *et al.* Report of the International Consensus Development Conference on female sexual dysfunction. *J Urol* 2000;163:889–93[8]

Dyspareunia: recurrent or persistent genital pain associated with sexual intercourse

Vaginismus: recurrent or persistent involuntary spasm of the musculature of the outer third of the vagina that interferes with vaginal penetration, which causes personal distress

Non coital sexual pain disorders: recurrent or persistent genital pain induced by non-coital sexual stimulation

Subtyping further differentiates the diagnosis of FSD according to

    the temporal onset: 'lifelong' versus 'acquired'
    the context-dependent dynamic: 'generalized' versus 'situational'
    the etiology: 'organic', 'psychogenic', 'mixed', or 'unknown'

FSD, female sexual disorders

satisfaction) and the interplay between biological, psychosexual and relational factors in female sexuality[1,8,9] (Figure 1).

PREVALENCE OF DYSPAREUNIA

Ten to fifteen percent of fertile, coitally active women and up to 39% of postmenopausal women complain of various degrees of dyspareunia[1,9]. This variation in clinical reporting is due to a number of factors: type of population considered (general, gynecological or sexological clinics, specialized in the medical approach to FSD); selection biases; quality of attention the clinician pays to such a complaint and to its solution; and most importantly, the quality of the clinician's listening to the disclosure and discussion of sexual complaints[1].

COMMUNICATION ON SEXUAL MATTERS

It's difficult to provide an effective intervention if there is no mention of a problem! FSD have been (and still are) the great absentees from the clinical consultation, due to both the lack of formal training in sexual medicine in most medical schools, and the uneasiness many

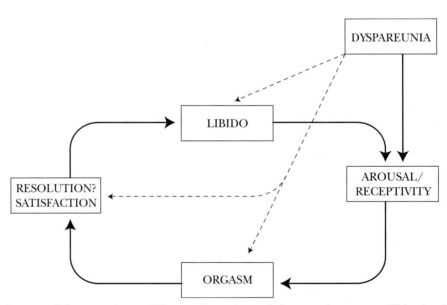

Figure 1 Impact of dyspareunia on different dimensions of the sexual response. This circular model, formulated by the presenting author, contributes to the understanding of: frequent overlapping of sexual symptoms reported in clinical practice (comorbidity), as different dimensions of sexual response are correlated from a physiopathologic point of view; potential negative or positive feedback mechanisms operating in sexual functions; and the *direct* inhibiting effect of dyspareunia on genital arousal and vaginal receptivity and the *indirect* inhibiting effect on orgasm, satisfaction and libido, with close interplay between biological and psychosexual factors

physicians feel when dealing with such an extremely sensitive matter[1,3,10,11]. Many physicians are also afraid of the 'waste of time' that opening a sexual issue might cause. However, on the contrary, it is dedicated time that can be rewarded with a higher satisfaction in the doctor–patient relationship, especially when the physician is able to give the appropriate answer to improve or, hopefully, solve the sexual problem he/she is listening to and caring about. The physician open to treating FSD should[1,4,10,12,13]:

(1) Gradually learn to be comfortable in asking questions about sexuality and responding to issues that arise from the questioning;

(2) be able to maintain a sensitive, non-judgemental approach;

(3) use precise questions within the limits imposed by tact, being aware that older cohorts of women may feel uneasy or even disrespected with the open language that may be in play with the younger cohorts;

(4) be sensitive to the optimal time to ask the most emotionally charged questions, maybe preferring open questions in the first visit (How do you feel? How are things at home? How's your sex life? Did you notice any change in your sexual interest since you became menopausal? etc);

(5) pay attention to non-verbal language (feeling-tone, facial expressions, posture, etc), which may be more informative about the emotional relevance of an issue than the simple meaning of words;

(6) assure the patient of the complete confidentiality of the issues discussed; and

(7) update regularly, as the field of female sexuality is finally having an outburst of interest both in basic and clinical research.

With a serene matter-of-fact attitude the physician will help the patient relax and become matter-of-fact too[10].

ETIOLOGY OF DYSPAREUNIA IN THE PERIMENOPAUSE

Sexual pain may be perceived in the introital area (introital or superficial dyspareunia), at mid-vagina (midvaginal dyspareunia), or deep in the pelvis (deep dyspareunia)[1,13]. Etiology may be multi-factorial (biologic, psychosexual and relational) and multi-systemic[13–17], as different systems (endocrine, vascular, muscular, immune, neurologic and pain-related) may contribute to the final perception of sexual pain[1,18,19].

Biological causes of introital and midvaginal dyspareunia

Hormonal etiology[1,3,4,15–17]

A hormonal cause of introital and midvaginal dyspareunia tops the list of factors (Table 2), as vaginal dryness is related to progressive (in premenopause) or definitive loss (in postmenopause) of an adequate concentration of vaginal estrogens. It is important to mention that vaginal estrogen concentration may be insufficient for adequate genital arousal and lubrication despite periods still being present[3,17]. Data from the Yale Midlife Study

Table 2 Leading biologic causes of dyspareunia in perimenopause

Introital and midvaginal
  Sexual hormone loss
  vulvovaginitis and vestibulitis
  vulvar dystrophy
  iatrogenic
  muscular
  vascular
  neurologic
  connective/immune
  traumatic
  pain-related disorders
Deep
  endometriosis
  pelvic inflammatory disease
  pelvic varicocele
  referred pain

indicated that 77% of women reported loss of sex drive, 58% had vaginal dryness and 39% suffered from dyspareunia[17]. This study also showed a relationship between serum estradiol levels and sex problems. With an arbitrary cut-off at 50 pg/ml, significantly more menopausal women with serum estradiol below this concentration reported problems of vaginal dryness, dyspareunia and pain than women whose estradiol levels were above 50 pg/ml[17]. Varying estrogenic receptor distribution may account for different tissue sensitivities and different symptom vulnerabilities in menopausal women[18]. Topical estrogens may be necessary in some clinical conditions to improve vaginal dryness: if the patient is prescribed extra-low contraceptive pills (with 15 µg of ethinylestradiol) in the pre-menopause, as on average one fifth of these patients may complain of vaginal dryness during this treatment; if she is on low-dose hormone replacement therapy (HRT) (Table 3); or if she is menopausal and not using HRT.

Vaginitis and vulvitis

Vaginitis and vulvitis may be frequent co-factors of acquired dyspareunia n the perimenopausal years[19–24]. The routine examination of vaginal pH, normally under 4.5 but which usually rises in hypoestrogenic conditions, may immediately give a biologic feedback on the vaginal environment and related ecosystem[17,24]. Gardnerella infections are more likely at a pH above 5, whilst saprophytic pathogens from colonic origin (Escherichia coli, Enterococcus faecalis) are usually in play at an even higher pH level, when the vagina is deprived of the majority of lactobacilli due to the loss of estrogens and increased pH[24]. When past vulvar vestibulitis syndrome (VVS) – the most frequent biological cause of dyspareunia at fertile age – is reported[1,19,20], special attention should be paid to diagnose potential recurrences, especially when sexually active women are using HRT[1,19]. Candida spp. infection may also be exacerbated when the woman starts HRT.

Vulvar dystrophy

Vulvar dystrophy is increasingly credited to be a full thickness-disorder, with a progressive reduction of all the tissue components. It is not limited to mucocutaneous lichen sclerosus[25], and is probably due to a genetic vulnerability accelerating hormone receptor loss. Tarcan and co-workers[26] proved that there is an age-dependent reduction of more than 50% of the cavernosal smooth muscle components from the first to the sixth decade of life, this being the basis of the increasingly reported difficulty in getting genitally aroused ('my clitoris is dead') up to orgasm.

Iatrogenic factors

Iatrogenic factors, that may be responsible for an acquired dyspareunia in the perimenopause: overzealous colporraphies and other pelvic surgeries[27–29] may be responsible for an anatomical narrowing of the introital area that may be incompatible with intercourse. Questions about ongoing sexual activity should be asked *before* every type of pelvic surgery, even in elderly patients, to prevent further comorbidity due to the wrong assumption that the patient was too old to have sex. Radiotherapy and/or radical surgery for cervical cancer may also cause a reduced vaginal receptivity due to shortening and retraction of the vagina[29]. With the exception of adenocarcinoma of the cervix (which is hormone dependent) there is no contraindication in treating patients cured of a

Table 3 Comparison of biological activity of different estrogens used for HRT. Reproduced with permission from Notelovitz M. *A Practical Approach to Postmenopausal Hormone Therapy. Obstetrics and Gynecology*, special edn. New York: MacMahon, 2002[3]

| | Estrogen dose | | |
	Low	Intermediate	High
17-β-Estradiol	0.5 mg	1 mg	2 mg
Esterified estrogens	0.3 mg	0.625 mg	1.25 mg
Combined equine estrogens	0.3 mg	0.625 mg	0.9 mg
Estradiol patch	25 µg	50 µg	100 µg

cervical squamous carcinoma with topical estrogens soon after surgery, especially if radiotherapy is prescribed[29]. This will reduce vaginal retraction, maintain a better mucosal and vascular trophism and, if combined with a timely rehabilitation of the pelvic floor, will help to maintain coital receptivity in these unfortunate women. Last but not least, as postmenopausal and elderly women are usually on multipharmacologic treatment, sexual side-effects of drugs contributing to dyspareunia through libido, arousal and/or orgasmic disorders should be considered[30].

Muscular factors

Muscular factors – namely a tightening of the pelvic floor – may become relevant in chronic dyspareunia, when the persistence of pain may cause a secondary defensive contraction of the levator ani, and even myalgia[1,31–33]. This may become an added cause of midvaginal dyspareunia and/or of post-coital cystitis[1]. Unwanted pain is the most powerful reflex inhibitor of perivaginal (and periurethral) arousal[1,19], increasing the vulnerability of the urethra and of the trigonal area, deprived of the protective effect of estrogen, thus further increasing mechanical trauma of intercourse without lubrication and without the protective vascular congestion of the periurethral vessel, which has a cavernosal structure in the lower third[34].

Vascular and metabolic factors

Vascular factors such as smoking, atherosclerosis and hypertension and metabolic disorders like diabetes with microangiopathy (and neuropathy) may all contribute to genital arousal disorders[1,6], in women and men, with vaginal dryness leading to dyspareunia.

Pain-related disorders

The most recent and exciting findings in dyspareunia, when caused by chronic VVS, indicate a specific pathology within the pain system, with an increased pain input from the introital area, a histologically proven increase in pain fibres[35–37], and a systemic lowering of the pain threshold[38]. This addresses the shift from nociceptive pain, when pain simply indicates an ongoing damage with tissue inflammation, to neuropathic pain, when pain is 'produced' and/or exacerbated within the pain system[39–41].

Neurologic diseases

The least frequent biologic factors are: neurological diseases including pudendal nerve entrapment syndrome[28,42,43], leading to dyspareunia, which may appear many years after coccygeal–sacral physical trauma or pelvic surgery; and multiple sclerosis.

Rare causes

Sjogren's syndrome[44], an auto-immune disease where antibodies attack components of the exocrine gland system; physical genital trauma and/or sexual abuse[45], infrequent but very traumatic in dystrophic genital conditions.

Psychosexual causes of introital and midvaginal dyspareunia

Psychosexual factors, mostly related to loss of libido, including arousal disorders; vaginismus, and/or orgasmic difficulties, either lifelong or acquired[1,4,46], are also a cause of dyspareunia.

Context-dependent causes of introital and midvaginal dyspareunia

Context-dependent factors, particularly relational, when either emotional intimacy is lacking, the relationship is abusive and or conflictual, or when chronic disregard to sufficient foreplay leads to penetration before the woman is adequately aroused and lubricated[1,4,46,47], are possible causes.

Frequent causes of deep dyspareunia

Pelvic endometriosis

Deep dyspareunia is the emerging symptom of pelvic endometriosis[48] recurring in cases of cyclic HRT. In women with previous endometriosis, and with a conserved uterus, low-dose continuous combined HRT (ccHRT) should be the first choice to avoid bleeding and recurrence of pain.

Pelvic inflammatory disease

Pelvic inflammatory disease (PID)[49] may cause lateral, deep pelvic pain. Once considered a disease of youth, PID is now to be considered, as modified sex habits may expose women of all ages to PID when they have unprotected sex with new partners.

Pelvic variocele

Pelvic variocele[1] is increasingly diagnosed as a cause of deep dyspareunia.

Levator ani myalgia

Deep pelvic pain may also be secondary to trigger point stimulation at the levator ani level, when the muscle is intensely myalgic[1,31–33].

HOW TO DIAGNOSE DYSPAREUNIA

When a woman seeks clinical help because of coital pain during intercourse in the perimenopause, the clinical approach should start with a few general questions (Table 4) helping to focus on the leading sexual complaint and sexual comorbidity. In this section, questions and answers will be presented in greater detail, to offer a meaningful clinical reasoning to be used when the patient complains of dyspareunia. A very careful clinical examination will complete the first-level diagnostic evaluation.

Table 4 Short form of a sexual history in perimenopause

How do you feel?
How's your sex life? Are you satisfied with it?
If your sex life is unsatisfying, what is the main complaint you have?
Do you feel a loss of sex drive (are you still interested in sex)?
Do you feel pain during or after the intercourse?
Do you feel an arousal/lubrication difficulty with vaginal dryness?
Do you have increasing difficulties in reaching orgasm?
If you have one or more of these disorders, did they appear or worsen after the menopause (or have they been lifelong)?
Do you have a stable relationship?
If yes, are you happy with it? And how is your partner's health (general and sexual)?
Do you feel that your sexual problem is more dependent on physical problems or lack of satisfaction in your relationship?
Are you personally interested in improving your sex life?

Clinical interview

(1) *When did you notice that intercourse was becoming painful? Did you always (lifelong) suffer from pain during intercourse, or is pain recent (acquired)?*

When lifelong, dyspareunia is usually caused by vaginismus[1] or coexisting life-long FSDs such as low libido[1,4,8,11–13] and arousal disorders[13,15,16] of psychosexual etiology. Lifelong dyspareunia may worsen until a complete avoidance of sex around the menopause because of hormonal loss. If pain prevents penetration, a severe vaginismus is probably revealed[1], occasionally during the first gynecological visit around the menopause, when menorrhagia or other acute symptoms necessitate examination.

(2) *If pain is recent (acquired), do you also suffer from vaginal dryness during intercourse? And from vaginitis? Do you suffer from cystitis-like symptoms, 24–72 hours after intercourse?*

Hormonal loss[3–5,13–19], altered vaginal eco-system[24] and a tightened pelvic floor[1,31–33] may concur with the clinical picture. All factors should be addressed for a full recovery.

(3) *Do you always feel pain during intercourse (general) or is it limited to some situations (situational)? In the latter case, which condition or situation precipitates it? In the case of a stable relationship, how is the quality of intimacy and couple satisfaction, besides sex? Does the partner suffer from any sexual problem: low libido, premature ejaculation, erectile deficit?*

Situational dyspareunia should focus the interview on the quality of the relationship[47,50], frustrated intimacy and love needs[46], potential conflicts[51], areas of disappointment, anger[50] and/or context-dependent worsening or precipitating factors. It also should open a window on the partner's sexuality[47], and on the potential collusion dynamics that may contribute to maintain the symptoms. Dennerstein and co-workers[47], in their 8-year prospective studies on women during the menopausal transition, found that 'feelings for partner' and 'partner's health and sexual problems' were the strongest predictors of sexual changes across the menopause, while the two symptoms more frequently recorded were loss of libido and arousal disorders. 'Symptom inducer and symptom carrier' scripts should also be gently explored[50,51].

(4) *If you avoid intercourse, is your sexual experience still pleasurable and satisfying or not? How is your sexual drive? Is arousal easy? Do you usually reach clitoral orgasm? Do you notice disappearance of lubrication when you try intercourse?*

These questions help to focus on the quality of sexual response, besides intercourse, and of intervening negative feedback on the sexual circuit (Figure 1). The presence of a dysfunctional sexual response, leading to sexual comorbidity, may suggest a mixed etiology, if organic factors are present as well. Worsening of the sexual response, after the onset of dyspareunia, addresses specifically the potent inhibitory effect of fear of pain on physical arousal[1,19,29].

(5) *How intense is the pain you feel?*

Focusing on the intensity and characteristics of pain is a relatively new approach in addressing dyspareunia issues[1,19,20,38]. Analogic scales, or other traditional quantitative or qualitative measures of pain and pain disorders, appear to be very useful for description and classification, particularly when vulvar vestibulitis is the leading cause of dyspareunia, as increasing input of pain signals[35–37] and a lowered central pain threshold are increasingly recognized as specific aspects of this disease.

(6) *When do you feel pain? Before, during or after intercourse?*

Pain before intercourse suggests a phobic attitude toward penetration or the presence of vestibulitis, if previous attempts at intercourse have caused a mechanic microtrauma of the introital mucosa[1,19]. Pain *during* intercourse is more frequently reported[20,52,53]. This information, combined with a description of the location of the pain, proves to be the most predictive of the organicity of pain[53]. Pain after intercourse, if introital, again suggests vestibulitis (in either fertile or postmenopausal women using HRT) because of the post-coital worsening irritation, hypertonic pelvic floor (the so called levator ani myalgia) or vulvo-vaginal dystrophia in the peri- and post-menopause[1,19].

(7) *Where does it hurt? At the entrance of the vagina, in the mid vagina or deep in the vagina?*

Meana and co-workers[52] observed that the location of the pain and its onset within an episode of intercourse were the strongest predictors of presence and type of organicity. Psychosocial variables such as situational factors, relationship adjustment and history of sexual abuse had no predictive value. Women with dyspareunia did not differ significantly from controls on these measures[52,53]. A different diagnostic – and cultural – approach, namely to consider dyspareunia as a sexual pain disorder, and not 'simply' a sexual disorder, is necessary to correctly address the many different issues covered by this comprehensive and yet elusive word[38,52].

PHYSICAL EXAMINATION

Inspection

Observation of the patient while she is awaiting examination, the degree of muscular tension, the presence of neurovegetative signs, or contracted postural attitudes should all be observed and reported on the clinical chart[1]. Careful inspection of the patient and of her external genitalia may help diagnosis in the case of superficial dyspareunia:

(1) Neurovegetative responses such as sweating, blushing, tachycardia, etc, are suggestive of a phobic attitude to coitus and often associated with vaginismus[1];

(2) Defensive general posture suggests a phobic aversion to coitus and/or long-lasting persistent pain. Muscular postural changes may become secondary sources of pain[19,31–33];

(3) Defensive contraction of the perineal muscle, with reduced distance fourchette–anus[1]; signs of inflammation, suggestive of vulvovaginitis[7,19] or vestibulitis[19–23]. Three signs will suggest the latter: variable reddening of the vestibular area (between clitoris, inner face of labia minora and fourchette), acute pain when touching at five and seven, looking at the introitus as a clockface, and defensive contraction of the perineal muscle at tentative insertion (mimicking what happens at intercourse)[1,19,52–54];

(4) Signs of vulvovaginal dystrophy in postmenopausal women[1,3,19,25];

(5) Retracted, painful scars of previous pelvic surgeries[27–29] or scars of vulvar traumas;

(6) Congested clitoris, in case of associated clitoralgia[19];

(7) Bartholinitis, painful surgical outcome of surgery on Bartholin glands[27], or inflamed Nuck's cyst (rare);

(8) Hemorrhoids, suggestive of colonic or pelvic floor dysfunction[27] that may be associated with repeated vaginitis or cystitis from colonic saprophytes[24], frequently associated with dyspareunia in the postmenopause.

Gynecological examination with semiology of pain

Accurate, delicate and respectful physical examination may indicate one or more specifically painful points, mimicking the pain the woman experiences during intercourse, in 90% of cases[52,54]. 'Where does it hurt?' This is the critical question. While gently and competently exploring all the possible sources of pain, the physician will not only build up a careful 'pain map'[1] based on solid anatomy and logic physiopathology but will also make a gesture of attention that is of outmost psychological value. After months or years of being told that 'pain is only in her mind', such a careful evaluation will create a very positive and trusting doctor–patient relationship[1]. If the partner is present in the consulting room, and if the woman agrees, explaining to him (or her) all the physical findings that might cause pain during the exploration (and likely, during penetration) is useful and positive for the couple's relationship. When the partner sees that there is a physical problem, with a medical diagnosis and a reasonably effective treatment, and that 'she is not just refusing sex or him (or her)', he/she becomes much more understanding and collaborative.

The examination might reveal or confirm:

(1) Acute pain at five and seven (vestibulitis) (Q tip test)[19,20,29,52–54];

(2) Tender or trigger points on retracted scars, or on superficial perineal muscles (mostly on the bulbocavernous muscle)[1,31–33];

(3) Congested, painful clitoris in case of associated clitoralgia[19];

(4) A narrow introitus after surgery (colporraphy, colpoperineorrhaphy)[27–29]. Retraction, pain, mucocutaneous and myofascial trigger points, vaginal anatomic outcome (introital caliber, vaginal length and post-repair elasticity), and the pelvic floor muscles' defensive hypertonus are frequent cofactors in introital and mid-vaginal dyspareunia after perineal surgery[31–33];

(5) A dry, dystrophic vagina[13,15–18];

(6) Spasm of the peri-vaginal muscles, with tender or trigger points in the mid-vagina, at the insertion of the levator ani on the spine, usually different in the two halves of the muscle[1,31–33]. Trigger points on the levator ani may cause referred deep pelvic pain and mimic deep dyspareunia. Sometimes the muscle presents a strong asymmetric spasm, suggestive of both local muscle pathologies or asymmetric spasms secondary to pelvic traumas[1]. Posterior palpation of the sacrum and coccyx *per vaginam* may confirm the presence of selective contractions or tension causing acute pain when touched;

(7) Acute provoked pain at bimanual deep exploration. Posterior pain when causing tension of the uterosacral ligaments may be suggestive of endometriosis[1,48], of which deep dyspareunia may be the emerging symptom, recurring in the case of cyclic HRT. In women with previous endometriosis, and with a conserved uterus, low-dose ccHRT should be the first choice to avoid bleeding. Lateral, deep pelvic pain may be more frequently caused by PID[49], sometimes by pelvic varicocele[55]; anterior pain, in the trigonal area, is more frequently present when dyspareunia is associated with post-coital cystitis, urgency and frequency[1]. As mentioned before, deep pelvic pain may also be secondary to trigger-point stimulation at the levator ani level[31–33].

Clinical interview and competent physical examination will contribute to an accurate etiologic diagnosis: organic, psychogenic or mixed. This latter group will be dramatically reduced if the classical medical steps in approaching pain disorders are respected and if a competent attitude to diagnose FSD is integrated with them.

TREATMENT

An integrated diagnosis of medical and psychosexual factors is preliminary to the effective treatment of dyspareunia, which requires physiopathologically oriented therapy of the physiologic factors and adequate attention to individual and couple psychosexual issues. Medical treatment of dyspareunia includes the following.

Topical hormonal treatment

This is the first choice to reduce pain caused by inadequate hormone-dependent genital arousal, particularly during and after the menopause.

Testosterone

Testosterone propionate powder 2% in petroleum jelly is applied to the external genitalia, daily or every other day, in very small quantities. This local treatment is effective in increasing the clitoral arousal, sensitivity and responsiveness. The same therapy applied to the vulva will relieve entry dyspareunia due to vulvar dystrophy. Testosterone is avidly absorbed from the peripheral tissues and if used frequently or for prolonged periods should be monitored by regular testosterone assays, to avoid supraphysiologic plasmatic levels and related side-effects[3].

Vaginal estrogens

Vaginal estrogens may offer rapid relief when dyspareunia is more dependent on vaginal dystrophy[1,13,15–18]. Topical estrogens may be the first line treatment in women who cannot have, or do not want, a systemic HRT. They should be prescribed even in the premenopause or during systemic HRT when symptoms or signs of vaginal dystrophy are present[24]. 17-β-Estradiol vaginal tablets may significantly improve atrophic vaginitis and related symptoms with a better compliance profile than the more powerful conjugated equine estrogen vaginal cream[56].

Systemic hormone replacement therapy

Systemic HRT is indicated in cases of sexual comorbidity (loss of libido and poor central arousal concomitant to the menopause)[1,5,12,15,16,57–60] or when other menopausal symptoms are complained of[3,5,17,29,47]. Estroandrogens are the treatment of choice when sexual comorbidity is reported, either in the form of injection or subcutaneous implant[5,57–59]. Testosterone patches are still under investigation[61]. Among the available oral treatments, tibolone, due to its androgenic action, seems to offer a very positive effect both on libido and central arousal and on peripheral genital arousal and orgasm, thus improving different dimensions of the sexual response and easing the sexual recovery when other organic etiologies of dyspareunia have been appropriately treated[60]. Progestins with androgenic properties like norethisterone do better still on the sexual response than the non-androgenic progestins. In tailoring treatment, the desire of the woman to maintain a good sexuality, or improve a fading one, should be considered for the optimal HRT choice. Two recent papers, on tibolone[62] and oral HRT containing norethisterone[63], suggest a significant positive effect on muscle trophism and motor competence. This impact could be beneficial also from the sexual point of view, both for the increased general well-being, which improves the vital energy and the sense of fitness, and specifically for the trophism of the pelvic floor, so important in female sexual function, although specific studies on this special aspect have not been performed so far. Systemic and

local HRT is being considered to reduce dyspareunia and improve the quality of life and overall sexuality of patients treated for genital cancer, with the exception of adenocarcinomata of the endometrium, of the cervix, and of the ovary[29,64].

Rehabilitation of the pelvic floor muscles

Rehabilitation of the pelvic floor muscles, defensively contracted in chronic coital pain, is of specific importance in the treatment of dyspareunia[1,65,66]. Stretching and relaxation of contracted muscles, self-massage with medicated oil (St. John's wort)[1] or electromyographic biofeedback[65,66], when available, may all relieve the muscle tension, reducing midvaginal dyspareunia and limiting the source of referred pain. In a prospective controlled study[54] of cognitive behavioral therapy, electromyographic biofeedback and vestibulectomy all proved to offer significant improvement in dyspareunia associated with VVS, by modifying different etiological factors contributing to pain. Special attention should be paid to systemic muscular involvement as part of a general defensive reaction when dyspareunia is associated with vaginismus[67].

Electroanalgesia

This should be recommended when introital hyperalgesia is due to chronic VVS[63]. Vestibulectomy, fashionable when the physiopathology of introital pain was not well understood, is to be considered after more conservative antalgic treatments[39,65,66].

Antalgic treatment

Antalgic treatment[39,68], both systemic and local, should be reserved for severe dyspareunia, usually associated with VVS or neurologic pain, when all previous treatments have failed. Systemic treatment may include tricyclics, like amytriptyline[68], aimed at modulating the serotonin and epinephrine imbalance associated with persisting pain, and anticonvulsants, like gabapentin[39], aimed at raising the threshold of the stimulus needed for nerves to fire, thus raising the central pain threshold. Presacral anethetic block of the ganglion impar (every 3 weeks, for up to 4 months) has recently been proposed[39] as an effective conservative second-line treatment when all previous treatments have failed.

Coexistent general medical conditions

Coexistent general medical conditions (vascular, metabolic, neurologic, immune) should be addressed to reduce the multisystemic etiology of dyspareunia[1].

CONCLUSION

Pain is rarely purely psychogenic; dyspareunia is no exception. As with all pain syndromes, usually it has one or multiple biologic etiologies. It deserves careful clinical attention, as it is the common emerging symptom of a variety of medical conditions that should be recognized and treated accordingly. Psychosexual factors (mostly low libido) lifelong or acquired because of the persisting pain, and arousal disorders, both lifelong and secondary to the inhibitory effect of pain, should be addressed in parallel, in order to give a comprehensive, integrated and more effective treatment. Psychodynamic issues, both personal or related to a couple's relationship, should be adequately addressed if present.

An interdisciplinary approach, with the contribution of different experts – gynecologists, sexologists, psychiatrists, pain therapists – is needed to give dyspareunia its full meaning, in respect of the individual complexity of sex pain experience. Gynecologists should enrich their clinical competence with a more active knowledge of the biologic basis of female sexual disorders that are rooted in their specialized domain, with an increasing competence in the physiopathology of sexual and pelvic pain. They are the physicians most suitable to offer the best first-line comprehensive diagnosis and treatment of sexual pain disorders.

References

1. Graziottin A. Dyspareunia. *J Sex Marital Ther* 2001;27:534–8
2. Diagnostic and Statistical Manual of Mental Disorders, 4th edn. Washington DC: American Psychiatric Association, 1994
3. Notelovitz M. *A Practical Approach to Postmenopausal Hormone Therapy. Obstetrics and Gynecology*, special edn. New York: MacMahon, 2002
4. Graziottin A. Loss of libido in the postmenopause. *Menopausal Med* 2000;8:9–12
5. Sands R, Studd J. Exogenous androgens in postmenopausal women. *Am J Med* 1995;98:76–9
6. Goldstein I, Berman JR. Vasculogenic female sexual dysfunction: vaginal engorgement and clitoral erectile insufficiency syndromes. *Int J Impotence Res* 1998;10:S84–S90
7. Barlow DH, Cardozo L, Francis RM, *et al.* Urogenital ageing and its effect on sexual health in older British women. *Br J Obstet Gynaecol* 1997;104: 87–91
8. Basson R, Berman J, Burnett A, *et al.* Report of the International Consensus Development Conference on female sexual dysfunction: definition and classification. *J Urol* 2000;163: 889–93
9. Lauman EO, Gagnon JH, Michaci RT, Michaels S. Sexual dysfunction in the United States: prevalence and predictors. *J Am Med Assoc* 1999;281:537–42
10. Andrews WC. Approaches to taking a sexual history. In Bachmann GA, ed. Menopause and Female Sexuality. *J Womens Health Gend Based Med* 2000;9(S1):S25–S32
11. Butcher J. ABC of sexual health. Female sexual problems II: sexual pain and sexual fears [clinical review]. *Br Med J* 1999;318:110–12
12. Bachmann GA. Menopause and female sexuality. *J Womens Health Gend Based Med* 2000;9(S1); S1–S3

13. Graziottin A. The biological basis of female sexuality. *Int Clin Psychopharmacol* 1998;13(Suppl 6):S15–S22

14. Masters WH, Johnson VE, Kolodny RC. *Heterosexuality.* Glasgow: Harper Collins, 1994

15. Levin RJ. The mechanism of human female sexual arousal. *Ann Rev Sex Res* 1992;3:1–48

16. Levin RJ. Measuring the menopausal genital changes: a critical account of laboratory procedures past and for the future. In Graziottin A, ed. *Menopause and Sexuality, Menopause Review IV.* Paris: Ed. Eska, 1999;49–57

17. Sarrel PM. Sexuality and menopause. *Obstet Gynecol* 1990;75:26–30

18. Gruber CJ, Tschugguel W, Schneeberg C, Huber JC. Production and action of estrogens. *N Engl J Med* 2002;346:340–52

19. Graziottin A, Castoldi E, Montorsi F, *et al.* Vulvodynia: the challenge of 'unexplained' genital pain. *J Sex Marital Ther* 2001;27:567–76

20. Bergeron S, Binik YM, Khalife S, Pagidas K. Vulvar vestibulitis syndrome: a critical review. *Clin J Pain* 1997;13:27–42

21. Reid R. The management of genital condylomas, intraepithelial neoplasia and vulvodynia. *Obstet Gynecol Clin North Am* 1996;23:917–91

22. Heller DS, Randolph P, Young A, *et al.* The cutaneous vulvar clinic revisited: a 5-year experience of the Columbia Presbyterian Medical Center Cutaneous Vulvar Service. *Dermatology* 1997;195:26–9

23. Kent HL. Epidemiology of vaginitis. *Am J Obstet Gynecol* 1991;165:1168–76

24. Caillouette JC, Sharp CE, Zimmermann GJ, Roy S. Vaginal pH as a marker for bacterial pathogens and menopausal status. *Am J Obstet Gynecol* 1997; 176:1270–7

25. Hagedorn M, Buxmeyer B, Schmitt Y, Bauknecht T. Survey of lichen sclerosus in women and men. *Arch Gynecol Obstet* 2002;266:86–91

26. Tarcan T, Park K, Goldstein I, *et al.* A histomorphometric analysis of age related structural changes in human clitoral cavernosal tissue. *J Urol* 1999;161:940–4

27. Wesselmann U, Burnett AL, Heinberg LJ. The urogenital and rectal pain syndromes [review]. *Pain* 1997;73:269–94

28. Shafik A. Pudendal canal syndrome as a cause of vulvodynia and its treatment by pudendal nerve decompression. *Eur J Obstet Gynecol Reprod Biol* 1998;80:215–20

29. Graziottin A. Sexual function in women with gynecologic cancer: a review. *It J Gynecol Obstet* 2001;2:61–8

30. Graziottin A, Maraschiello T. Airon, Ed. *Farmaci e Sessualità.* Milan, 2002

31. Travell J, Simons D. *Myofascial Pain and Dysfunction: The Trigger Points Manual, Volume 1.* Baltimore: Williams & Wilkins, 1983

32. Thompson JM. Tension myalgia as a diagnosis at the Mayo Clinic and its relationship to fibrositis, fibromyalgia and myofascial pain syndrome. *Mayo Clin Proc* 1990;65:1237–48

33. De Lancey JO, Sampselle CM, Punch MR. Kegel dyspareunia: levator ani myalgia caused by overexertion. *Obstet Gynecol* 1993;82:658–9

34. O'Connell HE, Hutson JM, Anderson CR, Plenter RJ. Anatomical relationship between urethra and clitoris. *J Urol* 1998;159:1892–7

35. Bohm-Starke N, Hilliges M, Falconer C, Rylander E. Increased intraepithelial innervation in women with vulvar vestibulitis syndrome. *Gynecol Obstet Invest* 1998;46:256–60

36. Bohm-Starke N, Hilliges M, Falconer C, Rylander E. Neurochemical characterization of the vestibular nerves in women with vulvar vestibulitis syndrome. *Gynecol Obstet Invest* 1999; 48:270–5

37. Bohm Starke N, Hilliges M, Brodda-Jansen G, *et al.* Psychophysical evidence of nociceptor sensitization in vulvar vestibulitis syndrome. *Pain* 2001;94:177–83

38. Pukall CF, Binik YM, Khalifé S, *et al.* Vestibular tactile and pain threshold in women with vulvar vestibulitis. *Pain* 2002;96: 163–75

39. Graziottin A, Vincenti E. Anthalgic treatment of intractable pain due to vulvar vestibulitis syndrome: preliminary results with oral gabapentin and anethetic block of ganglion impar [abstract]. *Proceedings of the Congress of the International Society for the Study of Women's Sexual Health (ISSWSH)*, Vancouver, October 10–14, 2002;51

40. Bonica J. Definitions and taxonomy of pain. In Bonica J, ed. *The Management of Pain.* Philadelphia: Lea & Febiger, 1990;18–27

41. Russo CM, Brose WG. Chronic pain. *Annu Rev Med* 1998;49:123–33

42. Turner MLC, Marinoff SC. Pudendal neuralgia. *Am J Obstet Gynecol* 1991;165:1233–6

43. Robert R, Prat Pradal D, Labat JJ, *et al.* Anatomic basis of chronic perineal pain: role of the pudendal nerve. *Surg Radiol Anat* 1998; 20:93–8

44. Mulherin DM, Sheeran TP, Kumararatne DS, *et al.* Sjogren's syndrome in women presenting with chronic dyspareunia. *Br J Obstet Gynaecol* 1997;104:1019–23

45. Jamieson DJ, Steege JF. The association of sexual abuse with pelvic pain complaints in a primary care population. *Am J Obstet Gynecol* 1997;177: 1408–12

46. Basson R. The female sexual response: a different model. *J Sex Mar Ther* 2000;26:51–65

47. Dennerstein L, Lehert P, Burger H, *et al.* Menoapuse and sexual functioning. In Studd J, ed. *The Management of the Menopause: The*

Millennium Review. Lancaster: Parthenon Publishing, 2000;203–10

48. Fukaya T, Hoshiai H, Yajima A. Is pelvic endometriosis always associated with chronic pain? A retrospective study of 618 cases diagnosed by laparoscopy. *Am J Obstet Gynecol* 1993;169:719–22

49. Sweet RL, Gibbs RS. Pelvic inflammatory disease. In Sweet R, Gibbs RS, eds. *Infectious Disease of the Female Genital Tract (Part 1)*. Baltimore: Williams & Wilkins, 1985;53–77

50. Clulow C, ed. *Adult Attachment and Couple Psychotherapy*. Hove (UK): Brunner Routledge, 2001

51. Miller MV. *Intimate Terrorism: the Deterioration of The Erotic Life*. New York: Norton & Company, 1995

52. Meana M, Binik YM, Khalife S, Cohen D. Dyspareunia: sexual dysfunction or pain syndrome? *J Nerv Ment Dis* 1997;185:561–9

53. Meana M, Binik YM, Khalife S, Cohen D. Biopsychosocial profile of women with dyspareunia. *Obstet Gynecol* 1997;90:583–9

54. Bergeron S, Khalifé S, Pagidas K, et al. A randomized comparison of group cognitive–behavioral therapy, surface electromyographic biofeedback and vestibulectomy in the treatment of dyspareunia resulting from VVS. *Pain* 2001;91:297–306

55. Beard RW, Highman JH, Pearce S, Reginald PW. Diagnosis of pelvic varicosities in women with chronic pelvic pain. *Lancet* 1984;2:946–9

56. Rioux JE, Devlin MC, Gelfand MM, et al. 17-beta estradiol vaginal tablets versus conjugated equine estrogen vaginal cream to relieve menopausal atrophic vaginitis. *Menopause* 2000;7: 156–61

57. Miller KK. Androgen deficiency in women. *J Clin Endocrinol Metab* 2001;86:2395–401

58. Davis S. Androgen replacement in women: a commentary. *J Clin Endocrinol Metab* 1999;84: 1886–91

59. Sherwin BB, Gelfand MM, Brender W. Androgen enhances sexual motivation in females: a prospective, cross-over study of sex steroid administration in surgical menopause. *Psychosm Med* 1987;47:339–51

60. Madelska K, Cummings S. Tibolone for post-menopausal women: systematic review of randomized trials. *J Clin Endocrinol Metab* 2002; 87:16–23

61. Shifren JL, Glenn D, Braunstein MD, et al. Transdermal testosterone treatment in women with impaired sexual function after oophorectomy. *N Engl J Med* 2000;343:682–8

62. Meewusen IB, Samson MM, Duursma SA, Verhaar HJ. Muscle strength and tibolone: a randomized, double-blind, placebo-controlled trial. *Br J Obstet Gynaecol* 2002;109:77–84

63. Sippila ML, Taaffe D, Cheng S, et al. Effects of hormone replacement therapy and high impact physical exercice on skeletal muscle in post-menopausal women: a randomized, placebo controlled study. *Clin Sci* 2001;101:147–57

64. Schindler AE. Hormone replacement therapy (HRT) in women after genital cancer. *Maturitas* 2002;41(Suppl. 1):S105–11

65. Glazer HI, Rodke G, Sewncionis C, Hetz R, Young AW. Treatment on vulvar vestibulitis syndrome with electromyographic biofeedback of pelvic floor musculature. *J Reprod Med* 1995; 40:283–90

66. McKay E, Kaufman RH, Doctor U, et al. Treating vulvar vestibulitis with electromyographic feedback of pelvic floor musculature. *J Reprod Med* 2001;46:337–42

67. van der Velde J, Laan E, Everaerd W. Vaginismus, a component of a general defensive reaction. An investigation of pelvic floor muscle activity during exposure to emotion-inducing film excerpts in women with and without vaginismus. *Int Urogynecol J Pelvic Floor Dysfunct* 2001;12: 328–31

68. Graziottin A. VVS: clinical approach. Proceedings of the congress of the International Society for the Study of Women's Sexual Health (ISSWSH), Vancouver, October 10–14, 2002; 82–8

24

Menopause and the internet

H. Currie and G. Cumming

'We are drowning in information and starving in knowledge.'

Rutherford D Rodgers

Today, compared with previous generations, health professionals are faced with an increasingly well-informed public. Furthermore, we can expect there to be even more dramatic changes in the interaction between the public and the medical profession over the next decade[1]. It is inevitable that informed 'patients' will have a much greater say in the management of all aspects of their health. Management of the menopause is no exception.

Health information has traditionally been obtained from health care professionals, magazines, books, telephone help lines, radio and television. More recently information is being sought from the internet. In the USA there has been a rapid growth of home PC use with 51% of households having one or more computers[2]. In the UK, under the auspices of 'anytime, anywhere learning', Bill Gates is aiming to ensure that every pupil in the UK has their own laptop within 5 years.

One of the most profound differences between use of the internet and traditional sources of health information is interactivity.

'What I hear, I forget
What I see, I remember
What I do, I remember always'

Confucius, 551– 479 BC

Confucius' dictum some 2500 years ago, describing the importance of interaction to aid learning, is as relevant today as it was then. Modern cognitive psychologists suggest that learning is facilitated if information is presented in more than one form simultaneously, which is easily achieved with computer technology.

There are essentially three models describing the patient–doctor relationship and decision-making[3]:

(1) *Paternalistic model*: the patient passively acquiesces to professional authority by agreeing to the doctor's choice of treatment.

(2) *Informed model*: the doctor leads and the communication is one way. The doctor communicates to the patient information on all relevant treatment options and the patient then makes an informed choice.

(3) *Shared model*: there is a two way exchange of information whereby both doctor and patient reveal treatment options and then agree on the chosen option.

Both the 'informed' and the 'shared' models of doctor–patient relationship are in keeping with this shift in patient understanding of health-related matters. It is recognized that this improved knowledge and better understanding of illness enables (or empowers) patients to make informed choices. This may in turn lead to less anxiety and better compliance with treatment resulting ultimately in improved health outcomes[4].

The challenges for those of us working in the complex area of the menopause include finding effective methods to educate both the public and the health professional and to help them keep up to date with the latest research. The internet is an ideal medium with which to achieve these aims: it is interactive, dynamic and uses learner-centred teaching. However, the difference between information and knowledge must be stressed. Communicating this to the public is important if the spectre of the patient presenting a mass of material downloaded from the internet is to be avoided!

In this chapter, we will review use of the internet by both patients and health professionals seeking health related information with particular emphasis on the menopause.

HOW MUCH IS THE INTERNET USED FOR HEALTH INFORMATION?

A recent survey by the independent research company Datamonitor, questioning 4531 adults in Europe and in the US[5], showed that of those that had researched information on health in the preceding 12 months, 57% had used the internet. In the age range 18–54, 32–34% of adults used the internet for health information; in the age range 55–64 this was 27%; not surprisingly, in the older age range (> 65), a lower figure of 14% sought health information from the internet. Younger users frequently looked for information for older family members.

The most common health topics searched for online are currently: 'living a healthy lifestyle', 'women's health', 'allergies' and 'cancer'. The general health sites and sites run by governments or institutions are more popular than those run by pharmaceutical companies because non-pharmaceutical sites are perceived as being more objective.

A poll by the market research company Harris Interactive in 2001[6] concluded that there are almost 100 million 'cyberchondriacs'

(internet users who seek health information) in America, 48 million in Japan, 31 million in Germany and 14 million in France.

The 2001 Pew research study, from the Pew Internet and American Life Project surveying Americans about their use of the internet for health information, entitled *Online Health Care Revolution*[7], showed that 55% of the internet-user population turned to internet sources to seek health information and that about 5.5 million Americans seek health information online per day.

A more recent report from the Canadian Inter@ctive Reid Report[8], based on 1000 telephone interviews and 1000 online interviews in 2002, showed that more Canadians had 'surfed' for online health information than any other online activity; 66% of online Canadians had searched for health-related information online, an increase from 55% in 2000. Females were more likely to have visited an online health site than males: 76 versus 56%.

Health professionals are also increasingly accessing the internet according to a study reported by the American Medical Association[9]. This study suggested that around 78% of American physicians now use the internet and over two-thirds of them go online daily, each spending an increasing amount of time online. Almost half of physicians surveyed feel that the internet has had a major impact on the way they practice medicine. In the UK, almost all general practitioners now have computers in their consulting rooms and are connected to the NHSnet[10]. In UK hospitals, 75% of hospital doctors have PCs with email and web access[11].

It has been stated that the 21st century will be the age of the net-empowered medical end-user, with the development of systems that will allow end-users to direct more of their medical care[12]. In menopause management, the internet provides an exciting opportunity to make available vast resources of up-to-date information from a variety of experts. We, as health professionals, should encourage and guide our patients to use the internet increasingly and effectively when seeking menopause information.

MENOPAUSE AND THE INTERNET

WHY DO PATIENTS USE THE INTERNET FOR HEALTH INFORMATION?

Patients use the internet mostly for research rather than for interaction with health professionals or for medicinal purchases. The Pew research study group[7] showed that only 9% of health website surfers had communicated with a doctor online and only 10% had used the net to purchase either medicine or vitamins.

It appears that patients navigate the internet's health websites very effectively – the Pew research study[7] found that 92% of health seekers questioned said that they found what they were looking for online, and 88% said the information they had found improved the way they took care of their health. Furthermore, a survey by Health on the Net Foundation[13] showed that 72% of American and 73% of European patients found information from the internet helpful because they became more knowledgeable.

The internet is able to provide an extensive range and variety of resources. It is easily accessible, can be viewed anonymously and is available 24 hours/day, 7 days/week, 52 weeks/year. This anonymity and convenience is greatly appreciated by patients: in the Pew research study[7], 80% of health seekers stressed the importance of accessing health information anonymously and 93% appreciated the ability to obtain health information when it is convenient for them.

Studies have consistently shown that > 50% of British women desire more menopause information[14] and the same proportion of women obtain such information from sources other than healthcare professionals[15]. This advice might be conflicting, unhelpful and incorrect.

Sadly, conflicting advice is also prevalent within the health profession, especially with respect to the merits or otherwise of the use of hormone replacement therapy (HRT). Not only might patients receive conflicting advice, but the consultation with the health professional is often rushed due to pressure of time. Patients therefore are understandably accessing health information from the internet and using this as a second opinion.

Although HRT has now been available for approximately 60 years, there is still great uncertainty among the health profession and the public regarding both the benefits and the absolute and relative risks of therapy. The recommendations regarding menopause management are in a state of flux and text books are inevitably soon out of date. It is only with the flexibility and ease with which information can be updated on the internet that women can obtain the latest information available.

A report in the *British Medical Journal* in 2001[16] showed that an interactive multimedia decision aid on HRT in primary care reduced decisional conflict, and enabled patients to play a more active part in decision-making without increasing anxiety. Such systems available on the internet can play an important part in achieving informed patient choice at low cost.

Large numbers of websites have been developed by patients themselves. These websites enable women to interact with each other by allowing them to share experiences and offer mutual support. This sharing of patient experiences is a very valuable aspect of care, the importance of which may not be appreciated by health professionals[17].

Concern has been expressed that information from the internet could adversely affect the doctor–patient relationship. Many doctors have felt intimidated or threatened when patients have produced printouts from the internet (internet printout syndrome, IPS). In contrast, 40% of respondents in the US, France and Japan, and 30% in Germany said that they thought their internet visits could improve the relationship with their doctor[6].

Brown[18] sees IPS as a tangible move towards equality in access to information that should be applauded and not seen as a threat to the health professions. All good health websites should aim not to replace interaction with a physician, but rather should aim to enhance it.

WHY DO HEALTH PROFESSIONALS USE THE INTERNET?

The internet is used by health professionals to communicate with colleagues and patients, for continuing medical education (CME), research, and most of all, to seek clinical information.

Websites are becoming integral in providing patients with general information regarding their local practice and/or hospital. Some hospital websites have developed the facility for patients to submit a question which is then answered by a physician within 10 or 15 minutes[19]. However communication with patients via the internet for purpose of diagnosis and/or treatment is potentially fraught with difficulties, principally concerning privacy, security and limited clinical information (incomplete medical history) issues. Recent guidelines from the eRisk Working Group for Healthcare[20] state that physicians should only consult online if they have previously established a professional relationship with the patient.

When seeking clinical information, Medline (www.medlineplus.gov) is frequently accessed by medical practitioners. This is the largest database indexing the literature published in clinical journals. Produced by the US National Library of Medicine, Medline contains approximately 11 million records and indexes approximately 4500 different journal titles from 70 countries, with at least 70% of medline entries including abstracts.

Knowledge of the menopause among health professionals is acknowledged as being inadequate, with only 63% of general practitioners and 27% of practice nurses being satisfied with their knowledge[21]. Searching for clinical information using databases such as Medline is therefore particularly relevant and fundamental to understanding and managing the menopause.

The uncertainty and confusion that currently surrounds menopause management was particularly highlighted following the release of the results of the Women's Health Initiative (WHI) study[22] in July 2002. An already controversial interpretation of the data was confused by often inaccurate and hyped media attention. This confusion was partly resolved by the rapid dissemination of the actual report via the internet which allowed physicians to form their own opinions and inform their concerned patients accordingly. The authors' website, www.menopausematters.co.uk, was able to produce a considered response to the WHI results which was available on the web the day after the media release. The hit rate to this site then quadrupled, giving an indication as to the value of such sites in rapidly disseminating information.

TYPES OF HEALTH AND MENOPAUSE WEBSITES

Health websites can be categorized according to their origin, authorship and/or funding[23] and, for the purpose of this chapter, can be divided into general health and menopause specific. The large range of types of websites contributes to the vast resources available on the internet.

Detailed information about the menopause is usually found on dedicated menopause websites. In contrast, the larger general health websites tend to include a limited amount of information specific to the menopause but often act as a portal whereby the surfer can be directed, with links, to more in-depth recommended sites.

Websites can be aimed at patients and/or health professionals but even those designed for health professionals usually contain information appropriate for patients also.

General health websites

General health websites that contain, and direct to, menopause information include:

Those sponsored by Government and healthcare providers

www.nhsdirect.nhs.uk and www.healthfinder. gov, UK and US government funded respectively, aiming to direct patients to high quality information sources; www.nelh.nhs.uk, the National Electronic Library for Health, providing access to two evidence-based sources of information: the Cochrane Library and Clinical Evidence; and www.medlineplus.gov from the US, produced by the National Library of Medicine, aimed at both patients and health professionals.

Medical organisations and societies

www.rcog.org.uk, Royal College of Obstetricians and Gynaecologists; www.rcgp.org.uk, Royal College of General Practitioners; www.bmj.com, British Medical Journal; and www.ama-assn.org, American Medical Association.

Independent websites

These may generate income through advertising, sponsorship or registration fees, and include: www.doctors.net.uk, aimed at UK doctors with > 80 000 doctors registered; www.patient. co.uk, developed by NHS GPs, providing a gateway to good quality UK sources of health information mainly targeted at non-medical people but has also become a valuable reference source for health professionals; www.medscape. com; www.obgyn.net; and www.medicdirect. co.uk

On these general health sites, menopause information is often included either in the form of a specific section, often included in 'women's health', by production of relevant articles from literature search or by recommended links to specific menopause sites. www.medscape.com in particular features a very comprehensive women's health section. Registered health professionals can regularly receive relevant peer reviewed articles from leading medical journals and conferences. In addition, a regular CME programme is available and topics covered have included menopause and osteoporosis.

Menopause-specific websites

Menopause-specific websites include:

Menopause organisations and societies

www.the-bms.org, The British Menopause Society; www.emas.obgyn.net, European Menopause and Andropause Society; www.imsociety. org, International Menopause Society; www. menopause.org, North American Menopause Society; and www.menopause.org.au, The Australasian Menopause Society.

These sites provide definitive menopause information, regular updates, journal reviews and links to other relevant sites. They are mainly intended for use by health professionals but the North American Menopause Society in particular has a very informative section for consumers. Information from these societies can of course be obtained from their hardcopy journals but additional benefits offered by their websites include easily accessible information for patients, feedback facilities and links to other useful resources.

An example of a local menopause group website is the Yorkshire Menopause Group: www.yorkshiremenopause.co.uk, providing general menopause information, review of relevant medical journal articles and local information pertaining to meetings and local guidelines.

Commercial websites

These include websites developed by companies involved with HRT or alternative products, using their website to promote their products, often offering the facility for patients to purchase products online. Several companies, in contrast, have developed non-promotional educational sites. Examples include: www. menopausefacts.co.uk and www.hrtinfo.co.uk, both sites developed for patients and health professionals.

Independent websites

Suh websites may be funded by sponsorship or by selling advertising, and include the authors' website: www.menopausematters.co.uk, an independent, clinician led site providing information for women and health professionals on the menopause and treatment options, and the editor's website; www.studd.co.uk, providing comprehensive information for patients and health professionals on menopause, HRT, osteoporosis and premenstrual syndrome in particular.

Patient-led/support websites

These are a rapidly developing aspect of health care and are proving extremely popular with patients. In an unpublished survey from a feedback questionnaire on the menopausematters. co.uk website, 70% of respondents requested further development of the site in the form of a bulletin board allowing sharing of experiences. Some examples are: www.howdyneighbor.com/menopaus; www.geocities.com/menobeyond; www.power-surge.com, and www.minniepauz. com (a humorous yet very informative website).

FINDING ONLINE MENOPAUSE INFORMATION

Search engines (or search directories) are the usual means by which information is retrieved from the internet. An internet search engine, rather than directly accessing a specific website, was the method used to find information by 81% of health seekers in the Pew research study[7].

The search engines can be general, whereby information is retrieved from the internet as a whole, or they can be targeted more specifically to retrieve information from health websites only. General search engines are now acknowledged as being the main access points to the internet. Different search engines can produce different results for the same enquiry and their results often complement one another.

Search engines use different criteria for ranking websites. These include rating by hit-rate and by the number of inbound links to a site.

General search engines include: www.google. com; www.yahoo.com; www.lycos.com; www. altavista.com; and www.netscape.com.

When using general search engines for retrieving menopause information, vast numbers of websites are usually identified. Typing in precise terms for the search request will reduce the number of sites identified. In using www.google.com, for example, specifying 'menopause' for the search identifies approximately 1.22 million sites in 0.06 seconds! If however, 'menopause symptoms' are used for the search, 273 000 sites are identified, and if the search term is refined further to 'menopause symptoms + HRT', 52 000 sites are listed[24].

Search engines specific to health websites include: www.hon.ch, Health On the Net, one of the oldest health-focused directories; UK focused search sites include www.omni.ac.uk, Organising Medical Networked Information – a filtering tool providing a gateway to evaluated quality resources in health and medicine, containing information on > 4500 sites; www. doctors.net.uk; www.nhsdirect.nhs.uk; and www.patient.co.uk. US-based search sites include healthfinder.gov; medlineplus.gov; www.medscape.com; www.medmatrix.org; and www.mdconsult.com.

Each of these medical search sites will provide information on the menopause with useful links when 'menopause' is the search term asked for. Compared with general search engines, fewer websites are suggested, thus simplifying the process of browsing.

Other ways of being directed to relevant menopause websites include advertising, recommendation of a site by peer review, for example BMJ netlines (which has featured both the BMS and the menopausematters.co.uk websites), and links from other sites.

QUALITY OF HEALTH AND MENOPAUSE WEBSITES

The quality of health information available on the internet is extremely variable and much debate surrounds how quality on the web should be ensured and measured, or 'kite marked'. Many researchers, organizations and website developers are now exploring ways of helping people to find high-quality information on the internet.

The Pew research study showed that 86% of health surfers are concerned about getting health information from an unreliable source online, though 52% of users who had visited health sites thought that 'almost all' or 'most' health information on the internet is credible.

Little, if any, information is available examining quality of the menopause websites specifically, but the following considerations apply equally to menopause and general health websites.

Since 1996, many organizations have developed tools for rating health websites, but a paper published in the *British Medical Journal*[25] illustrates how underdeveloped this utility is at present. This study, examining instruments used to rate quality of health information, concluded that many incompletely developed rating instruments continue to appear on health websites even though the organisations that gave rise to those instruments no longer exist.

Nevertheless, kite-marking must become credible to enhance public and professional confidence in health websites. Tools used for rating the quality of health information on the internet were very clearly described by Wilson[26] and include the following.

Quality label – self applied

This is demonstrated by the display of a logo or symbol on the website. The presence of the label signifies that the website follows certain principles and the label can only be displayed after submission of a formal application and acceptance by the label provider. The oldest and best-known quality label is provided by the Health On the Net (HON) Foundation (www.hon.ch) and is used by more than 3000 websites. Principles of the HON code of conduct include: authority, complementarity, confidentiality, attribution, justifiability, transparency of authorship, transparency of sponsorship and honesty in advertising and editorial policy[27].

Some menopause websites including www.menopause.org and menopausematters.co.uk display the HON label.

Quality label – externally applied

This is the most advanced approach for quality rating and systems currently being developed. One such project is the European Union Project MedCERTAIN (MedPICS Certification and Rating of Trustworthy Health Information on the Net – www.medcertain.org), which aims to educate users and encourage information providers to label their services, while monitoring and evaluating these labels to prevent misuse. NHS Direct Online is also developing a star rating system[28].

Gateways or filters

Organisations that evaluate and then recommend health websites act as gateways or filters, directing consumers and health professionals to quality health websites. Examples include UK-based OMNI (www.omni.ac.uk), NHS Direct Online (www.nhsdirect.nhs.uk) and www.patient.co.uk, and US-based www.healthfinder.gov.

Inbound links

Endorsement of a website by linkage from another site is often seen as a marker of quality. Since the search engine www.google.com ranks websites in part by the number of inbound links to a site (reputation), high ranking in a Google search suggests good quality. Hernandez-Borges and colleagues found there to be a positive correlation between the number of inbound links to a health website and the likelihood of that site conforming to the quality criteria of the Health on the Net code[29].

Other factors by which users judge a website include ease of use, speed to download, layout and design, readability and inclusion or not of banner advertising. According to Eysenbach and Kohler[30], consumers may assess online health information in a different way than is assumed, and in fact consumers assess credibility of a site by primarily looking for the source and a professional design. Unpublished results from the menopausematters.co.uk website questionnaire showed that almost all respondents are confident with information on a health website if it is written by health professionals.

CONCLUSIONS

Management of the menopause in the third millennium must encompass the principles of the shared model of the doctor–patient relationship. The internet and e-health provides an unparalleled opportunity to:

Educate women and health professionals;
Empower; and
Enable women everywhere to take a much more active part in the management of their menopause. Discussion with their health professional then becomes a process of a dialogue rather than a monologue.

'Hope in life comes from the interconnections among all the people in the world. We believe that if we all work for what we think individually is good, then we as a whole will achieve more power, more understanding, more harmony as we continue through the journey. . . '

Tim Berners-Lee, Weaving the Web – The Past, Present and Future of the World Wide Web by its Inventor[31].

References

1. Eaton L. A theme issue for medics and an increasingly health informed public. *Br Med J* 2002;325:984
2. Home Computers and internet use in the United States: August 2000. US Department of Commerce Economics and Statistics Administration, US Census Bureau. Available from: *http://www.census.gov* (accessed 25 February 2003)
3. Charles C, Whelan T, Gafini A. What do we mean by partnership in making decisions about treatment? *Br Med J* 1999;319:780–2
4. Kenny T, Wilson RG, Purves IN, *et al.* A PIL for every ill? Patient information leaflets (PILs): a review of past, present and future use. *Fam Pract* 1998;15:471–9
5. Who is looking for health information online? A Segmentation Analysis of the Online Consumer. Available from: *http://www.datamonitor.com/~899 25589d63946318c8dad77113b23fb~/technology/reports/product_summary.asp?pid=BFHC0470* (accessed 25 February 2003)
6. Harris Poll 2001. Available from: *http://www.harrisinteractive.com/harris_poll/index.asp?PID=229* (accessed 25 February 2003)
7. Fox S, Lee R. The online healthcare revolution: how the web helps Americans take better care of themselves. The Pew Internet and American Life Project, Washington, DC, 2000. Available from: *http://www.pewinternet.org/reports/toc.asp?Report=26* (accessed 25 February 2003)
8. Ipsos-Reid. Searching for online health information is the number one online activity in Canada. Ipsos-Reid's Canadian Inter@ctive Reid Report, 2002. Available from: *http://www.ipsos-reid.com/media/dsp_displaypr_us.cfm?id_to_view=1696* (accessed 25 February 2003)
9. American Medical Association. AMA study: physicians' use of Internet steadily rising, 2002. Release available from: *http://www.ama-assn.org/ama/pub/article/1616-6473.html* (accessed 25 February 2003)
10. NHS Information Authority. NHS connect programme. Birmingham: NHSIA, 2002. Available from: *http://www.nhsia.nhs.uk/nhsnet/pages/connecting/nhsconnect* (accessed 25 February 2003)
11. Equal waiting. Michael Cross. The Guardian, Thursday 28th November 2002
12. Ferguson T. From patients to end users. *Br Med J* 2002;324:555–6
13. Health on the Net Foundation. Evolution of internet use for health purposes – Feb/Mar 2001. Available from: *http://www.hon.ch/Survey/Feb/ Mar2001/survey.html* (accessed 25 February 2003)
14. Hope S, Wager E, Rees M. Survey of British women's views on the menopause and HRT. *J Br Men Soc* 1998;4:33–6
15. Hope S, Rees M. Why do British women start and stop hormone replacement therapy? *J Br Men Soc* 1995;1:26–8

16. Murray E, Davis H, SeeTai S, *et al.* Randomised controlled trial of an interactive multimedia decision aid on hormone replacement therapy in primary care. *Br Med J* 2001;323:490–3

17. Ferguson T. Online patient-helpers and physicians working together: a new partnership for high quality healthcare. *Br Med J* 2000; 321:1129–32

18. Brown H. View from the front line–internet printout syndrome (IPS). He@lth Information on the Internet, 2000. Available from: *http://www.wellcome.ac.uk/en/images/hiotil3_pdf_2260.pdf* (accessed 25 February 2003)

19. On-line cancer treatment forums. Available from: *http://www.meds.com/mol/forums.html* (accessed 25 February 2003)

20. New guidelines remove risk from doctor–patient email. Available from: *http://www.medem.com/corporate/xl_corporate_medeminthenews_detail.cfm?Extranet PressNewsKey=135* (accessed 25 February 2003)

21. Roberts P-J, Sibbald B. Menopause healthcare provision: the views of women, general practitioners and practice nurses. *J Br Men Soc* 2000;6:154–8

22. Writing Group for the Women's Health Initiative investigators. Risks and benefits of estrogen plus progestin in healthy postmenopausal women. Principal results for the Women's Health Initiative randomized controlled trial. *J Am Med Assoc* 2002;288:321–33

23. Brown H. *Information for Patients. Medicine and the Internet, Third Edition.* Oxford: Oxford University Press, 2002;169–77

24. Google search. *http://www.google.com/search* (accessed 26 February 2003)

25. Gagliardi A, Jadad A. Examination of instruments used to rate quality of health information on the internet: chronicle of a voyage with an unclear destination. *Br Med J* 2002;324:569–72

26. Wilson P. How to find the good and avoid the bad or ugly: a short guide to tools for rating quality of health information on the internet. *Br Med J* 2002;324:598–600

27. Health on the Net Foundation. HON code of conduct (HONcode) for medical and health web sites. Available from: *http://www.hon.ch/HONcode?Conduct.html* (accessed 25 February 2003)

28. Eaton L. NHS Direct Online explores partnerships with other health organisations. *Br Med J* 2002;324:568

29. Hernandez Borges AA, Macias Cervi P, Torres Alvorez de Arcaya ML, *et al.* Rate of compliance with the HON code of conduct versus number of inbound links as quality markers of pediatric web sites. Proceedings of the 6th World Congress on the Internet in Medicine, Udine, Italy, Nov 29–Dec 2, 2001

30. Eysenbach G, Kohler C. How do consumers search for and appraise health information on the world wide web? Qualitative study using focus groups, usability tests, and in-depth interviews. *Br Med J* 2002;324:573–6

31. Berners-Lee T. Weaving the Web: The Past, Present and Future of the World Wide Web by Its Inventor. New York: Texere, 1999:227

25

Nutrition and the menopause

S. Palacios and C. Rueda

INTRODUCTION

The menopause is a stage in a woman's life characterized by a series of hormonal changes and clinical alterations, reflecting a decline in ovarian function. The hormonal deprivation which this implies sets off various events related to the normal aging process, putting women into a framework whereby there is a greater risk of suffering certain diseases. For this reason, medicine has been seeking to offer a better quality of life to the older woman, and, as a result, has advanced in its knowledge of diseases and problems arising from hypoestrogenism, focusing attention on hormone replacement therapy (HRT) and alternative treatments. Without doubt, this line of research has been the mainstay of current knowledge regarding the menopause. However, it is fundamental to know, in depth, important aspects of a woman's health such as her life-style and especially her diet.

A good, healthy diet, which is maintained throughout life and especially during certain stages such as the menopause, will help prevent the occurrence of various diseases. Because the older population is increasing in number, the normal aging process and its impact on metabolic and nutritional functions should be made known. Understanding the metabolic changes occurring in this stage of life is the first step towards improved knowledge of nutritional requirements that form part of a normal diet for the older woman. In addition, the majority of diseases presenting during the menopause stem from a metabolic alteration which could be prevented by a healthy diet.

The concept of a healthy diet goes beyond the importance of avoiding an excessive consumption of fats and carbohydrates. The benefits of calcium, fiber, soya, essential fatty acids and alcohol in small doses in preventing many health problems mean that there is a need to know and understand their actions, giving as much, if not more, importance to these nutrients as to any medicaments. A balanced diet forms part of a life-style that a woman should follow in the search for a better quality of life.

METABOLIC CHANGES IN THE POSTMENOPAUSAL WOMAN

Energy balance

The diminished metabolic activity that occurs in the postmenopausal woman is a consequence of the natural aging process, and therefore a risk factor in terms of health problems often experienced at this stage of life.

The principal cause of death in the Western woman is cardiovascular disease. Hyperlipidemia, hypertension and obesity are the most important factors related to this disease, and should form the basis from which to fight against its occurrence[1]. A healthy, balanced diet should be the principal goal, and, to achieve this, it is very important to control weight. The loss of muscular mass and increased redistribution of peripheral fat in women have the immediate consequence of a drop in estrogen production. This results in a greater prevalence of overweight women than men in the age group 45–55 years, and consequently the risk of obesity in women of this age is also greater. Obesity is the manifestation of a dysfunction of the body-weight control system which impedes adjustment of the fatty masses reserve to its optimum size[2,3]. The problem lies in an imbalance of control between energy ingested and that consumed in metabolic processes[4,5]. The basal energetic requirements diminish by 2% per decade during adult life. If this is not compensated, this slight drop in energy requirement could lead to an increase of 1–1.5 kg in weight per year, i.e. 10–15 kg each decade[3].

Therefore, a special effort should be made to maintain an adequate energy balance; this is achieved by a healthy diet and regular physical exercise, helping to avoid excess weight which is a main risk factor for many health problems.

Metabolism of calcium

Plasma calcium levels depend on the balance between calcium ingested and bone resorption, intestinal absorption and tubular renal resorption on the one hand, and calcium loss in bone formation on the other. After the menopause, and especially from the age of 60 onwards, there is a major deterioration of the balance of calcium associated with the following factors[3]:

(1) Hypercalciuria;

(2) Diminished intestinal calcium absorption;

(3) Decrease in 1,25-dihydroxy-vitamin D;

(4) Diminished ingestion of calcium.

The alteration in the metabolism of calcium is perhaps the main risk factor which can be corrected to prevent osteoporosis in the menopause. To achieve this, it is most important to have a diet that provides the level of calcium necessary to balance the ingestion and loss of this mineral. Foods rich in calcium are the best source of intake, because they contain a high amount of elemental calcium, engender a high degree of absorption and have a relatively low cost compared with the total nutritional value[3,6].

ROLE OF CORRECT DIET IN PREVENTION OF DISEASE

Cardiovascular disease

Taking into account the change in energy metabolism that occurs in the postmenopause, and knowing that cardiovascular disease is a multifactorial problem, a knowledge of nutritional aspects related to this disease is the first step in medical management in terms of primary and secondary prevention. Apart from diet, both physical exercise and healthy life-style are the axes upon which prevention of cardiovascular disease should turn. Changes in life-style recommended by the National Cholesterol Education Programme (NCEP) in the USA[7], to prevent coronary disease, are focused on three basic points:

(1) Reduce daily intake of saturated fats (< 7% of total calories) and cholesterol (< 200 mg/day);

(2) Reduce weight;

(3) Increase physical activity.

Among the foods closely related to the incidence of cardiovascular disease, fats seem to occupy the most important place and especially when they are associated with hyperlipidemia. The effect of ingested fat on the cardiovascular system depends not only on the quantity but also on the type and degree of saturation, in such a way that saturated fats and cholesterol favor cardiovascular disorders and polyunsaturates help to prevent these disorders.

The relationship between polyunsaturated fatty acids and saturated fats can be expressed as an index (P/S) of the hyperlipidemic capacity of fats; this indicates that those fats with a P/S index higher or equal to 0.5 are hypercholesterolemic, i.e., 1 g of saturated fat has a hyperlipidemic power double that of 1 g of polyunsaturated fat[3].

Due to the metabolic changes that occur with hypoestrogenism and that determine a risk in terms of altered levels of lipoproteins in the menopause, a diet low in fats should be a general guideline for all women who reach this stage in life. Dietary recommendations foused on reducing low-density lipoprotein (LDL), established by the NCEP[7], are the following:

Saturated fats   Recommended intake: less than 7% of total calories.

Polyunsaturated fats   Recommended intake: up to 10% of total calories.

Monounsaturated fats   Recommended intake: up to 20% of total calories.

Total fats   Recommended intake; Between 25 and 35% of total calories.

Carbohydrates   Recommended intake: 50–60% of total calories. Carbohydrates should be derived from cereals, especially wholemeal, fruits and vegetables.

Fibre   Recommended intake: 20–30 g/day.

Proteins   Recommended intake: Approximately 15% of total calories.

Cholesterol   Recommended intake: less than 200 mg/day.

The Spanish Society for the Study of Obesity (SEEDO), in agreement with nutritional guidelines directed at preventing cardiovascular disease, has designed several diet models, which include not only recommended foods but also foods not recommended in a routine diet (Table 1).

Osteoporosis

During the menopause a series of metabolic changes in calcium are produced, which could finally lead to a negative balance of calcium, bone loss and osteoporosis. All women in this stage of life, independent of the risk factors they may have for this disease, should follow a life-style and diet focused on preventing bone loss and fractures[3,6]. Calcium requirements increase after the age of 50 and particularly in the postmenopausal woman, owing mainly to diminished intestinal absorption of this mineral and the kidneys' weakened ability to conserve it. Both of these effects are a response to the decreased levels of circulating estrogens[8].

The daily intake of calcium in the diet of peri- and postmenopausal women, recommended by the US National Institutes of Health, is based on the total content of this mineral in all foods. To achieve maximum calcium absorption in the diet, not only should food that contains elemental calcium (such as dairy products and their by-products) be taken into account, but also the food in a diet that could inhibit calcium absorption, such as that which contains oxalic acid (spinach) or some cereals rich in fiber (wheat bran). The primary source of calcium should be food rich in this mineral, because of the greater intestinal absorption which these engender. The minimum dietary requirement of this mineral is 1200 mg daily. Calcium supplements and fortified food products could be an alternative for those women who are unable to achieve the basal requirements in their normal diet[6,8].

Vitamin D (calciferol) is a liposoluble vitamin whose fundamental physiological role is to assure the plasmatic levels of calcium and phosphates necessary to achieve favorable conditions for mineralization of bones, as well as maintaining the homeostasis of the plasmatic concentration of calcium. The principal source of vitamin D is ultraviolet rays from solar light. Adequate exposure to sunlight can avoid vitamin D deficiency. This vitamin is also found in food, especially fish liver oil, animal fats, egg yolks or supplementary foods. The recommended daily intake of this vitamin is 400 IU/day for women between 50 and 70 years of age and 600 IU/day for women older than 70. Those women who have little exposure to sunlight should take 800 IU daily[6].

It is quite clear that calcium can reduce bone mineral loss, especially during the first 5 years after the menopause, and it also reduces fractures, above all in the older woman. However, calcium alone or together with vitamin D is not as effective a therapy as HRT, selective estrogen receptor modulators (SERMs) or

Table 1 Dietary recommendations in the prevention of arteriosclerosis. Adapted with permission from Astorga R, Bellido D, Campillo JE, *et al.* Consenso SEEDO (Sociedad Española para el estudio de la Obesidad) 2000 para la evaluación del sobrepeso y la obesidad y el establecimiento de criterios de intervención terapéutica. *Med Cclin* 2000;115:587–97[5]

Permitted*	In moderation*	Not recommended*
First course		
Vegetables, root vegetables, legumes, Italian pasta, cereals, bread, potato	pasta made with egg, olives, avocado, cold pasta	packet or tinned soups, potato chips, pizza
Dairy products/eggs		
Milk (skimmed), fat-free youghurt, low-fat cheese, egg white	milk with added vegetable fat, whole egg, cottage cheese	full-fat milk or yoghurt, cream cheese, smoked cheese, cheese spreads
Meat		
Chicken, turkey, rabbit, veal hamburger, cold meats such as turkey	beef, pork, lamb, cured ham	duck or goose, paté, cold meats, ham, sausage, salami
Fish		
White, blue fish, tinned, fresh or smoked	tinned in oil, salted cod, seafood	fish-roe
Oils and fats		
Olive, sunflower, corn, soya[†], mayonnaise, made from skimmed milk	margarine, peanut butter, mayonnaise made with egg	butter, lard, coconut oil
Desserts		
Fruit, fruit juices, plums, currants, sultanas, dates, flans (no eggs), water ices	nuts, jam, honey, tinned fruit in syrup, toffees, sweets, nougat	chocolate, cakes, pastries[‡], ice-creams, egg flan, pancakes[‡]
Drinks		
Mineral water, soda water, soft drinks (diet), tea, infusions, wine or beer (once a day)	soft drinks with sugar	Liquors

*Permitted: every day, in moderation: two or three times/week, not recommended: exceptionally; [†]not more than 40 ml/day; [‡]if vegetable oil is used in the preparation, these can be consumed in moderation

bisphosphonates in the treatment of osteoporosis. Nevertheless, calcium and vitamin D are essential components when treating this disease in combination with all antiresorptive agents.[6,8]

Cancer

In women, cancers with the highest death rates are those of the breast, colon–rectum and lung[3]. Many of the risk factors related to carcinogenesis are associated in some way with nutritional aspects. In the same way as with all diseases of multifactorial origin, cancer is susceptible to prevention through changes in life-style and diet. In the light of today's evidence, the prevention of colorectal cancer is supported by studies in animals and intervention trials which have demonstrated the protective role of fiber in the incidence of this type of cancer. However, the magnitude of reduction in the risk of cancer, in relation to a diet rich in fiber has not yet been defined. Apparently, not only is food rich in fiber in the diet important, but also the length of time of this habit. Epidemiological studies suggest that immigrant populations to countries with 'industrial diets' experience a delay in the appearance of colon cancer of 10–20 years. Because the incidence of this disease clearly increases with age, with its higest peak after the age of 60, a fiber-rich diet as a protective measure againt this type of cancer should be initiated a minimum of 20 years before reaching this peak[9]. The majority of intervention trials have demonstrated a protective effect against colon cancer of a fiber-rich diet, 3–4 times greater than that of a diet with the average consumption of fiber of the North American population (11.1 g/day). This fiber could come from vegetables, fruits, cereals and legumes[9]. Apart from fiber intake, other factors should be considered, such as life-style, to prevent this disease. These include decreasing consumption of fats (total, animal and saturated fats) and red meat, reducing obesity, and eliminating consumption of alcohol and tobacco[9].

Regarding breast cancer, a higher prevalence can be observed in industrialized countries, with the exception of Japan[3]. If the diet in Oriental countries influences the lesser incidence of breast cancer, there are still no conlusive data pointing towards effective prevention with soya and its by-products, soya being the food on which these cultures base their diets. However, it has been observed that obesity, above all after the menopause, is a risk factor for breast cancer, probably because of the higher production of estrone in fatty tissue. This indicates, indirectly, that a diet focused on reducing obesity, together with a healthy life-style, might be the correct behavior for prevention of this disease during the menopause[3,4].

NUTRITIONAL SUPPLEMENTS

Beyond the possible benefits that food supplements can bring, it is important to take into account that balanced diet at any age is a key factor in obtaining a healthy life-style. This concept is still valid during the menopause, given that all women are exposed to health risks at this stage in their lives. Nevertheless, more and more data show an interesting profile in terms of prevention of certain health problems; including various dietary supplements such as soya, omega-3 fatty acids and alcohol in small doses, among others. In the future, objective data will be available about the nutritional value of these supplements and diet for the postmenopausal woman.

Isoflavones

The effects of isoflavones have been studied in many clinical trials, not only in animals but also in humans. The studies with the most rigorous methodologies have found some benefits of these components derived from soya for the postmenopausal woman. Difficulties in obtaining conclusive data have arisen because of variations especially in the populations studied, the soya products used and, above all, the durations of exposure to these[10].

Based on the effects of isoflavones on the climacteric symptoms studied, and on the prevention of diseases seen in the postmenopause, the favorable action of these components on the lipid profile is the most important epidemiologic evidence. Some isoflavone supplements have been shown to be effective by improving levels of high-density lipoprotein (HDL), as well as levels of LDL and total cholesterol and arterial compliance. In October 1999, the Food and Drug Administration (FDA) approved the daily intake of soya protein (25 g) as a dietary complement in low-saturated-fat and low-cholesterol diets, as an element that reduces risks of coronary disease[10–12].

As part of a healthy diet, consumption of soya and its by-products is recommended, together with foods originating from plants, fiber, antioxidants and a low intake of saturated fats and cholesterol. Nevertheless, it is too soon to make specific recommendations about the role of a diet rich in isoflavones for the prevention of chronic diseases. Based on results from various studies and a consensus opinion[10], the dietary recommendations for isoflavones are the following:

(1) The optimum reduction of cholesterol requires approximately 50 mg daily of

isoflavones; its equivalent corresponds approximately to 25 g daily of soya protein. This in turn is in line with the recommendation made by the FDA. Some evidence indicates that daily consumption of 40–80 mg of isoflavones is necessary to obtain the effects on arterial compliance, as the minimum for antioxidant effects is 10 mg daily. To date, there are no solid recommendations regarding coronary disease prevention.

(2) A limited number of studies recommend a minimun of 50 mg daily of isoflavones to obtain benefit for bone mass. However, as in the above-mentioned case of coronary disease, there are no conclusive data relating to prevention of osteoporosis.

(3) Various studies recommending an intake of isoflavones to benefit vasomotor symptoms in the menopause suggest 40–80 mg daily[10].

n-3 fatty acids

With aging there is an increase in the quantity of total fat in the organism which could lead to obesity, associating this with the development of many chronic diseases such as arterial hypertension, diabetes, cardiovascular disease, altered biliary tract, etc. Fat is the component that contributes the most calories to a diet, and this contribution plays an important role[3].

Among fats consumed in a diet, monounsaturates contain the fewest total calories, followed by polyunsaturates and saturates; the replacement of saturated fats by monounsaturated and polyunsaturated fats is a way to reduce the risk of cardiovascular disease. However, diets with a high content of polyunsaturated fats could increase LDL susceptibility to oxidation, potentially contributing to the pathology of arteriosclerosis[13].

Supplements of fish oil, whose principal components are n-3 fatty acids (eicosapentaenoic acid, EPA and docosahexaenoic acid, DHA), have been studied independently and compared with other polyunsaturated fatty acids in terms of their role as cardiovascular protectors.

Studies carried out to date, without being conclusive, have compared polyunsaturated fatty acids with EPA and DHA, showing that the latter two do not increase the oxidization of LDL, exercising in this manner a protective action on atheromatosis[13]. On the other hand, the effects of the n-3 fatty acids in postmenopausal women have been studied, with and without HRT, where their actions have had a favorable influence on cardiovascular risk factors, especially in the reduction of concentrations of triacyl glycerol and the ratio triacylglycerol/HDL, in both women using HRT and those who did not receive HRT[14]. In addition, it has been possible to evaluate the effects of fatty acids in fish oil, as part of diets used in the treatment of dyslipidemia, and also their effects on insulin sensitivity, with improvements in these parameters when n-3 fats were added to the diet compared with when they were not present[15].

Alcohol

Alcohol cannot be considered as part of the list of nutritional supplements in a healthy diet. However, the consumption of alcohol in low doses is a recommendation in many diet plans, due to its preventive function in relation to cardiovascular disease[3,5]. Moreover, the moderate ingestion of alcohol has been seen to improve insulin sensitivity in patients who are not diabetic. Results noted during clinical trials have demonstrated that the consumption of 30 g daily of ethanol improves response to insulin by 7%, at the same time reducing triglyceride concentration by 10%[16]). This function could be beneficial in obtaining an adequate metabolic profile in the postmenopausal woman.

Given that alcohol is toxic for the liver, recommended daily intake should be no more than 40 g of ethanol per day (two glasses). In women, it is advisable to consume less, as they are more susceptible to the toxic effect of alcohol[5,16]. To obtain the content in grams of pure ethanol, the following formula should be applied: grams of ethanol = ml × 'degrees' × 0.8/100, where 'degrees' refers to the alcoholic grading of the drink. For example, 200 ml of wine of 11%, grams of ethanol = $200 \times$ '11' $\times 0.8/100 = 17.6$ g.

RECOMMENDATIONS IN NUTRITION

The objective of nutritional recommendations is to achieve a balanced diet that allows an adequate supply of calcium to be maintained, the correct weight, and avoidance of diseases related to incorrect diet such as an increase in cholesterol or triglycerides, or arterial pressure, among others. The recommended intakes of the various food groups should be in the following proportions:

Fats: Of total energy ingested, fats represent 30–35%, distributed as one-third in the form of animal fat and two thirds vegetable.

Carbohydrates: Also, 50–60% of calories consumed should be supplied in the form of carbohydrates. Total intake in the menopausal woman should be about 1700 kcal/day. These recomendations can vary substantially in relation to physical activity[5].

Table 2 indicates a model diet, which includes the various food groups, and their proportions, in a nutritional guideline for women after the menopause.

CONCLUSIONS

To maintain good health, women during the menopause should aim for an adequate life-style and habits, fundamentally that of achieving a balanced diet. To reach this goal, the healthy diet should consist of dairy products, fruit, vegetables, whole-grain cereals, fish, chicken, fiber and low consumption of fats, especially saturated. Results obtained in clinical trials with a high standard of evidence suggest that nutritional components of a healthy diet can influence the prevention of diseases that are most frequent in the postmenopausal woman, such as osteoporosis, cardiovascular disease and cancer of the colon.

Table 2 Nutritional recommendations. Data from reference 5

Food group	Recommendations
Cereal and by-products (bread, rice or pasta)	consume daily; provide carbohydrates
Vegetables, root vegetables, fruit and soya	five or seven portions daily
Milk and by-products	four daily portions
Legumes (chick peas, lentils, beans)	two portions per week
Eggs	no more than three per week
Fish, chicken and lean meat	three to five portions of fish per week, four of chicken (preferably without skin) and three of lean meat
Oil	olive oil is highly recommended: in overweight women, consume in moderation
Sweets	owing to their high contents of animal fat and simple sugar, restricted intake is recommended: once or twice per week
Alcohol	no more than 30 g daily of ethanol (two glasses of wine or beer)

References

1. *Nutritional strategies efficacious in the prevention or treatment of hypertension.* Nutrition Screening Initiative, 1998. Available at: http://www.guideline.gov

2. Beaton GH. Criteria of an adequate diet. In Shils ME, Young UR, eds *Modern Nutrition in Health and Disease,* 7th edn. Philadelphia: Cea and Febinger, 1988:649–65

3. Palacios N. Alimentación y nutrición en la mujer postmenopáusica Climaterio y Menopausia. In Palacios S, ed. *Climaterio y Menopausia.* Mipral, 1993:294–306

4. *AACE/ACE position statement on the prevention, diagnosis and treatment of obesity.* American Association of Clinical Endocrinologists, Clinical Guidelines. 1998. Available at http://www.guideline.gov

5. Astorga R, Bellido D, Campillo JE, *et al.* Consenso SEEDO (Sociedad Española para el estudio de la Obesidad) 2000 para la evaluación del sobrepeso y la obesidad y el establecimiento de criterios de intervención terapéutica. *Med Clin* 2000;115:587–97

6. The North American Menopause Society. Management of postmenopausal osteoporosis. *Menopause* 2002;9:84–101

7. *Third report of the National Cholesterol Education Program (NCEP) Expert Panel on Detection, Evaluation, and Treatment of High Blood Cholesterol in Adults (Adult Treatment Panel III).* Department of Health and Human Services, Public Health Service, National Institutes of Health, National Heart, Lung and Blood Institute, 2001. Available at: http://www.guideline.gov

8. The North American Menopause Society. The role of calcium in peri- and postmenopausal women: consensus opinion of The North American Menopause Society. *Menopause* 2001; 8:84–95

9. American Gastroenterological Association. Medical position statement: impact of dietary fiber on colon cancer ocurrence. *Gastroenterology* 2000;118:1233–4

10. The North American Menopause Society. The role of isoflavones in menopausal health: consensus opinion of The North American Menopause Society. *Menopause* 2000;7:215–29

11. Goodman-Gruen D, Silverstein D. Usual dietary isoflavone intake is associated with cardiovascular disease risk factors in postmenopausal women. *J Nutr* 2001;131:1202–6

12. Squadrito F, Aaltavilla D, Morabito N, *et al.* The effect of the phytoestrogen genistein on plasma nitric oxide concentrations, endothelin-1 levels and endothelium dependent vasodilation in postmenopausal women. *Artherosclerosis* 2002; 163:339–47

13. Higdon JV, Du SH, Lee YS, Wu T, Wander RC. Supplementation of postmenopausal women with fish oil does not increase overall oxidation of LDL *ex vivo* compared to dietary oils rich in oleate and linoleate. *J Lipid Res* 2001;42:407–18

14. Stark KD, Park EJ, Maines VA, Holub BJ. Effect of a fish-oil concentrate on serum lipids in postmenopausal women receiving and not receiving hormone replacement therapy in placebo-controlled, double-blind trial. *Am J Clin Nutr* 2000;72:389–94

15. Mori TA, Bao DQ, Burke V, *et al.* Dietary fish as a major component of a weight-loss diet: effect on serum lipids, glucose, and insulin metabolism in overweight hypertensive subjects. *Am J Clin Nutr* 1999;70: 817–25

16. Davies MJ, Baer DJ, Judd JT, *et al.* Effects of moderate alcohol intake on fasting insulin and glucose concentrations and insulin sensitivity in postmenopausal women: a randomized controlled trial. *J Am Med Assoc* 2002;287:2559–62

26

Alternative therapies for postmenopausal women

L. Speroff

INTRODUCTION

It was surprising news in 1998 when it was reported that 42% of adults had used some alternative therapy[1,2]. About 60% – $12 of $21 billion – spent on such therapies in the US in 1997 was in the form of cash payments. In 1997, 18.4% of prescription users also took herbal remedies and/or high dose vitamins; less than 40% of patients disclosed this use to physicians[1,2]. In 1998, those numbers were astounding, but today, our own awareness of what is happening makes these numbers less surprising. This is now a worldwide phenomenon. The growth of sales has slowed, but overall sales remain at a high level. Unfortunately, most studies of alternative therapy treatments are of short duration, and safety data on long-term use are lacking.

Why are herbs and botanicals not regulated? The promotion of many of these treatments relies on a network of alternative providers, authors, and compounding pharmacies. In the US, the Dietary Supplement Health and Education Act of 1994 deregulated the industry by classifying dietary supplements as neither foods nor drugs. Thus, manufacturers of dietary supplements are not required to demonstrate that they are safe or effective.

Besides a lack of regulation, there are many other problems associated with herbs and botanicals. The products vary in the amount and purity of active ingredients. A famous study performed by *Consumer Reports*[3] indicated that the actual content of commercial preparations varied from 5 to 140% of the labeled amounts. There are no long-term data regarding health consequences. And very importantly, there is enormous variation in the plants themselves because of genetic, harvest year, and processing differences, and in individual metabolism of the products.

PHYTOESTROGENS

'Phytoestrogens' is a descriptive term applied to non-steroidal compounds that have estrogenic activity or are metabolized into compounds with estrogen activity. Phytoestrogens are classified into three groups: isoflavones, lignans, and coumestans[4,5] (Table 1). They are present in about 300 plants, especially legumes, and bind to the estrogen receptor. Soybeans – a rich source of phytoestrogens – contain isoflavones, the most common form of phytoestrogens, mainly genistein and daidzein, and a little glycitin. These isoflavones are concentrated in the portion of the seedlings just below the seed leaves with some in the first layer of leaves.

Isoflavones exist in plants bound as glycoside conjugates attached at the 3 position, called glycones. The carbohydrate component requires gut bacteria to remove the sugar moiety to produce active compounds, the aglycones. Individual variability in gastrointestinal microflora and absorption rates influences the

Table 1 Phytoestrogens

1. Isoflavones (genistein, daidzein, glycitin)
   Soybeans, lentils, chickpeas (garbanzo beans)
2. Lignans
   Flaxseed, cereals, vegetables, fruits
3. Coumestans
   Sunflower seeds, bean sprouts

bioavailability of isoflavones. Bochanin and formononetin are methylated precursors that are metabolized to genistein and daidzein. Red clover and lentils contain significant amounts of these precursors. The isoflavones are in the active, deconjugated forms in fermented soy foods like miso and tempeh. The concentration of isoflavones in tofu is highly variable.

The phytoestrogens are characterized by mixed estrogenic and antiestrogenic actions, depending on the target tissue. Variations in activity may also be due to the fact that the soy phytoestrogens have a greater affinity for the estrogen receptor-β compared with estrogen receptor-α, although the affinity for the beta receptor is still only 35% that of estradiol[6]. Despite a low affinity for the α receptor, circulating levels many times that of steroidal estrogens produce the potential for biologic activity.

You can eat soybeans every day and never see a bean (Table 2). Soybeans are defatted to produce soy flour. Soy flour is then prepared to remove the carbohydrates. Ninety-five per cent of soy flour is toasted and used as animal feed. Alcohol washing is used to get a taste-free product, but alcohol extraction removes the phytoestrogens[8]. SUPRO, known as 'isolated soy protein', from Protein Technologies International, the major supplier for commercial products and research, is extracted by aqueous washing and retains the isoflavones. SoySelect® (Indena, Milan, Italy) and Healthy Women® (Johnson and Johnson, US) are alcohol extracts. Oil and margarine have only traces of isoflavones; the conjugates are not soluble in oil.

The reason why most of the soybean crop is devoted to animal feed and oil is because what is left after removing lipids is totally bland. The solution is to mix soybeans with other foods, such as beans and soups. Unfortunately they require standing in water for about 12 hours, and simmering for 2–3 hours in order to be cooked.

The average Japanese intake of isoflavones is about 50 mg per day[9]. The rest of Asia has an average consumption of about 25–45 mg per day; Western consumption is less than 5 mg per day[10,11].

Table 2 Food derived from soybeans

Soy milk – the liquid obtained from cooked soybeans; lacks calcium and vitamin D; cooked to destroy protease inhibitor activity

Tempeh – fermented beans, originated in Indonesia. Fermented with bacteria, shaped into cakes, and refrigerated. As perishable as tofu

Miso – soybeans mixed with grain, fermented and made into a paste, used in many ways. A Japanese product. Fermented products hydrolyze the glycoside conjugates and are rich in aglycones

Tofu – made like cheese by coagulating soy milk to form curds, which are then pressed. A Chinese product over 1000 years old. Highly susceptible to bacterial contamination. Twenty-eight percent of tofu tested was unacceptable in terms of standards for freshness, and 16% contained coliform bacteria; most was displayed at unsafe (warm) temperatures[7]

Soy sauce – made from fermented soybeans and aged using yeast and *Lactobacillus*. Invented by the Chinese

Soy protein isolate – used in infant formulas

Soy protein concentrate – ingredient in many foods

TVP – textured vegetable protein, an American product, is made from soy protein isolate or concentrate. Used as a meat substitute

ALTERNATIVE THERAPIES FOR HOT FLUSHING

A belief that Asian women report fewer menopausal symptoms has been an underlying force in the promotion of isoflavones. However, this apparent difference in the prevalence of symptoms comparing Asia and the West may reflect cultural differences and not actual experience.

The study of hot flushing requires randomization to placebo treatment because placebo treatment is associated with an average 51% reduction in hot flush frequency[12]. An Italian study using SUPRO found a 45% reduction in flushing with 60 g isolated soy protein daily (76 mg isoflavones), compared with a 30% reduction in the placebo group[13]. Two other studies, both with 50 mg/day isoflavones, found a similar 15% reduction in the number of flushes compared with placebo[14,15]. Another placebo-controlled short-term trial found a greater reduction in flushes with 70 mg isoflavones daily[16]. In a randomized, crossover study of a high dose of isoflavones, 150 mg/day, for flushes in breast cancer survivors, the treated group and the placebo group demonstrated equal effects[17]. The dose was 150 mg isoflavones per day, similar to three glasses of soy milk daily. An Australian study randomized women to 118 mg/day isoflavones or placebo and after 3 months could detect no difference in hot flushing, libido, vaginal dryness, or any of a long list of symptoms[18]. In a randomized study in Iowa, no differences were found in hot flush frequency comparing isoflavone-rich soy protein with a whey protein control[19]. And finally, another randomized trial of breast cancer survivors found no difference comparing placebo with 90 mg isoflavones daily[20].

Promensil is an extract of red clover (*Trifolium pratense*) containing formononetin, biochanin, daidzein, and genistein. Formononetin and biochanin are metabolized to daidzein and genistein, respectively. Red clover is a legume used to enrich nitrogen levels in soils. Promensil is produced by Novogen in Australia and marketed by Solvay in the US. A 500 mg tablet contains 200–230 mg of dried extract, which contains 40 mg of isoflavones. The recommended dose is one tablet daily

Two randomized, placebo-controlled studies of the effect of Promensil on hot flushes were reported in 1999[21,22]. Neither demonstrated a significant difference compared with the placebo group. In one of the reports, four times the recommended dose (four tablets daily) also had no effect[22]. On the other hand, an appropriately designed Dutch study, using two tablets daily, detected a significant reduction of flushing in a 12-week period of time[23].

Why do these randomized, blinded, and placebo-controlled trials lack agreement? The most reasonable explanation is that isoflavones have a modest impact on hot flushing, detectable only in women with frequent and severe flushing. A major clinical response should not be expected.

One randomized, placebo-controlled trial examined the effect of dong quai on hot flushing[24]. No estrogenic effects could be detected on flushing, endometrium, or vagina. Ginseng has the same impact on menopausal symptoms as placebo treatment[25]. Similarly vitamin E supplementation is ineffective for hot flushing[26].

Evening primrose is often recommended for mastalgia, PMS, and menopausal symptoms. Oil of evening primrose is extracted from the seed; it provides linoleic and gamma-linoleic acids (precursors of prostaglandin E). Appropriately blinded and controlled studies have failed to find any differences comparing primrose oil with placebo[27–29].

Black cohosh is also called black snakeroot and bugbane. 'Remifemin' is commercially available, an alcoholic extract of the root. Black cohosh contains formononetin. A tablet contains 2 mg; the dose is two tablets bid or 40 drops of liquid extract bid. Most reviewers of black cohosh refer to an article on black cohosh that is itself a review[30]. Under a heading of clinical trials, there are eight human studies:

(1) An essay in German in 1960 recounting one physician's experience with 517 patients[31];

(2) A German report from 1982; Remifemin, 40 drops bid, for 6–8 weeks, no controls. An

improvement in menopausal symptoms was observed in approximately 80% of the patients;

(3,4) Two open studies, again in Germany, one with 36 patients and one with 50. These 3-month studies indicated improvement in 4 weeks. There were no placebo control groups;

(5) An open study of 60 patients in whom black cohosh was compared with estrogen; not surprisingly, both reduced symptoms;

(6) There was one randomized double-blind study of 80 women with three treatments: black cohosh, estrogen, and placebo. But this was a study designed to study vaginal response, not flushing[32];

(7) A randomized study of symptoms compared estriol, conjugated estrogens, estrogen and progestin, or Remifemin, but there was no placebo group; and

(8) An open study compared results with a placebo group, but this was a study of gonadotropin response, not symptoms[33].

On the basis of this evidence, the author concluded: 'The positive influence of Remifemin on the profile of menopausal ailments has been established in open and in controlled investigations using established and validated testing procedures'. A review of the actual reports does not sustain this conclusion. In another appropriate study – a randomized, placebo-controlled trial of black cohosh in breast cancer survivors – the hot flush response in the treated group was found to be identical to that in the placebo group[34].

The serotonin uptake inhibitor class of antidepressants has been found to be very effective for the treatment of hot flushes in breast cancer survivors, including hot flushes associated with tamoxifen treatment[35–38]. The potency of this class of agents is impressive. Titering the treatment to achieve the lowest effective dose is easily accomplished. This is now the treatment of choice for flushing women who will not or cannot take estrogen.

ALTERNATIVE THERAPIES TO PREVENT CARDIOVASCULAR DISEASE

The cardiovascular story with phytoestrogens received a large boost in 1995, when a meta-analysis concluded that an intake of an average of 47 g soy protein per day lowered total cholesterol and low-density lipoprotein (LDL) cholesterol[39]. This was supported by Clarkson's studies in the monkey indicating that isoflavone increased high-density lipoprotein (HDL) cholesterol, enhanced vasodilatation, and decreased atherosclerosis[40].

Only intact soy protein has a beneficial effect on lipids. Separation of the protein component from dietary soy protein removes the effect. This effect depends on the inhibition of cholesterol absorption by the non-isoflavone protein[41,42]. The mechanism involves upregulation of the LDL receptor and catabolism of LDL cholesterol, leading to an increase in bile excretion. The soy peptide binds bile acids and prevents resorption. Alcohol extraction removes the isoflavones from soy protein and causes a loss of the beneficial effect on atherosclerosis in monkeys[43]. Thus, both the isoflavone portion and the protein component are required for a full cardiovascular effect.

Non-alcohol-washed soy protein extract has been extensively studied in monkeys. This preparation lowers total and LDL cholesterol and raises HDL cholesterol[44,45] produces coronary artery vasodilatation[46], inhibits reduction in coronary flow after collagen-induced platelet aggregation and serotonin release[47], and inhibits atherosclerosis, but not as robustly as estrogen[40,45,48].

In women, soy protein reduces total and LDL cholesterol, does not affect triglycerides or HDL cholesterol; and ethanol-extracted soy protein has no effect[49–52]. The minimal dose is about 60 mg isoflavones daily, which is present in 25 g soy protein/day[53]. LDL cholesterol needs to be above the normal of 130mg/dl in order to have an effect. A double-blind crossover study of healthy men and women could detect no effect of phytoestrogens (80 mg isoflavones per day) on lipids or brachial vasodilatation[54]. In a 12-week study of women with type 2 diabetes mellitus, dietary supplementation of 30 g soy protein (132 mg isoflavones) daily improved insulin resistance and glucose control, in addition to lowering total and LDL cholesterol levels[55]. Promensil, in a 10-week study, had no effect on lipids (it only contains isoflavones, no protein) but did improve arterial compliance[56].

The US Food and Drug Administration (FDA), in October 1999, authorized the use of health claims on the association between soy protein and reduced risk of coronary heart disease (CHD) on food labels and in food labeling: 'based on the totality of publicly available scientific evidence, soy protein included in a diet low in saturated fat and cholesterol may reduce the risk of CHD by lowering blood cholesterol levels'[57].

Remember that you need both protein and isoflavones for a cardiovascular effect. Isoflavones by themselves have no effect on lipids[15,56,58]. Protein without isoflavones has no effect on vasodilatation and atherosclerosis[43]. The FDA has stated that there is insufficient evidence to allow them to exclude alcohol-washed products from the health claim, but it makes sense that a combined protein–isoflavone product is best. Even in older women with moderate hypercholesterolemia, a high intake of soy phytoestrogens (purified isoflavones without protein) had no effect on the lipid profile[59]. And also remember, that there is probably no effect on the lipids in individuals who already have a normal profile.

It will require appropriate clinical trials to determine how phytoestrogens compare with estrogens, and the efficacy, safety, and correct dosage (studies thus far recommend a daily intake of 60 g soy protein). In addition, the intake of sufficient soy to produce a clinical response is not easy, handicapped by gastro-intestinal symptoms, a major alteration in diet or the use of an unpalatable supplement, and great variability in plant contents and products (due to processing). Also, individuals demonstrate great variability in absorption and metabolism. A user-friendly preparation needs to be developed that minimizes individual variability in response.

ALTERNATIVE THERAPIES TO PREVENT BONE LOSS

Phytoestrogens are effective in preventing bone loss in rats, but not in monkeys[60–62]. In women, studies have demonstrated at best a slight effect on spinal bone, but no effect on hip bone[50,63,64]. Flaxseed supplementation had no effect on biomarkers of bone metabolism[65]. The difference between hip fracture incidence in Japanese and American women may be due to structural and/or genetic differences, not dietary intake[66].

Ipriflavone is a synthetic isoflavone; it is methylated dehydroxydaidzein, which is metabolized to daidzein. It was developed by Chiesi Pharmaceuticals in Parma, Italy. It is marketed in the US over the counter as Twinlab® (Twin Laboratories, Hauppauge, NY); each tablet contains 150 mg ipriflavone combined with calcium (375 mg), vitamin D (187 IU), soy isoflavones (40 mg) and boron (3 mg). The Italian product is pure ipriflavone. The recommended dose is 600 mg per day, two tablets bid taken with meals. With the US product, this means more calcium than is needed. Studies with ipriflavone have demonstrated prevention of bone loss over a year[67–70]. Overall the effect on bone is not as great as that observed with the standard dose of estrogen or alendronate; perhaps not great enough to yield a benefit. A 4-year randomized trial in Europe assessed the effect of ipriflavone on bone density, urinary markers, and vertebral fractures in 474 women and could find no difference in the treated group compared with the placebo group[71].

PHYTOESTROGENS AND COGNITION

Phytoestrogens upregulate cognition markers and improve memory in rats equally when compared with estrogen[72,73]. There is one human study, and the results are disturbing. Men, in a National Institutes of Health study begun in 1965, reported their tofu consumption[74]. Cognition was tested in 1991–93 when the men were aged 71–93. Higher midlife tofu consumption (two or more servings per week) was associated with poor cognitive test performance, enlargement of ventricles, and low brain weight.

PHYTOESTROGENS AND THE BREAST

In the parts of the world where soy intake is high, there is a lower incidence of breast, endometrial, and prostate cancers[75]. For example, a case–control study concluded that there was a 54% reduced risk of endometrial cancer, and another case–control study indicated a reduction in the risk of breast cancer, in women with a high consumption of soy and other legumes[76,77]. Daidzein and genistein urinary excretion are low in Australian women who develop breast cancer[78]. High soy and tofu consumption and high urinary excretion of isoflavones have been reported to be associated with a lower risk of breast cancer in Singapore, China, and Australia[77,79–81]. These studies have supported the belief that high phytoestrogen intake protects against breast cancer. It is by no means certain, however, that there is a direct effect of soy intake[82]. Indeed, a 6-month study of the impact of administered soy protein on breast secretions in premenopausal and postmenopausal women revealed increased breast secretions with the appearance of hyperplastic epithelial cells[83]. Epithelial hyperplasia based on cytology in breast secretions was demonstrated in 7 of 24 (29.2%) subjects.

Genistein increases epidermal growth factor in immature rat mammary tissue, and it has been hypothesized that early exposure to genistein promotes early cell differentiation leading to breast glands that are more resistant to the development of cancer[84]. On the other hand, using the chemically induced rat breast cancer model, no evidence of isoflavone inhibition of tumor development has been detected[85]. In monkeys treated for 6 months, no proliferation was reported in either endometrium or mammary tissue[86,87].

One hypothesis speculates that phytoestrogens protect the breast by decreasing exposure to the more potent endogenous estrogens. However, the evidence does not support this idea. High-dose treatment (100 mg of daidzein plus 100 mg genistein) does lower estradiol and dehydroepiandrosterone sulfate levels in premenopausal women, and increases cycle length[88]. However these are extremely high doses. One study reported that treatment with Asian soy foods (approximately 32 mg isoflavones per day) was associated with a 9.3% significant decrease in luteal serum estradiol levels, but there were no other changes, including follicular phase estradiol, progesterone, and sex hormone-binding globulin (SHBG) levels, or cycle length[89]. Interestingly the reduction in luteal estradiol was observed only in Asian participants in whom urinary excretion of isoflavones was higher than non-Asians[89]. These same investigators reported that a high intake of the soy protein alone (with the isoflavones removed) reduced estradiol and progesterone levels throughout the cycle[90]. Other studies have found no effects on estradiol, follicle stimulating hormone (FSH), luteinnizing hormone (LH), or SHBG in premenopausal women[91], and most importantly, no effects on circulating hormones in postmenopausal women[92,93]. The lack of an effect on gonadotropin levels is important, depriving the clinician of a method to assess dosage.

Catecholestrogens (2-hydroxy estrogens) have long been proposed as a metabolite pathway that could be protective, or at least antiestrogenic. Hydroxylation in the 2 position produces an inactive metabolite. In one study, eight premenopausal women treated with a soy milk supplement increased their urinary excretion of 2-hydroestrone by an average of 47%[94]. However, another could detect no change in 2-hydroxyestrogen[91].

In response to soy, no significant increase in nipple aspirate levels of genistein and daidzein could be detected[95]. However, an indication of estrogenic stimulation occurred, as measured by pS2 (a protein upregulated by estrogen) levels, but there was no evidence of an effect on epithelial cell proliferation, estrogen and progesterone receptors, apoptosis, or mitosis. Thus, no antiestrogenic effect could be detected, and at best there was a very weak estrogen effect. In another study, 48 women with normal breasts received a 60 g soy supplement for 14 days, and in these women lobular epithelial proliferation and progesterone receptor expression increased, an indication of estrogen stimulation[96]. Some argue that the key to a beneficial impact on breast may be early exposure, and a sudden increase late in life of dietary phytoestrogens may be harmful.

SUMMARY OF PHYTOESTROGEN EFFECTS

There is agreement that phytoestrogens have no effects on the uterus or vagina[14,15,21,22,24,86,87,92,93,97]. A beneficial effect on vaginal dryness and dyspareunia cannot be expected; however, a proliferative stimulus on the endometrium is not an unwanted consequence of phytoestrogen supplementation.

Currently the recommended intake expected to have some effect on CHD is 50–60 mg isoflavones per day, an amount that is in 25 g of soy protein aqueous extract. A beneficial impact on CHD in women with abnormal lipid profiles is to be expected, a consequence of a decrease in total and LDL cholesterol and an increase in vascular reaction. The size of the effect is unknown. Excess intake can cause gastrointestinal upset and flatulence, inhibition of enzymes necessary for the digestion of proteins, possibly obstruction of mineral uptake, and weight gain.

GINKGO AND ALZHEIMER'S DISEASE

In a meta-analysis of over 50 reports on Ginkgo and Alzheimer's disease, only four studies indicating some benefit, with only 212 treated subjects and 212 control subjects, were deemed worthy[97]. Recent randomized trials, however, have failed to demonstrate any beneficial effects on Alzheimer's disease, learning, memory, attention, verbal fluency, or concentration[99,100].

ST. JOHN'S WORT AND DEPRESSION

St. John's wort has been reported to be comparable to tricyclic antidepressants in treating mild-to-moderate depression, based on eight appropriate trials[101]. This is the conclusion of two other meta-analyses[102,103]. All studies have been short-term, about 4–6 weeks in duration, and with small numbers. The treatment consists of a 300 mg plant extract in tablet form, administered tid. Two large, American 8-week trials found no difference between treatment and placebo[104,105].

The FDA issued an alert in February, 2000, that St. John's wort may interact with drugs known to be metabolized by the cytochrome P450 pathway: theophylline, digoxin, immune suppressants, and oral contraceptives[106]. St. John's wort activates an orphan receptor that induces the expression of metabolic enzymes[107]. In clinically depressed individuals being treated with prescription antidepressants, manic reactions can result (the central serotonergic syndrome).

ESTRIOL

Interest in estriol can be traced to Lemon's report in 1975 that estriol limited the growth of breast tumors in the chemical-induced rat tumor model[108]. However, it is usually overlooked that estradiol worked equally well in that model. Estriol treatment of postmenopausal women has no overall effect on lipids and no effect in the prevention of myocardial infarction[109,110]. Estriol, without concomitant progestin treatment, does increase the risk of endometrial cancer with the long-term oral use of 1–2 mg per day[111]. At least two studies have been unable to demonstrate prevention of bone loss with the administration of 2 mg estriol daily[112,113]. And one case–control study found no reduction in hip fractures with estriol compared with a lower risk with estradiol[110].

A major factor in the potency differences among the various estrogens (estradiol, estrone,

Table 3 Clinical effects of phytoestrogens

Flushes	Modest
Coronary heart disease	Weak
Bone	None
Cognition	Unknown
Breast	May be protective
Endometrium	No effect
Vagina	No effect

estriol) is the length of time the estrogen–receptor complex occupies the nucleus. The higher rate of dissociation with the weak estrogen (estriol) can be compensated for by continuous application to allow prolonged nuclear binding and activity. Estriol has only 20–30% affinity for the estrogen receptor compared with estradiol; therefore, it is rapidly cleared from a cell. But if the effective concentration is kept equivalent to that of estradiol, it can produce a similar biologic response[114]. In pregnancy, where the concentration of estriol is very great, it can be an important hormone, not just a metabolite. Thus, higher estriol levels are not necessarily protective. Indeed, antagonism of estradiol occurs only within a vary narrow range of the ratio of estradiol to estriol, a range rarely encountered either physiologically or pharmacologically[115]. Below this range, estradiol is unimpeded, above this range estriol itself exerts estrogenic activity.

TRANSDERMAL PROGESTERONE

Transdermal (or percutaneous) progesterone has been promoted by John Lee, who reviewed his patient records, and reported in 1990 that 63 of 100 women treated daily with 20 mg of transdermal progesterone cream increased their spinal bone density[116]. Two English randomized, blinded, placebo-controlled studies used two to four times the recommended dose and reported blood levels of about 1 ng/ml, supported by very low urinary pregnanediol levels[117,118]. An American study achieved progesterone blood levels of 2–3 ng/ml with application twice daily[119]. An Italian one-year study did not measure blood levels, but could detect no effects on bone density, lipid profiles, or depression scores[120]. These studies indicate very little systemic absorption (the levels do not reach normal luteal phase concentrations) with great variability.

An Australian study of 16, 32, or 64 mg transdermal progesterone administered daily could detect no significant absorption, and most importantly, no endometrial response, and no effect on flushes, lipids, bone, moods, or sexuality[121,122]. Incidentally, this study found salivary progesterone levels to be so variable that they had no meaning. Progesterone cream can produce high salivary levels, without a significant change in serum or urinary levels (the mechanism is unknown)[123,124]. Red cell levels (championed by Lee) reflect serum levels[124]. Clinicians and patients should be aware that transdermal progesterone will not protect the endometrium against the risk of endometrial cancer associated with estrogen therapy.

Wild Yam creams are marketed as progesterone precursors or balancing formulas. Yam contains diosgenin, a plant steroid that can be converted to progesterone in a chemical laboratory, but not in the human body. Predictably, a wild yam cream has no effects on a wide range of measurements in postmenopausal women[125]. Some do contain progesterone, added by the manufacturer. Creams with less than 0.016% progesterone can be sold over the counter.

DEHYDROEPIANDROSTERONE (DHEA)

Adrenal androgen production decreases dramatically with aging. The mechanism is not known, but it is not due to the loss of estrogen at menopause, nor can it be reversed with estrogen treatment[126]. The impressive decline (75–85%) in circulating levels of dehydroepiandrosterone (DHEA) that occur with aging (greater in men than in women) has stimulated a search for a beneficial impact of DHEA supplementation. Animal studies (in animals that do not even synthesize DHEA) have suggested that DHEA administration enhances the immune system and protects against many conditions associated with aging.

The only proven function of DHEA and its sulfate, DS, is to provide a pool of prohormone for conversion to androgens, and ultimately estrogens. By age 70 or 80, the circulating levels in men and women are about 10% of peak levels that occur between 20 and 30 years of age. It is this decline that has prompted the promotion of DHEA supplementation[127]. However, DHEA supplementation does not produce improvements in menopausal symptoms, mood, libido, cognition, or memory; but does increase testosterone and decrease HDL cholesterol[128].

Although low levels of DHEA and DS have been reported to be associated with increased risk of cardiovascular disease in men, in women conflicting results are found in cross-sectional data. In a longitudinal study of 236 women, higher levels of DHEA and DS in middle-aged women correlated with an *increased* risk of cardiovascular disease[129].

DHEA supplementation, 50 mg per day, produced reproductive levels of DS in elderly men, did not change levels of testosterone and dihydrotestosterone, and raised estradiol and estrone levels, although still within normal range[130]. In women, 25 mg or 50 mg per day increased testosterone levels, decreased SHBG levels, and produced adverse effects on the lipid profile[131,132]. Exogenously administered DHEA is converted to potent androgens and estrogens. Potential long-term effects include hirsutism, alopecia, voice changes, prostate and breast effects, and an increased risk of CHD.

CONCLUSION

In closing, let me suggest a clinical approach that I have found to be effective. I believe it is appropriate to inform a patient that when she uses preparations lacking in data regarding safety and efficacy, she is experimenting with her own body. Of course, every patient has the right to do so, but we have the obligation to provide this admonishment. An impressive number of patients will appreciate this advice and conclude that they would rather not be the subject of experimentation.

There is only one medicine

Anything claiming to treat or prevent health problems must withstand the rigor of scientific studies of efficacy and safety. Anything with the potential to affect health must be subject to this requirement. Those treatments that pass this testing will become part of our medical practice; those that fail will fall by the wayside. The simplicity and correctness of this argument are so overwhelming, this will be the future of alternative therapies.

Suggested website

Columbia Rosenthal Center for Alternative and Complementary Medicine at http://cpmcnet. columbia.edu/dept/rosenthal

References

1. Astin JA. Why patients use alternative medicine: results of a national study. *J Am Med Assoc* 1998;279:1548–53
2. Eisenberg DM, Davis RB, Ettner SL, *et al.* Trends in alternative medicine use in the United States, 1990–1997: results of a follow-up national survey. *J Am Med Assoc* 1998;280: 1569–75
3. *Consumer Reports.* New York: Consumers Union, March 1999;44–8
4. Murkies AL, Wilcox G, Davis SR. Phyto-estrogens. *J Clin Endocrinol Metab* 1998;83: 297–303
5. Tham DM, Gardner CD, Haskell WL. Potential health benefits of dietary phytoestrogens: a review of the clinical, epidemiological, and mechanistic evidence. *J Clin Endocrinol Metab* 1998;83:2223–35
6. Kuiper GGJM, Carlsson B, Grandien K, *et al.* Comparison of the ligand binding specificity and transcript tissue distribution of estrogen receptors alpha and beta. *Endocrinology* 1997; 138:863–70
7. Ashraf HR, White M, Klubek B. Microbiological survey of tofu sold in a rural Illinois county. *J Food Prot* 1999;62:1050–3
8. Anderson RL, Wolf WJ. Compositional changes in trypsin inhibitors, phytic acid, saponins and isoflavones related to soybean processing. *J Nutr* 1995;125(Suppl):581S–88S

9. Messina M. Isoflavone intakes by Japanese were overestimated (letter to the editor). *Am J Clin Nutr* 1995;62:645

10. Coward L, Barnes NC, Setchell KDR, Barnes S. The isoflavones genistein and daidzein in soybean foods from American and Asian diets. *J Agric Food Chem* 1993;41:1961–7

11. Cassidy A, Bingham S, Setchell KDR. Biological effects of a diet of soy protein rich in isoflavones on the menstrual cycle of premenopausal women. *Am J Clin Nutr* 1994;60:333–40

12. MacLennan AH, Henry D, Hills S, Moore V, eds. *Oral Oestrogen Replacement Therapy Versus Placebo for Hot Flushes*. Oxford: Cochrane Library Update Software, 2000

13. Albertazzi P, Pansini F, Bonaccorsi G, *et al.* The effect of dietary soy supplementation on hot flushes. *Obstet Gynecol* 1998;91:6–11

14. Scambia G, Mango D, Signorile PG, *et al.* Clinical effects of a standardized soy extract in postmenopausal women: a pilot study. *Menopause* 2000;7:105–11

15. Upmalis DH, Lobo R, Bradley L, *et al.* Vasomotor symptom relief by soy isoflavone extract tablets in postmenopausal women: a multicenter, double-blind, randomized, placebo-controlled study. *Menopause* 2000;7:236–42

16. Faure ED, Chantre P, Mares P. Effects of a standardized soy extract on hot flushes: a multicenter, double-blind, randomized, placebo-controlled study. *Menopause* 2002;9: 329–34

17. Quella SK, Loprinzi CL, Barton DL, *et al.* Evaluation of soy phytoestrogens for the treatment of hot flashes in breast cancer survivors: a North Central Cancer Treatment Group trial. *J Clin Oncol* 2000;18:1068–74

18. Kotsopoulos D, Dalais FS, Liang Y-L, *et al.* The effects of soy protein containing phytoestrogens on menopausal symptoms in postmenopausal women. *Climacteric* 2000;3: 161–7

19. St. Germain A, Peterson CT, Robinson JG, Alekel DL. Isoflavone-rich or isoflavone-poor soy protein does not reduce menopausal symptoms during 24 weeks of treatment. *Menopause* 2001;8:17–26

20. Van Patten CL, Olivotto IA, Chambers GK, *et al.* Effect of soy phytoestrogens on hot flashes in postmenopausal women with breast cancer: a randomized, controlled clinical trial. *J Clin Oncol* 2002;20:1449–55

21. Baber RJ, Templeman C, Morton T, *et al.* Randomized placebo-controlled trial of an isoflavone supplement and menopausal symptoms in women. *Climacteric* 1999;2: 85–92

22. Knight DC, Howes JB, Eden JA. The effect of Promensil™, an isoflavone extract, on menopausal symptoms. *Climacteric* 1999;2:79–84

23. van de Wijer PHM, Barentsen R. Isoflavones from red clover (Promensil®) significantly reduce menopausal hot flush symptoms compared with placebo. *Maturitas* 2002;42: 187–93

24. Hirata JD, Swiersz LM, Zell B, *et al.* Does dong quai have estrogenic effects in postmenopausal women? A double-blind, placebo-controlled trial. *Fertil Steril* 1997;68: 981–86

25. Wiklund IK, Mattsson LA, Lindgren R, Limoni C. Effects of a standardized ginseng extract on quality of life and physiological parameters in symptomatic postmenopausal women: a double-blind, placebo-controlled trial. Swedish Alternative Medicine Group. *Int J Clin Pharmacol Res* 1999;19:89–99

26. Barton DL, Loprinzi CL, Quella SK, *et al.* Prospective evaluation of vitamin E for hot flashes in breast cancer survivors. *J Clin Oncol* 1998;16:495–500

27. Khoo SK, Munro C, Battistutta D. Evening primrose oil and treatment of premenstrual syndrome. *Med J Aust* 1990;153:189

28. Collins A, Cerin A, Coleman G, Landgren B-M. Essential fatty acids in the treatment of premenstrual syndrome. *Obstet Gynecol* 1993;81: 93–8

29. Chenoy R, Hussain S, Tayob Y, *et al.* Effect of oral gamolenic acid from evening primrose oil on menopausal flushing. *Br Med J* 1994;308: 501–3

30. Lieberman S. A review of the effectiveness of *Cimicifuga racemosa* (Black Cohosh) for the symptoms of menopause. *J Womens Health* 1998;7:525–9

31. Brucker A. Essay on the phytotherapy of hormonal disorders in women. *Med Welt* 1960; 44:223

32. Stoll W. Phytotherapy influences atrophic vaginal epithelium. *Therapeutikon* 1987;1:23

33. Duker EM, Kopanski HJ, Wuttke W. Effects of extracts from *Cimicifuga racemosa* on gonadotropin release in menopausal women and ovariectomized rats. *Planta Med* 1991;57:420

34. Jacobson JS, Troxel AB, Evans J, *et al.* Randomized trial of black cohosh for the treatment of hot flashes among women with a history of breast cancer. *J Clin Oncol* 2001;19:2739–45

35. Plouffe LJ, Trott EA, Sanal S, *et al.* Sertraline (Zoloft) for the management of hot flashes in women on tamoxifen: a randomized controlled pilot trial (abstract). *Menopause* 1997;4:262

36. Loprinzi CL, Pisansky TM, Fonseca R, *et al.* Pilot evaluation of venlafaxine hydrochloride for the therapy of hot flashes in cancer survivors. *J Clin Oncol* 1998;16:2377–81

37. Loprinzi CL, Quella SK, Sloan JA, *et al.* A randomized evaluation of fluoxetine (Prozac) for treating hot flashes in breast cancer

survivors (abstract). *Am Soc Clin Oncol* 2000, San Antonio

38. Stearns V, Isaacs C, Rowland J, *et al.* A pilot trial assessing the efficacy of paroxetine hydrochloride (Paxil®) in controlling hot flashes in breast cancer survivors. *Ann Oncol* 2000;11: 17–22

39. Anderson JW, Johnstone B, Cook-Newell ME. Meta-analysis of the effects of soy protein intake on serum lipids. *New Engl J Med* 1995; 333:276–82

40. Clarkson TB, Anthony M, Morgan TM. Inhibition of postmenopausal atherosclerosis progression: a comparison of the effects of conjugated equine estrogens and soy phytoestrogens. *J Clin Endocrinol Metab* 2001;86:41–7

41. Greaves KA, Parks JS, Williams JK, Wagner JD. Intact dietary soy protein, but not adding an isoflavone-rich soy extract to casein, improves plasma lipids in ovariectomized cynomolgus monkeys. *J Nutr* 1999;129:1585–92

42. Greaves KA, Wilson MD, Rudel L, *et al.* Consumption of soy protein reduces cholesterol absorption compared to casein protein alone or supplemented with an isoflavone extract or conjugated equine estrogen in ovariectomized cynomolgus monkeys. *J Nutr* 2000;130:820–6

43. Anthony MS, Clarkson TB, Williams JK. Effects of soy isoflavones on atherosclerosis: potential mechanisms. *Am J Clin Nutr* 1998;68: 1390S–3S

44. Anthony MS, Clarkson TB, Hughes Jr CL, *et al.* Soybean isoflavones improve cardiovascular risk factors without affecting the reproductive system of peripubertal Rhesus monkeys. *J Nutr* 1996;126: 43–50

45. Anthony MS, Clarkson TB. Comparison of soy phytoestrogens and conjugated equine estrogens on atherosclerosis progression in postmenopausal monkeys (abstract). *Circulation* 1998;90:829

46. Honoré EK, Williams JK, Anthony MS, Clarkson TB. Soy isoflavones enhance coronary vascular reactivity in atherosclerotic female macaques. *Fertil Steril* 1997;67:148–54

47. Williams JK, Anthony MS, Clarkson TB. Interactive effects of soy protein and estradiol on coronary artery reactivity in atherosclerotic, ovariectomized monkeys. *Menopause* 2001;8: 307–13

48. Clarkson TB, Anthony MS. Effect of hormone replacement therapy on internal carotid artery atherosclerosis of postmenopausal monkeys (abstract). *Circulation* 1998;97:830

49. Crouse JR, 3rd., Morgan T, Terry JG, *et al.* A randomized trial comparing the effect of casein with that of soy protein containing varying amounts of isoflavones on plasma concentrations of lipids and lipoproteins. *Arch Intern Med* 1999;159:2070–6

50. Potter SM, Baum JA, Teng H, *et al.* Soy protein and isoflavones: their effects on blood lipids and bone density in postmenopausal women. *Am J Clin Nutr* 1998;68(Suppl):1375S–9S

51. Washburn S, Burke GL, Morgan T, Anthony M. Effect of soy protein supplementation on serum lipoproteins, blood pressure, and menopausal symptoms in perimenopausal women. *Menopause* 1999;6:7–13

52. Merz-Demlow BE, Duncan AM, Wangen KE, *et al.* Soy isoflavones improve plasma lipids in normocholesterolemic, premenopausal women. *Am J Clin Nutr* 2000;71:1462–9

53. Teixeira SR, Potter SM, Weigel R, *et al.* Effects of feeding 4 levels of soy protein for 3 and 6 wk on blood lipids and apolipoproteins in moderately hypercholesterolemic men. *Am J Clin Nutr* 2000; 71:1077–84

54. Simons LA, von Konigsmark M, Simons J, Celermajer DS. Phytoestrogens do not influence lipoprotein levels or endothelial function in healthy, postmenopausal women. *Am J Cardiol* 2000;11:1297–301

55. Jayagopal V, Albertazzi P, Kilpatrick ES, *et al.* Beneficial effects of soy phytoestrogen intake in postmenopausal women with type 2 diabetes. *Diabetes Care* 2002;25:1709–1714

56. Nestel PJ, Pomeroy S, Kay S, *et al.* Isoflavones from red clover improve systemic arterial compliance but not plasma lipids in menopausal women. *J Clin Endocrinol Metab* 1999;84:895–8

57. Food and Drug Administration. Food labeling: health claims; soy protein and coronary heart disease. *Federal Register* 1999;64:57700–33

58. Hodgson JM, Puddey IB, Beilin LJ, *et al.* Supplementation with isoflavonoid phytoestrogens does not alter serum lipid concentrations: a randomized controlled trial in humans. *J Nutr* 1998;128:728–32

59. Dewell A, Hollenbeck CB, Bruce B. The effects of soy-derived phytoestrogens on serum lipids and lipoproteins in moderately hypercholesterolemic postmenopausal women. *J Clin Endocrinol Metab* 2002;87:118–21

60. Arjmandi BH, Birnbaum R, Toyal NV, *et al.* Bone-sparing effect of soy protein in ovarian hormone-deficient rats is related to its isoflavone content. *Am J Clin Nutr* 1998;68 (Suppl):1364S–8S

61. Jayo MJ, Anthony MS, Register TC, *et al.* Dietary soy isoflavones and bone loss: a study in ovariectomized monkeys (abstract). *J Bone Miner Res* 1996;11(Suppl 1):S228

62. Lees CJ, Ginn TA. Soy protein isolate diet does not prevent increased cortical bone turnover in ovariectomized macaques. *Calcif Tissue Int* 1998;62:557–8

63. Alekel DL, Peterson C, St. Germain A, Hanson K. Isoflavone-rich soy isolate exerts significant bone-sparing in the lumbar spine of peri-menopausal women (abstract). *Am Soc Bone Miner Res* Annual Meeting 1999

64. Gallagher JC, Rafferty K, Wilson MD, Haynaska V. The effect of soy protein on bone metabolism (abstract). *N Am Men Soc* Annual Meeting 1999

65. Lucas EA, Wild RD, Hammond LJ, *et al.* Flax-seed improves lipid profile without altering biomarkers of bone metabolism in post-menopausal women. *J Clin Endocrinol Metab* 2002;87:1527–32

66. Nakamura T, Turner CH, Yoshikawa T, *et al.* Do variations in hip geometry explain differences in hip fracture risk between Japanese and white Americans? *J Bone Miner Res* 1994;9:1071–6

67. Melis GB, Paoletti AM, Cagnacci A. Ipriflavone prevents bone loss in postmenopausal women. *Menopause* 1996;3:27–31

68. Gennari C, Agnusdei D, Crepaldi G, *et al.* Effect of ipriflavone – a synthetic derivative of natural isoflavones – on bone mass loss in the early years after menopause. *Menopause* 1998;5:9–15

69. de Aloysio D, Gambacciani M, Altieri P, *et al.* Bone density changes in postmenopausal women with the administration of ipriflavone alone or in association with low-dose ERT. *Gynecol Endocrinol* 1997;11:289–93

70. Gambacciani M, Ciaponi M, Cappagli B, *et al.* Effects of combined low dose of the isoflavone derivative ipriflavone and estrogen replacement on bone mineral density and metabolism in postmenopausal women. *Maturitas* 1997;28:75–81

71. Alexandersen P, Toussaint A, Christiansen C, *et al.* Ipriflavone in the treament of post-menopausal osteoporosis. A randomized controlled trial. *J Am Med Assoc* 2001;285:1482–8

72. Pan Y, Anthony M, Clarkson TB. Effect of estradiol and soy phytoestrogens on choline acetyltransferase and nerve growth factor mRNAs in the frontal cortex and hippocampus of female rats. *Proc Soc Exp Biol Med* 1999;221:118–25

73. Pan Y, Anthony M, Watson S, Clarkson TB. Soy phytoestrogens improve radial arm maze performance in ovariectomized retired breeder rats and do not attenuate benefits of 17β-estradiol treatment. *Menopause* 2000;7:230–5

74. White LR, Petrovitch H, Ross GW, *et al.* Brain aging and midlife tofu consumption. *J Am Coll Nutr* 2000;19:242–55

75. Adlercreutz H, Mazur W. Phyto-oestrogens and western diseases. *Ann Med* 1997;29:95–120

76. Goodman MT, Wilkens LR, Hankin JH, *et al.* Association of soy and fiber consumption with the risk of endometrial cancer. *Am J Epidemiol* 1997;146:294–306

77. Ingram D, Sanders K, Kolybaba M, Lopez D. Case-control study of phyto-oestrogens and breast cancer. *Lancet* 1997;350:990–4

78. Murkies A, Dalais FS, Briganti EM, *et al.* Phytoestrogens and breast cancer in post-menopausal women: a case control study. *Menopause* 2000;7:289–96

79. Lee HP, Gourley L, Duffy SW, *et al.* Dietary effect on breast cancer risk in Singapore. *Lancet* 1991;337:1197–200

80. Wu AH, Ziegler RG, Horn-Ross PL, *et al.* Tofu and risk of breast cancer in Asian-Americans. *Cancer Epidemiol Biomarkers Prev* 1996;5:901–6

81. Zheng W, Dai Q, Custer LJ, *et al.* Urinary excretion of isoflanonoids and the risk of breast cancer. *Cancer Epidemiol Biomarkers Prev* 1999;8:35–40

82. Messina MJ, Persky V, Setchell KDR, Barnes S. Soy intake and cancer risk: a review of the *in vitro* and *in vivo* data. *Nutr Cancer* 1994;21:113–31

83. Petrakis NL, Barnes S, King EB, *et al.* Stimulatory influence of soy protein isolate on breast secretion in pre- and postmenopausal women. *Cancer Epidemiol Biomark Prev* 1996;5:785–94

84. Lamartiniere CA. Protection against breast cancer with genistein: a component of soy. *Am J Clin Nutr* 2000;71(Suppl):1705S–7S

85. Cohen LA, Zhao Z, Pittman B, Scimeca JA. Effect of intact and isoflavone-depleted soy protein on NMU-induced rat mammary tumorigenesis. *Carcinogenesis* 2000;21:929–35

86. Foth D, Cline JM. Effects of mammalian and plant estrogens on mammary glands and uteri of macaques. *Am J Clin Nutr* 1998;68(Suppl):1413S–17S

87. Foth D, Cline JM, Romer T. Effect of isoflavones on mammary gland and endometrium of post-menopausal macaques (*Macaca fasicularis*). *Zentralbl Gynakol* 2000;122:96–102

88. Lu L-JW, Anderson KE, Grady JJ, Nagamani M. Effects of soya consumption for one month on steroid hormones in premenopausal women: implications for breast cancer risk reduction. *Cancer Epidemiol Biomark Prev* 1996;5:63–70

89. Wu AH, Stancyzk FZ, Hendrich S, *et al.* Effects of soy foods on ovarian function in premeno-pausal women. *Br J Cancer* 2000;82:1879–86

90. Lu LW, Anderson KE, Grady JJ, Nagamani M. Effects of an isoflavone-free soy diet on ovarian hormones in premenopausal women. *J Clin Endocrinol Metab* 2001;86:3045–52

91. Martini MC, Dancisak BB, Haggans CJ, *et al.* Effects of soy intake on sex hormone metabolism in premenopausal women. *Nutr Cancer* 1999;34:133–9

92. Baird DD, Umbach DM, Lansdell L, *et al.* Dietary intervention study to assess estrogenicity of dietary soy among postmenopausal women. *J Clin Endocrinol Metab* 1995;80:1685–90

93. Duncan AM, Underhill KE, Xu X, *et al.* Modest hormonal effects of soy isoflavones in postmenopausal women. *J Clin Endocrinol Metab* 1999;84:3479–84

94. Lu LJ, Cree M, Josyula S, *et al.* Increased urinary excretion of 2-hydroxyestrone but not 16alpha-hydroxyestrone in premenopausal women during a soya diet containing isoflavones. *Cancer Res* 2000;60:1299–305

95. Hargreaves DF, Potten CS, Harding C, *et al.* Two-week dietary soy supplementation has an estrogenic effect on normal premenopausal breast. *J Clin Endocrinol Metab* 1999;84:4017–24

96. McMichael-Phillips DF, Harding C, Morton M, *et al.* Effects of soy-protein supplementation on epithelial proliferation in the histologically normal breast. *Am J Clin Nutr* 1998;68(Suppl): 1431S–5S

97. Balk JL, Whiteside DA, Naus G, *et al.* A pilot study of the effects of phytoestrogen supplementation on postmenopausal endometrium. *J Soc Gynecol Invest* 2002;9:238–42

98. Oken BS, Storzbach DM, Kaye JA. The efficacy of ginkgo biloba on cognitive function in Alzheimer disease. *Arch Neurol* 1998;55:1409–15

99. van Dongen MC, van Rossum E, Kessels AG, *et al.* The efficacy of ginkgo for elderly people with dementia and age-associated memory impairment: new results of a randomized clinical trial. *J Am Geriatr Soc* 2000;48:1183–94

100. Solomon PR, Adams F, Silver A, *et al.* Ginkgo for memory enhancement. A randomized controlled trial. *J Am Med Assoc* 2002;288:835–40

101. Gaster B, Holroyd J. St. John's wort for depression: a systematic review. *Arch Intern Med* 2000;160:152–6

102. Kim HL, Streitzer J, Goebert D. St. John's wort for depression: a meta-analysis of well-defined clinical trials. *J Nerv Ment Dis* 1999;187:532–8

103. Linde K, Mulrow CD. St John's wort for depression. *Cochrane Database Syst Rev* 2000; CD000448

104. Shelton RC, Keller MB, Glelenberg A, *et al.* Effectiveness of St John's Wort in major depression. A randomized controlled trial. *J Am Med Assoc* 2001;285:1978–86

105. Hypericum Depression Trial Study Group. Effect of *Hypericum perforatum* (St John's Wort) in major depressive disorder. A randomized controlled trial. *J Am Med Assoc* 2002;287: 1807–14

106. Food and Drug Administration. Risk of drug interactions with St. John's wort and indinavir and other drugs. *FDA Public Health Advisory,* Feburary 10, 2000

107. Moore LB, Goodwin B, Jones, SA, *et al.* St. John's wort induces hepatic drug metabolism through activation of the pregnane X receptor. *Proc Natl Acad Sci USA* 2000;97:7500–2

108. Lemon HM. Estriol prevention of mammary carcinoma induced by 7,12-dimethylbenz(a)-anthracene. *Cancer Res* 1975;35:1341–53

109. Takahashi K, Okada M, Ozaki T, *et al.* Safety and efficacy of oestriol for symptoms of natural or surgically induced menopause. *Hum Reprod* 2000;15:1028–36

110. Grodstein F, Stampfer MJ, Falkeborn M, *et al.* Postmenopausal hormone therapy and risk of cardiovascular disease and hip fracture in a cohort of Swedish women. *Epidemiology* 1999; 10:476–80

111. Weiderpass E, Baron JA, Adami HO, *et al.* Low-potency oestrogen and risk of endometrial cancer: a case-control study. *Lancet* 1999;353: 1824–8

112. Lindsay R, Hart DM, MacLean A, *et al.* Bone loss during oestriol therapy in postmenopausal women. *Maturitas* 1979;1:279–85

113. Devogelaer JP, Lecart C, Dupret P, *et al.* Long-term effects of percutaneous estradiol on bone loss and bone metabolism in postmenopausal hysterectomized women. *Maturitas* 1998;28: 243–9

114. Katzenellenbogen BS. Biology and receptor interactions of estriol and estriol derivatives *in vitro* and *in vivo. J Steriod Biochem* 1984;20:1033

115. Melamed M, Castraño E, Notides AC, Sasson S. Molecular and kinetic basis for the mixed agonist/antagonist activity of estriol. *Mol Endocrinol* 1997;11:1868–78

116. Lee JR. Osteoporosis reversal: the role of progesterone. *Clin Nutr Rev* 1990;10:384–9

117. Cooper A, Spencer C, Whitehead MI, *et al.* Systemic absorption of progesterone from Progest cream in postmenopausal women. *Lancet* 1998;351:1255–6

118. Carey BJ, Carey AH, Patel S, *et al.* A study to evaluate serum and urinary hormone levels following short and long term administration of two regimens of progesterone cream in postmenopausal women. *Br J Obstet Gynaecol* 2000;107:722–6

119. Burry KA, Patton PE, Hermsmeyer K. Percutaneous absorption of progesteorne in postmenopausal women treated with trans-dermal estrogen. *Am J Obstet Gynecol* 1999;180: 1504–11

120. Leonnetti HB, Longo S, Anasti JN. Trans-dermal progesterone cream for vasomotor symptoms and postmenopausal bone loss. *Obstet Gynecol* 1999;94:225–8

121. Wren BG, McFarland K, Edwards L, *et al.* Effect of sequential transdermal progesterone cream on endometrium, bleeding pattern, and plasma

progesterone and salivary progesterone levels in postmenopausal women. *Climacteric* 2000;3: 155–60

122. Wren BG, Champion SM, Willetts K, *et al.* Transdermal progesterone and its effect on vasomotor symptoms, blood lipid levels, bone metabolic markers, moods, and quality of life for postmenopausal women. *Menopause* 2003; 10:13–18

123. O'Leary P, Feddema P, Chan K, *et al.* Salivary, but not serum or urinary levels of progesterone are elevated after topical application of progesterone cream to pre- and postmenopausal women. *Clin Endocrinol* 2000;53:615–20

124. Lewis JG, McGill H, Patton V, Elder PA. Caution on the use of saliva measurements to monitor absorption of progesterone from transdermal creams in postmenopausal women. *Maturitas* 2002;41:1–6

125. Komesaroff PA, Black C, Cable V, Sudhir K. Effects of wild yam extract on menopausal symptoms, lipids and sex hormones in healthy menopausal women. *Climacteric* 2001;4: 144–50

126. Slayden SM, Crabbe L, Bae S, *et al.* The effect of 17β-estradiol on adrenocortical sensitivity, responsiveness, and steroidogenesis in postmenopausal women. *J Clin Endocrinol Metab* 1998;83:519–24

127. Baulieu EE, Thomas G, Legrain S, *et al.* Dehydroepiandrosterone (DHEA), DHEA sulfate, and aging: contribution of the DHEAge Study to a sociobiomedical issue. *Proc Natl Acad Sci USA* 2000;97:4279–84

128. Barnhart KT, Freeman E, Grisso JA, *et al.* The effect of dehydroepiandrosterone supplementation to symptomatic perimenopausal women on serum endocrine profiles, lipid parameters, and health-related quality of life. *J Clin Endocrinol Metab* 1999;84:3896–902

129. Johannes CB, Stellato RK, Feldman HA, *et al.* Relation of dehydroepiandrosterone and dehydroepiandrosterone sulfate with cardiovascular disease risk factors in women: longitudinal results from the Massachusetts Women's Health Study. *J Clin Epidemiol* 1999; 52:95–103

130. Aarlt W, Haas J, Callies F, *et al.* Biotransformation of oral dehydroepiandrosterone in elderly men: significant increase in circulating estrogens. *J Clin Endocrinol Metab* 1999;84: 2170–6

131. Morales P, Katz DF, Overstreet JW, *et al.* The relationship between the motility and morphology of spermatozoa in human semen. *J Androl* 1988;9:241

132. Casson PR, Santoro N, Elkind-Hirsch KE, *et al.* Postmenopausal dehydroepiandrosterone (DHEA) administration increases insulin-like growth factor-I (IGF-I) and decreases high density lipoprotein (HDL): a six month trial. *Fertil Steril* 1998;70:107–10

Index

affective and anxiety disorders, 95–109
  case report examples, 104–105
  subtypes and hormonal effects, 104
  see also depression
alcohol
  BMD effects, 153
  as nutritional supplement, 258–259
alendronate, osteoporosis treatment, 154
alternative therapies, 261–274
Alzheimer's disease
  ginkgo therapy, 267
  HRT, 6
amenorrheic HRT regimens, reference period of
  observation, 163
American Medical Association website, 247
androgenization, progestin therapy, 55
androgens
  depression, 100–101
  HRT future development, 7, 9
aneuploidy, age relationship, 187, 192
angiotensin-converting enzyme (ACE) inhibitors,
  CVD therapy, 24
antalgic therapy, dyspareunia, 238
antifibrinolytic drugs, CVD therapy, 24
anxiety disorders *see* affective and anxiety disorders;
  depression
arteriosclerosis, dietary recommendations, 256
assisted reproduction technology (ART)
  early ovarian aging, 185–198
  see also in vitro fertilization
Australasian Menopause Society website, 247
autoimmune diseases, 179–180

Battey's operation, PMS, 120, 121
beta-blockers, CVD therapy, 24
bisphosphonates, osteoporosis treatment, 154–155
black cohosh therapy, 263–264
bladder function, hormonal effects, 29
bleeding patterns, HRT, 159–174
  intrauterine levonorgestrel systems, 135–136
  withdrawal requirements, 159
bone mineral content, 140
bone mineral density (BMD), 139–149
  clinical use, 139–149
    diagnosis, 141–143
    prognosis, 143–146
  GnRH effects, 121–122
  hip as fracture diagnostic reference site, 142

measurement techniques, 139–146
osteoporosis diagnosis, 151–153
PET, 224
population variations, 143
brain, gonadal steroid effects, 104
breast
  breast density
    endogenous and exogenous hormone
      influence, 70–73
    evaluation, 69–70
    mammographic classification, 68–69
    mammography, 67–76
  breast disease, benign, progestin therapy, 54
  breast pain, progestin therapy, 54
  cell proliferation assessment, 61–62
  fine needle aspiration biopsy, 61
  mammographic density, 62–64, 67–76
  progestogen effects, 59–66
breast cancer
  BRCA1/2 gene, mammographic appearance, 74
  cell proliferation regulation, 61–62
  dietary considerations, 257
  estrogen deficiency management, 6–7
  estrogen role, 79–80
  HRT, 59–60, 77–83
    post-cancer, 80–82
    risk factors, 3–4, 6, 14, 19–20, 73
    users *vs* non-users, 81
  mammographic breast density, 62–64, 67–76
  phytoestrogens, 266–267
  progestin therapy, 55
  prognosis and early detection, 67–68
British Medical Journal website, 247
British Menopause Society website, 247
broad-band ultrasound attenuation (BUA), BMD,
  140

calcitonin, osteoporosis treatment, 155
calcium
  dietary considerations and recommendations,
    254–256
  metabolism, 254
  supplementation, osteoporosis, 155
calendar of premenstrual experiences (COPE),
  PMS, 113
cancer, dietary considerations, 256–257
Cancer and Steroid Hormone (CASH) study, OCs
  and ovarian cancer relationship, 87–88

cardiovascular disease
  DHEA, 269
  dietary recommendations, 254–256
  HRT, 17–26
    risk factors, 3, 17–20
  life style changes, 22–24
  phytoestrogens, 264–265, 267
  primary prevention, 4–5
  secondary prevention, 5
cervical cancer, vaginal retraction, 232–233
cigarette smoking, BMD effects, 153
cognition
  HRT protection, 6
  phytoestrogens, 265–266
collagens
  FACIT, 42
  hormonal effects, 30
  urogenital, 41–48
colorectal cancer
  dietary recommendations, 256–257
  HRT benefits, 14, 20
computerized tomography (CT), BMD, 140
conjugated equine estrogen (CEE), 2–8, 63, 159, 199
connective tissue
  component organization, 42
  fibrous components, 41–43
  genitourinary prolapse, 47
  HRT effects, 45
  metabolism, 44–45
  ultrastructure, 41–42
  see also collagen
continuing medical education, internet, 246
contraception
  intrauterine levonorgestrel systems, 54
  see also oral contraceptives
coronary heart disease, HRT risks, 14–15

danazol, ovulation suppression, 114
deep vein thrombosis, transdermal HRT, 201
dehydroepiandrosterone (DHEA)
  depression, 100–101
  HRT future development, 7
  supplementation, 268–269
dehydroepiandrosterone sulfate (DHEAS)
  depression, 100–101
  neuroactive properties, 97
depression
  hormone effects, 119–129
    correlational studies, 99–101
    domino theory, 102
    epidemiological studies, 97–99

    perimenopause, 125–127
    PMS, 121–125
    postnatal depression, 123–125
    therapeutic studies, 101–103
  perimenopause, 125–127
  St John's wort, 267
diabetes, soy protein effects, 264–265
dietary considerations, 253–260
  cardioprotection, 24
  see also nutrition
doctor–patient relationship, internet issues, 243–244, 245
drug reactions, dyspareunia, 233
dual energy absorptiometry (DPA), BMD, 139–140
dual energy X-ray absorptiometry (DXA)
  BMD, 140, 152
  osteoporosis diagnosis, 141
    hip as reference site, 142
    inaccuracies, 141
  osteoporosis prognosis, 143–144
dyslipidemia, transdermal HRT, 201
dysmenorrhea, premenopause, progestin therapy, 53–54
dyspareunia, 229–241
  classification, 229–230
  diagnosis, 234–235
  etiology, 231–234
  examination, 235–237
  introital and midvaginal, biological causes, 231–233
  muscular factors, 233
  prevalence, 230
  sexual comorbidity, 229–230
  treatment, 237–239
  vascular and metabolic factors, 233
  vulvar vestibulitis syndrome, 232, 233

Edinburgh Postnatal Depression Score (EPDS), transdermal estrogen therapy in postnatal depression, 124–126
education, continuing medical education, internet, 246
elastin, 44
electroanalgesia, vulvar vestibulitis syndrome, 238
endometrial cancer
  ERT, 77–83
  estriol risk factor, 267
  hyperplasia, tamoxifen-induced, MLI protective effects, 134–135
  neoplasia
    HRT risk factor, 167
    irregular bleeding with HRT, 170

ultrasound evaluation, 169
vaginal estrogens, 215–216
progestin therapy, 53, 55
survival, ERT users *vs* non-users, 78–79
endometrial polyps
HRT bleeding patterns, 164–165
SIS evaluation, 169
endometriosis
pelvic, dyspareunia, 233–234
progestin therapy, 54
endometrium
continuous progesterone effects, 133–135
histology
COCs, 163–164
dyssynchronous endometrium, 164
endometrial retardation, 163
investigations, 167–169
energy balance, dietary considerations, 253–254
epithelial ovarian tumors, OC protective effects,
90
estradiol
biological availability, HRT administrations,
205–206
post-HRT parenteral administration, 206, 207
vaginal administration, 215, 216, 218
see also pulsed estrogen therapy
estriol
alternative menopausal therapy, 267–268
endometrial cancer risk, 267
vaginal administration, 216
estrogen deficiency
lower urinary tract symptoms, 30–31
urogenital atrophy, 27
estrogen receptors
bladder function, 29
lower urinary tract function, 29
urethra, 29
urogenital atrophy, 28–31, 29
estrogen replacement therapy *see* hormone
replacement therapy
estrogens
antidepressant and anxiogenic properties, 96,
99–100, 104
breast cancer risk, 79–80
CEE, 7–8, 63, 159, 199
metabolism, 214–215
natural and synthetic, dosage and
administration, 199–200
ovulation suppression, 114
PMS, 121–123
postnatal depression, 123–125
vaginal administration, 204–205, 213–220
dyspareunia treatment, 237

estrone levels, post-HRT parenteral administration,
206, 207, 210
ethnicity
effects on HRT bleeding patterns, 164
endometrial neoplasia, 167
etidronate, osteoporosis therapy, 154
European Menopause and Andropause Society
guidelines, 24–25
website, 247
evening primrose oil, alternative menopausal
therapy, 263
exercise
BMD effects, 153
cardioprotection, 22
extracellular matrix (ECM), 41–45

fats and lipids
cardiovascular risk association, 254–255
dietary recommendations, 255–256, 258
lipoproteins, HRT effects, 203–204
metabolism, postmenopause, 135
fatty acid n-3 supplements, 258
female sexual disorders *see* dyspareunia
fiber intake, colorectal cancer prevention, 256–257
fibroids, HRT bleeding patterns, 165–166
fibronectin, 44
fibrous connective tissue *see* collagens; connective
tissue
fine needle aspiration biopsy, 61
fish oil supplements, 258
fluoxetine, PMDD, 114
follicle stimulating hormone (FSH)
follicle growth phase, 189
HRT parenteral administration, 206, 208
follicles
age related depletion, 185–187
ovarian responsiveness and biological age, 190
resting pool, response to IVF, 189–190

gastrointestinal problems, HRT parenteral
administration, 201, 206
genitourinary prolapse, connective tissue, 47
geographical location
endometrial neoplasia, 167
HRT bleeding pattern, 164
ginkgo, Alzheimer's disease, 267
glycosaminoglycans (GAGs), 43
gonadotropin-releasing hormone (GnRH)
add-back therapy, 116, 121–122
bone demineralization, 121–122
HPA axis effects, 178–179

ovulation suppression, 113–114
government and healthcare providers, websites, 246–247

health information, internet, 244–245
Health on the Net
    website, 248
    website quality label, 249
healthcare provider websites, 246–247
hepatic disorders, HRT parenteral administration, 201, 206
HERS (Heart and Estrogen/progestin Replacement Study), 1, 5, 19–23, 159–160
hip fracture, HRT benefits, 14, 20
hormone replacement therapy (HRT)
    adenocarcinoma, 77
    administration methods, 8
        advantages and disadvantages, 213–214, 216
        continuous combined regimens, 131–132, 159–160, 163, 170
        efficacy and tolerance, 199–211
        intranasal, 202
            see also pulsed estrogen therapy
        oral, 199–200
        percutaneous, 200–202
        transdermal, 8, 200–202
        vaginal, 32, 33–35, 170, 217–218
    animal model studies, 61–62
    bleeding patterns, 159–174
        intrauterine levonorgestrel systems, 135–136
    breast cancer, 73, 77–83
    breast density, 62–64
    cardiovascular disease, 4–5, 17–26
    cognitive function protection, 6
    conjugated equine estrogens (CCE), 7–8, 63, 159, 199
    connective tissue effects, 45
    depression, 101–103, 119–129
    dosage, efficacy and tolerance, 199–211
    dyspareunia, 233–234, 237–238
    endometrial cancer, 77–83, 167
    estrogen–progestogen combination, 60–62
    future developments, 1–11
    HERS trial, 1, 5, 19–23, 159–160
    immune system effects, 176–177, 179, 181, 182
    osteoporosis treatment, 153–154
    ovarian cancer association, 90–91
    plasma lipoproteins, 203–204
    PMS induction, treatment strategies, 115–116
    progesterone, 103
    risks, 2–4, 6, 73, 90–91
    transdermal, 122–126, 268

urinary incontinence, 31–32, 45–47
urinary tract infection, 31, 33–34
urogenital atrophy, 34–35
urogenital collagen turnover, 41–49
WHI trial, 2–5, 13–16, 19–23, 159–160
WISDOM trial discontinuation, 15
    see also intrauterine levonorgestrel systems; pulsed estrogen therapy (PET)
hormone responsive mood disorders (HRMD), 119
hormones
    brain effects, 104
    CNS effects, 95
    dyspareunia, 231–232
    immune system interactions, 177–179
    mood changes
        correlational studies, 99–101
        therapeutic studies, 101–103
        see also depression
    neuroactive and psychoactive properties, 96–103
    non-immune regulation, 176
    urogenital atrophy, 28–31
hot flushing, phytoestrogens, 263–264
hyaluronan, 43
hypercalcemia, calcitonin, 155
hypertriglyceridemia, HRT parenteral administration, 201–207
hypothalamic–pituitary–adrenal (HPA) axis, immune/inflammatory response, 177–179, 181
hypothalamic–pituitary–gonadal (HPG) axis, immune/inflammatory response, 177–178
hysterectomy
    as PMS treatment, 123, 127
    urogenital atrophy, 28
hysteroscopy, abnormal bleeding investigation, 168, 169

ibandronate, osteoporosis treatment, 155
immune system
    adaptive/specific immunity, 176
    age-related changes, 175
    cellular immunity, 176–177
    gender responses, 179
    HPA axis regulation, 177–179, 181
    HRT benefits, 181, 182
    humoral immunity, 176
    menopausal changes, 179
        postmenopausal, 175–183
    natural/innate immunity, 176
    neuroendocrine interaction, 177
    overview, 176–177
    sex hormone interactions, 177–179
    T-helper lymphocytes, 175, 176, 181

thymic involution, 175
see also autoimmune diseases
in vitro fertilization (IVF)
   age-related success rates, 187–188
   ovarian reserve, 187–189
   resting follicular pool, 189–190
incontinence, urinary, 28, 30–32
   HRT, 31–32, 45–47
   see also urogenital atrophy
integrins, 44
interleukins
   age-related changes, 175
   immune system response, 176–179
International Menopause Society website, 247
internet
   continuing medical education, 246
   health information, 244–245
   menopause management, 243–251
   printout syndrome, 245
   search engines, 248
   see also websites
intrauterine levonorgestrel systems, 131–138
   contraception, 54
   endometrial effects, 133–135
   fitting requirements, 136
   HRT-induced PMS, 116
   lipid and lipoprotein metabolism, 135
   pharmacokinetics, 134
   PMS treatment, 122–123
   progestogenic effects, 136–137, 170
   structure, 132–133
   tamoxifen-induced endometrial hyperplasia,
      135
   vaginal bleeding disturbances, 52–53, 135–136
ischemic heart disease, CEE, 159
isoflavones
   hot flushing, 263–264
   soybeans, 261
   supplements, 257–258

Kupperman index
   HRT parenteral administration, 201, 206, 209
   PET administration, 223

levator ani myalgia, dyspareunia, 234
levonorgestrel *see* intrauterine levonorgestrel
   systems
lifestyle changes, BMD effects, 153
liver disease, transdermal HRT, 201, 206
luteinizing hormone (LH), HRT parenteral
   administration, 206, 208

lymphocytes, 175, 176
   HRT benefits, 181

magnetic resonance imaging (MRI), BMD, 140
mammography
   breast density, 62–64, 67–76
      breast cancer diagnosis, 67–68
      breast cancer risks, 74–75
      classification, 68–69
   sensitivity and specificity, 73–74
matrix metalloproteinases (MMPs), extracellular
   matrix degradation, 44
MedCERTAIN website information quality label,
   249
medical organisations and societies websites, 247
Medical Research Council (MRC), WISDOM trial
   discontinuation, 15
Medline website, 246, 247
menopausal levonorgestrel intrauterine systems
   (MLIs) *see* intrauterine levonorgestrel systems
menopause
   CVD, 18–19
   defined, 98
   mood changes, 95–109
   perimenopause
      defined, 98
      depression
         HRT, 126–127
         progesterone, 100
      immune system function, 181
      PET efficacy, 223
   PMS, 111–117
   postmenopause, transdermal HRT, 268
   premenopause, defined, 98–99
   surgical, depression, 98
menorrhagia, premenopause, progestin therapy,
   52–53
menstruation
   bleeding pattern assessment, 160–162
      amenorrheic HRT, 163
      diary interpretation, 161
      intermenstrual bleeding, 161
      pictorial chart, 162
      severity, 161–162
   disorders, progestin therapy, 52–53
   HRT regulation, 159–174
   see also bleeding patterns
metabolic changes, postmenopause, 253–254
micturition, hormonal effects, 28–31
Montgomery Asberg Depression Rating Scale
   (MADRS), estrogen therapy in postnatal
   depression, 125

mood changes
    menopause, 95–109
    see also affective and anxiety disorders;
        depression
myocardial infarction (MI), C-reactive protein
    levels, 23

National Electronic Library for Health website, 247
National Health and Nutrition Examination Survey
    (NHANES) III, BMD reference ranges, 143
National Osteoporosis Society statement, HRT and
    WHI study, 13–16
neuroendocrine system, immune system
    interaction, 177, 182
neurotransmitters, PMS, 114–115
NHS website, 246
North American Menopause Society website, 247
Nurses' Health Study
    CHD reduction, 24
    OCs and ovarian cancer relationship, 86
nutrition, 253–260
    BMD effects, 153
    disease prevention, 254–257
    food group recommendations, 259
    supplements, 257–259

obesity, 253–254
    breast cancer risk, 257
oocyte quality and quantity, age-related
    deterioration, 187
oophorectomy
    CVD risk, 19
    PMS therapy, 114
    see also Battey's operation;
        salpingo-oophorectomy
oral contraceptives (OCs)
    breast epithelial proliferation, 61
    combined oral contraceptives (COCs),
        endometrial histology changes, 163
    mammographic breast density, 72–73
    ovarian cancer relationship, 85–94
    progestins, 54
        ovarian cancer relationship, 90
Organising Medical Networked Information
    website, 248
osteoporosis, 151–158
    BMD definition, 141
    BMD diagnostic techniques, 142–145
    BMD intervention thresholds, 145–146
    BMD prognostic techniques, 143–146
    definition, 151
    diagnosis, 151–153
    dietary recommendations, 255–256
    etiology, 151
    HRT, 5–6
    personal and financial outcomes, 151
    PET, 224
    phytoestrogens, 265
    progestin therapy, 55
    SERMs, 8–9
    transdermal HRT, 201
    treatment, 153–156
ovarian aging, early
    ART, 185–198
    defined, 192
    primary prevention, 193–194
    reproductive milestones, 185–187
    screening, 193
ovarian cancer
    HRT risk factor, 90–91
    OC protective effects, 85–94
    progestin therapy, 55
ovarian cycle syndrome, defined, 121
ovarian cysts, OC protective effects, 90
ovarian reserve, ART assessment, 187–189, 192–193
ovarian stimulation
    poor response
        defined, 190
        menopause association, 190–191
ovulation suppression
    GnRH analogs, 113–114
    PMS, 113–114
Oxford Family Planning Association study, OCs and
    ovarian cancer relationship, 86

parathyroid hormone (PTH), osteoporosis
    treatment, 155
pelvic floor muscle rehabilitation, dyspareunia
    treatment, 238
pelvic inflammatory disease, dyspareunia, 234
pelvic surgery, dyspareunia, 232
phytoestrogens, 261–267
    bone loss, 265
    breast cancer, 266–267
    cardiovascular disease, 264–265
    classification, 261–262
    cognition, 265–266
    hot flushing, 263–264
postmenopausal hormone therapy (PHT) *see*
    hormone replacement therapy
postnatal depression, 123–125
premenstrual dysphoric disorder (PMDD)
    defined, 111–112

fluoxetine, 114
premenstrual symptoms, 111
premenstrual syndrome (PMS), 111–117
   calendar of premenstrual experiences, 113
   defined, 111
   estrogens, 120–123
   etiology, 113
   GnRH analog therapy, 122
   HRT induced, 115–116
   neurotransmitters, 114–115
   ovulation association, 113
   ovulation suppression, 113–114
   progesterone, 114–115
   progestogen intolerance, 127
   symptoms and diagnosis, 112–113
   transdermal HRT, 122–124
progesterone
   anxiolytic effects, 97, 104
   depression, perimenopause, 100
   metabolic pathway, 103
   neuronal effects, 96–97
   PMS, 114, 115
      cyclical symptoms, 121
      HRT-induced, 115–116
   withdrawal symptoms, 97
progesterone receptor expression, 60
progestins
   classification, 51
   HRT future development, 7
   mechanism of action, 52
   premenopause, 51–57
   premenstrual syndrome, dysmenorrhea, 53–54
progestogens
   anti-estrogenic effects, 131–132
   breast cancer therapy, 60
   breast effects, 59–66
   endometrial changes, 164
   estrogen attenuation, 122
   HRT bleeding patterns, 52–53, 164
   HRT compliance, 115, 122
   intolerance, 127
   intrauterine systems, 131–138
      adverse effects, 136–137
   lipid and lipoprotein metabolism alterations,
      135
   lower urinary tract symptoms, 30–31
proteoglycans (PGs), 43–44
psychosexual factors, dyspareunia, 233
pudendal nerve entrapment syndrome,
   dyspareunia, 233
PUFAs, cardioprotection, 24
pulmonary embolism, HRT risks, 20
pulsed estrogen therapy (PET), 221–227

bone turnover and BMD, 224
breast safety, 224–225
dosage and administration, 225
endometrial safety, 225
mode of action, 222–223
nasal tolerance and safety, 225
perimenopause symptom effects, 223–224
pharmacokinetics, 222

quantitative computed tomography (QCT), BMD
   estimation, 152
quantitative ultrasound (QUS), BMD, 140, 152

raloxifene
   cardioprotection, 9
   osteoporosis therapy, 154
randomized clinical trials (RCTs), HRT and CVD
   relationship biases, 22–23
red clover, menopausal therapy, 263
reproductive milestones
   age of rapid decline and menopause, 190–192
   fixed time intervals, 185–187, 190
research, internet, 243–251
rheumatoid arthritis, hormone association, 180, 181
risedronate, osteoporosis therapy, 154
Royal College of General Practitioners
   study of OCs and ovarian cancer relationship,
      85–86
   website, 247
Royal College of Obstetricians and Gynaecologists,
   website, 247

St John's wort, depression, 267
saline instillation sonohysterography (SIS),
   abnormal bleeding investigation, 168, 169
salpingo-oophorectomy, bilateral
   as PMS treatment, 127
   transdermal estrogen treatment, 123
selective estrogen receptor modulators (SERMs)
   HRT, 8–9, 116
   osteoporosis treatment, 154
selective serotonin reuptake inhibitors (SSRIs)
   hot flushing, 264
   HRT synergy, 102
   PMS, 114
sexual abuse, dyspareunia, 233
single energy X-ray absorptiometry (SXA), BMD,
   140
single photon absorptiometry (SPA), BMD,
   139–140

Sjogren's syndrome, dyspareunia, 233
soybean protein
    cardiovascular disease therapy, 264
        food derivatives, 262
        isoflavones, 261
        supplements, 257–258
spinal fracture, HRT benefits, 14
statins, CVD therapy, 24
stress urinary incontinence, HRT effects, 45–47
stroke, HRT risks, 3, 14, 15, 20
strontium ranelate, osteoporosis treatment, 136
sulfated neuroactive steroids, 97

T-helper lymphocytes, 175, 176, 181
tamoxifen, endometrial hyperplasia induction, MLI
    protective effects, 135
testosterone
    dyspareunia treatment, 237
    estrogen combination, PMS treatment, 122
    HRT future development, 7
thromboembolism
    HRT risk, 2, 3, 14
    SERM as risk factor, 154
    transdermal HRT, 8, 201
thrombophlebitis, HRT parenteral administration,
    201, 206–207
thymic involution, 175
tibolone
    HRT, 8
    PMS treatment, 116

ultrasonography
    abnormal bleeding investigation, 168, 169
    endometrial thickness, 169
    levonorgestrel intrauterine systems, 132
    velocity, BMD, 140
urethra, hormonal effects, 29
urinary incontinence see incontinence, urinary
urinary tract
    estrogen deficiency, 30–31
    hormonal effects, 29
urinary tract infection
    estrogen management, 31, 33–34
    intravaginal estriol therapy, 216, 217
urogenital atrophy, 27–40
    economic considerations, 28
    estrogen management, 34–35
    estrogen receptors, 28–31
    hormonal effects, 30
    vaginal estrogens, 213–216
urogenital collagen turnover, HRT, 41–49

urogenital prolapse, 28
US Walnut Creek Study, OCs and ovarian cancer
    relationship, 85
uterine cancer, ultrasound evaluation, 169

vaginal atrophy see urogenital atrophy
vaginal dryness, dyspareunia, 231–232
vaginal estrogen therapy, 204–205, 213–220
    silicone ring administration, 216–218
vaginismus, 230
vaginitis, 232
variocele, pelvic, 234
vasomotor symptoms, progestin therapy, 54
venous disorders, HRT parenteral administration,
    201, 206
vitamin D
    dietary recommendations, 255
    supplementation, 155
vulvar dystrophy, 232
vulvar vestibulitis syndrome
    antalgic therapy, 238
    dyspareunia, 232, 233
    electroanalgesia, 238
vulvitis, 232

websites
    alternative therapies, 269
    commercial, 247
    general health, 246–247
    government and healthcare providers,
        246–247
    health and menopause, 246
    independent, 247–248
    information quality, 248–249
        HON label, 249
    links, 249
    medical organizations and societies, 247
    Medline, 246, 247
    menopause-specific, 247
    patient-led/self-support, 248
    search engines, 248
weight control, 253–254, 257
WHI (Women's Health Initiative) trial of HRT, 2–5,
    13–16, 19–23, 159–160
wild yam creams, postmenopausal therapy, 268
World Health Organization Collaborative Study of
    Neoplasia and Steroid Contraceptives, OCs and
    ovarian cancer relationship, 88

zolendronate, osteoporosis treatment, 155